Rural Health Services: Organization, Delivery, and Use

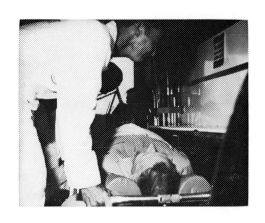

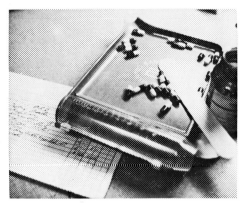

North Central Regional Center for Rural Development

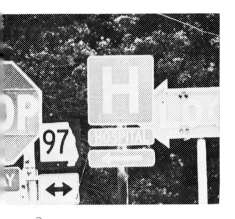 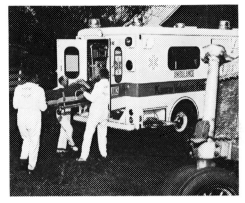

Rural Health Services:
Organization, Delivery, and Use

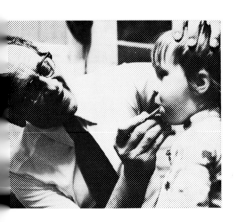

Iowa State University Press / **AMES** / 1976

Volume Editors: **Edward W. Hassinger** and **Larry R. Whiting**

Photos on cover and title page courtesy of Donald F. Haydon, University of Missouri, and Lyman C. Greiner, Iowa State University

Composed and printed by
The Iowa State University Press

First Edition, 1976
Second printing, 1978

Library of Congress Cataloging in Publication Data
Main entry under title:

Rural health services.

    Includes bibliographies and index.
    1. Rural health services—United States. 2. Health planning—United States.
3. United States—Rural conditions. I. Hassinger, Edward Wesley. II. Whiting,
Larry R. III. North Central Regional Center for Rural Development.
RA445.R87   362.1'0973   75–45496
ISBN 0–8138–1465–0

CONTENTS

v

PREFACE

RURAL HEALTH and the delivery of health services are many-faceted problems, and solutions are similarly varied. The general approach of this volume is to describe the present situation, analyze that situation, and discuss specific means for meeting the problems—all within the historical and situational context of rural society.

The chapters cover a wide range of topics reflecting the diverse backgrounds of the authors. Many begin by stating the problem of rural health in nearly identical terms but then advance to in-depth and sometimes novel discussions. In arranging the chapters we have proceeded from general situations to specific considerations of solutions, with a final chapter that looks to the future. We believe it is especially appropriate that Dr. Milton Roemer has the introductory chapter, since he was coauthor of the pioneer work in rural health which remains as the only comprehensive and detailed statement on this subject.

The editors wish to express appreciation to the authors for their cooperation and forebearance in the sometimes heavy demands of the editing process. In behalf of the North Central Regional Center for Rural Development, we also wish to extend our appreciation to the Farm Foundation, Chicago; the Cooperative State Research Service, USDA, Washington, D.C.; the Department of Rural and Community Health, American Medical Association, Chicago; and the National Center for Health Services Research, Public Health Service, Rockville, Maryland. Thanks must be given Judy Anderson, who functioned as an assistant volume editor. Finally we gratefully acknowledge a special debt to Daryl Hobbs, University of Missouri, for his guidance and encouragement of this publication effort.

EDWARD W. HASSINGER
University of Missouri
LARRY R. WHITING
Iowa State University

vii

Rural Health Services: Organization, Delivery, and Use

CHAPTER ONE

HISTORICAL PERSPECTIVE OF HEALTH SERVICES IN RURAL AMERICA

MILTON I. ROEMER, MD

AS THE United States has become increasingly urbanized, the quality of life of the people "left behind" in the rural areas has become a matter of national concern. Included in that quality is the availability of health services. The organized social actions taken to provide or improve health services for rural people have been along numerous paths; they have emanated from both governmental and private initiative at local, state, or national levels and have been interwoven with the larger sociopolitical trends of our society.

EARLY IDENTIFICATION OF NEEDS. The notion that rural life had its health handicaps, in spite of fresh air and sunshine, was expressed as early as 1862 in the first report of the Commissioner of Agriculture to President Abraham Lincoln (15). Dr. W. W. Hall reported high incidence of insanity among farm people, of respiratory disease, of the hazards of miasmas around farmhouses, of gastrointestinal problems associated with the use of outdoor privies, and of the longevity of farmers which, he said, "is not so great as we might suppose." Definite statistical evidence of rural morbidity rates did not accumulate until some years later. Mortality in rural populations, age-adjusted, was lower than in urban populations in 1900 and probably still is, though the differential has declined. The need for health services, however, has never been defined by death rates alone (42). Social actions have been stimulated by the problems of disease, pain, suffering, and disability and by the concept of applying medical science to human welfare, regardless of mortality tables.

MILTON I. ROEMER, MD, is Professor of Health Services Administration, University of California, Los Angeles.

After the Civil War America developed rapidly with the expansion to the West, the rise of industry, and the growth of large cities. Thousands of immigrants came from Europe, providing a work force for the factories and, with weak social programs, became congested in urban slums. In this atmosphere the prominent issue in health service was to prevent the spread of communicable disease in the cities through better environmental sanitation; later, with the rise of bacteriology, immunizations were developed, along with more standardized policies on isolation and quarantine. The public health movement, which took shape in those years, was essentially urban. The classical Shattuck Report of 1850, giving rise 20 years later to the first state health department (Massachusetts), was obviously written from the perspective of Boston (51).

It was not until about 1910 that the first health departments for systematic promotion of preventive service were organized on a county rather than a city basis. But even these Kentucky, North Carolina, and Washington units were largely oriented to the main towns within the county borders. The first local health department with a full-time health officer, established in a county that contained no incorporated place of 2,500 or more, was in Robeson County, South Carolina, in 1912 (33). The work of the Rockefeller Sanitary Commission after 1909, tackling hookworm infestation in southern counties, underscored the need for proper excreta disposal on farms as well as in city tenements (2).

Official legal action in the way of sanitary ordinances had been taken somewhat earlier. In one rural county of West Virginia, a county board of health—with the duty of enforcing various ordinances—was established in 1891 (43). The first county health officer was evidently not appointed until 1909, but he was simply a local practicing physician who was assigned certain legal duties. It was not until 1929 that a full-time health officer was appointed and paid to serve the county, with his office all too typically in the basement of the county courthouse.

By the end of World War I the United States acquired a powerful economic and political position in the world, and several movements for improved health service began to take shape throughout the nation. With the advantage of hindsight we can identify these as movements along several distinct paths such as organized disease prevention, health manpower, hospital development, and improved financing of medical care. Each of these movements has had clear implications for rural areas, and some were specifically focused on rural needs. Obviously there were close interrelationships among the parallel paths. Since community action came first in the sphere of disease prevention, this movement should be considered first.

ORGANIZED PREVENTION OF DISEASE. The goal of American public health leadership after 1920 became the achievement of "coverage" of all the nation's 3,070 counties with full-time health departments—that is, public health agencies with a scope wide enough to warrant a full-time director. In 1914 there had been 14 such counties, in 1920 there were 109, in 1930 there were 505 (21). This relatively rapid growth was doubtless a reflection of the importance attached in those years to control of the still-common communicable diseases through both personal preventive and environmental sanitation measures.

The enactment of the Sheppard-Towner act in 1921 contributed to the strengthening of rural county health departments by providing for the first time federal grants to the states for supporting maternal and child health stations. The rural birth rate then, as now, was higher than the urban; giving immunizations to babies, along with counseling mothers on infant feeding and child-rearing, was obviously a worthy social objective in the small towns and villages (32). Perhaps reflecting the appreciation of rural public health needs mounting in these years, in 1925 the American Public Health Association (APHA) changed the name of its Committee on Municipal Public Health Practice (founded in 1920) to simply the Committee on Administrative Practice (CAP) (68). However, during the conservative era of Herbert Hoover, with the emphasis on private enterprise and local government, the Sheppard-Towner program of health grants was terminated in 1929.

The massive economic depression that began in late 1929 was a setback for rural as well as urban preventive health efforts. Government attention became focused on relief for the destitute. It took the Social Security Act of 1935 to give a new boost to preventive services. While many social leaders urged a health insurance title in the act, President Roosevelt did not wish to get embroiled in the issue of socialized medicine; instead Titles V and VI were included (48). Title V in effect reinstated federal grants to the states for maternal and child health services; Title VI gave grants for all other types of public health services. Since city governments generally had greater revenue resources of their own, these funds were used largely to build up preventive programs in the more rural counties. The variable matching formulas of these grants yielded relatively greater assistance to the poorer states of the South. They also facilitated strengthening of most state health departments, whose consultation and standard-setting practices (e.g., state sanitary codes) were probably of greatest relevance to rural areas that lacked strong local public health agencies of their own.

By 1942, after the first seven years of these federal health grants, about 1,800 counties had achieved full-time public health coverage; there were still 1,250 counties, mostly rural, without such protection (20). Part of the rural problem was the small population base, let alone poverty, of many counties. As part of the postwar planning that came with World War II, therefore, the APHA proposed a plan for consolidating the public health tasks of several adjacent rural counties into multicounty districts and also the merging of city and county health departments. The goal was to achieve nationwide public health coverage through about 1,200 units (9). This general strategy has succeeded in attaining public health agency coverage today in about 80 percent of the nation's counties and a higher proportion of the rural population (61).

The scope of public health services has generally widened in the United States to include mental health, chronic disease detection, accident prevention, and other activities beyond communicable disease control; but this broader policy seldom applies to the small health departments in rural districts. Moreover, there are many vacancies among these units in the poorer states where health officer salaries are low (41). The main foot soldiers of rural public health work are the public health nurses and the sanitarians, who have doubtless played a significant role in the reduction of infant mortality and cases of enteric fevers. The ratio of public health nurses per 100,000 population, nevertheless, is still substantially lower in the more rural states in spite of the greater drain on their time caused by travel.

Newer preventive programs in which rural health departments have played a significant role have included family planning and a wider scope for child health to include some treatment services. In the southeastern states, with large black populations, birth-control advisory services have been offered by rural health departments for longer than elsewhere; the small Roman Catholic constituencies and the rapid growth of black compared with white populations may account for this. The recently funded wider-scope MIC (maternity and infant care) and C & Y (children and youth) health care programs are typically found in the large city slums, where medical schools or medical centers are at hand—seldom in rural districts. Fluoridation of water supplies to prevent dental caries is another measure that is dependent on efficient public water systems and seldom found in small towns and not at all in open-country areas.

While the coverage of rural counties with official public health services has shown great improvement since 1910, the scope of services offered has not been very impressive. The "basic six" of the APHA program of 1945 (identified with Dr. Haven Emerson) are still the usual boundaries: communicable disease control, environmental sanitation, maternal and child health preventive services, and health education, plus two instrumentalities of these—vital statistics and laboratory services. Even within these boundaries the impacts have been small, probably because of meager manpower resources and the timid leadership of most rural health departments.

IMPROVED DISTRIBUTION OF HEALTH MANPOWER. Perhaps the most obvious health service deficiency perceived by rural people is a shortage of doctors. This shortage has not always existed; a physician writing from the rural South in 1843 complained of greater competition than in the New England states because of there being "twice the number of doctors that the community needed" (44). But when the output of doctors was greatly reduced following the Flexner revolution in medical education (1910) and the smaller number of new graduates began to flock to the cities (with their greater wealth, more opportunities for specialization, and many cultural advantages), the lack of rural doctors—as well as other health personnel—became a prominent issue.

The first social actions to cope with this problem were taken by small towns themselves. In response to this issue the New Hampshire Legislature in 1923 enacted a statute that read:

> Towns may at any annual meeting vote to raise such sums of money as they may deem necessary towards support of a resident physician in such towns which, in the absence of such appropriation, would be without the services of such physician (29).

These tax funds could be used to pay the doctor for health services to school children or to the poor, so as to supplement his earnings from private practice; sometimes they would be used for a direct subsidy on top of private earnings to reach a guaranteed annual income. Other direct actions by rural communities have included inducements of a rent-free house, an automobile, or ready-made office facilities. Petitions for a doctor signed by hundreds of citizens have been launched to offer an enticing welcome (39). Private industrial firms in isolated areas—mines, public utilities, or lumber companies—have secured doctors for their workers and dependents by paying them salaries from funds raised through wage reductions or management contributions.

Another approach was attempted in the 1930s by the Commonwealth Fund, which gave fellowships to medical students on the condition that they would practice in a rural location for a certain number of years. The results were discouraging, however; after the period of obligation was finished, nearly all these young doctors left the rural town for a larger city. The same idea was launched by state governments on a larger scale a little later. In 1942 Virginia passed a law to

provide tuition and fellowships for the complete medical education
of rural youths who would agree to return to a rural community
designated by the State Health Department as needing a doctor. In
the later 1940s about ten other states, mostly in the South, enacted
similar programs.

The financial extent of this rural medical fellowship support has
never been very great, and it has fluctuated from year to year. When
I wrote to Virginia's State Health Commissioner in 1967 to inquire
about the results of 20 years of this effort, he replied:

> It is hard to evaluate the effectiveness of the program. Certainly it has
> not been a great boon to [medical] practice in the rural areas; on the
> other hand, it has helped to fill a monetary need for these students (50).

A proper evaluative study of state government efforts to attract young
doctors to rural areas might well be conducted; the general evidence
of persistently lower doctor-population ratios in rural counties suggests
they have not been very successful.

In 1953 a state medical society set out to tackle the problem by
giving advice and assistance to rural communities in establishing small
private clinics to attract doctors. The Tennessee State Medical Association claimed some success in this approach (24). In 1959 the Sears
Roebuck Foundation invested in this project—lending money to small
towns, along with free architectural plans to build modern private
medical quarters (26). However, it has been observed that the purely
private entrepreneurial base of this program has led to instability;
when the doctor decides to move away, the clinic building may be sold
to an insurance agent or a beauty shop operator (22).

For some years the American Medical Association, through its
Council on Rural Health Services, has provided an information service
on communities needing doctors. Since 1948 the AMA also has held a
series of National Conferences on Rural Health, publicizing this and
other approaches to the problem.

More fundamental attacks on the rural shortage of doctors have
been the many actions (especially since the end of World War II) to
increase the total national output of physicians, along with many other
types of health workers. As long as the overall supply of health manpower is less than the mounting demand, one must expect that the
least attractive areas—whether central city slums or rural districts—
will get the leanest pickings. Social actions to increase the output
of all types of health manpower have been taken largely by government at both state and national levels.

In 1945 there were 77 approved medical schools in the United
States; since then the trend of reduction initiated by the Flexner report
has been reversed, so there are now about 115. Most of the new

schools were established by state governments, and all of them with public subsidy. Moreover, most schools—both public and private— have increased their enrollments and numbers of graduates (5). This increase was still not enough to accommodate the expanding need of the nation's hospitals for interns and residents, and matters would have been and would still be much worse if it were not for a large inflow of graduates from foreign medical schools.

The expansion of health manpower education, so important for rural areas, depended on an increasing flow of subsidy from the federal government. In spite of initial opposition to such subsidy by the AMA—for fear of federal domination of the professional schools—the need became so glaring that by the mid-1960s general consensus had been achieved. The National Advisory Commission on Health Manpower in 1967 advocated not only greatly increased numbers of virtually all types of health personnel but also increased rationalization of the delivery system so that "new categories of health professionals" could be effectively used (37).

Such new categories of medical assistants—dating from the Russian feldsher of the 1870s—have always been considered especially relevant for thinly settled rural districts. In the 1960s several dozen grant programs were initiated under the auspices of different federal agencies to subsidize the training of many types of health manpower (58). In 1971 a comprehensive health manpower act achieved integration of several of these federal grant programs. Today we see scores of new training programs for physician assistants, Medex personnel, nurse practitioners, pediatric associates, anaesthetic technicians, midwives, and others being developed by universities and hospitals with encouragement from both the government and the private health professions.

Other countries have long used another approach for getting doctors into rural areas—invoking national authority. In Mexico, for example, most medical degrees are awarded by the National University of Mexico, with a condition that the new graduate spend a period of "social service" in a rural district; recently this was increased from six months to one year. Iran uses the military conscription laws as a vehicle for getting manpower to outlying areas through a Rural Health Service Corps. The Soviet Union has long required a three-year period of rural service for most, though not all, new graduates (12). While the United States has not gone as far as these foreign examples, the National Health Service Corps, set up under the Emergency Health Personnel Act of 1970, has been a step in this direction. Under this law physicians, dentists, nurses, and some other health professionals are brought into a federal program which in effect meets military obligations. They are then sent to communities of need, mostly rural, where they serve the poor without charge and others on a fee basis; sometimes they work in organized health units and sometimes in traditional private offices. Of about 5,000 communities estimated to need such assistance, a few hundred have so far been helped (17).

Improvement of the rural health manpower supply has also been tackled through various indirect approaches. Provision of modern hospitals has been one basic strategy advanced often as a means of attracting new doctors. Promotion of better medical incomes through various forms of health insurance—social or voluntary—has been another strategy. Regionalized systems and group medical practice have been other mechanisms to render settlement in a rural community less isolated and more stimulating.

FACILITIES. The importance of general hospitals for good medical care is too obvious to elaborate, but until about 1930 the initiative and financial resources for their construction were entirely dependent on local effort. This did not apply to hospitals for long-term care of mental disorder or tuberculosis, which were built by state governments since the late 19th century, nor to a special "charity-hospital" system for the poor in Louisiana. For day-to-day management of serious illness, however, the community general hospitals of the nation required entirely local initiative—usually by voluntary bodies (religious or nonsectarian) and sometimes by local government, especially in rural counties. This resulted in a severe imbalance of hospital bed-population ratios between urban and rural districts, since the latter have always had weaker economic resources.

In the early 1930s the Commonwealth Fund launched a program to help rural communities build small general hospitals through a two-thirds subsidy of the cost of construction and equipment (54). Fourteen hospitals were built under this program; later other foundations, such as the Kellogg in Michigan and the Duke Endowment in North Carolina, gave other forms of capital assistance to rural hospitals.

It took the Great Depression to bring federal government resources to bear on this problem. Under the New Deal's PWA (Public Works Administration) and WPA (Work Projects Administration), assistance was given to the construction or improvement of hundreds of hospitals, although mainly in larger cities. During World War II the Community Facilities Act also provided federal grants to support hospital construction in congested areas created because of war production or military training (28). Some of this construction, which also established health centers for housing public health agencies, was in small towns definitely serving rural people.

A nationwide overview of hospital needs, which emphasized the deficiencies of rural areas, was first taken as part of postwar planning during World War II. The leadership of the U.S. Public Health Service in those years was extremely important, especially the imaginative role of Dr. Joseph W. Mountin. In 1945 he and his colleagues published the first national survey of hospital bed supply in relation to population in all the counties of the nation, along with theoretical proposals for action needed to achieve rural-urban equity (30). Health service areas were defined in which peripheral (rural), intermediate and base hospitals should ideally exist. In tandem with this governmental work, a voluntary national Commission on Hospital Care was established in 1944, mainly through the initiative of the American Hospital Association and aided by private foundations. This body's report on hospital care in the United States appeared in 1946 (6).

These studies laid the technical basis for the National Hospital Survey and Construction (Hill-Burton) Act of 1946. This legislation provided grants to the states to subsidize hospital construction in areas of greatest need, the latter to be determined by surveys in each state with design of a state master plan (64). The law and regulations under it required that a ranking of priorities be established through which areas of greatest deficiency from the optimal standard of bed need would get assistance first. Inevitably this meant that the maximum aid went to building hospitals in rural districts. It also is noteworthy that the Hill-Burton act aided hospitals under both governmental and voluntary nonprofit sponsorship—in fact, mainly the latter—so that the public-private partnership concept was being implemented 20 years before passage of the Partnership for Health Act of 1966. Important conditions of the grants were that certain standards of hospital design be met and that every state receiving aid had to enact a hospital licensure program to assure continuation of proper hospital maintenance and professional practices.

Largely because of the Hill-Burton influence, the hospital resources of rural America have been greatly improved, both in quantity and quality. Between 1946 and 1966 the disparity in bed supply between the predominantly rural and predominantly urban states was largely eliminated. In fact, in 1964 the Hill-Burton act was amended to give grants for modernization of facilities, which was designed to channel more support into the deteriorating hospitals of the larger cities. Over the years the law has been repeatedly amended to adjust to newly perceived needs for chronic disease facilities, new types of health centers, research in hospital service, and areawide planning (i.e., below the level of the state government).

The trend in hospital use by rural people over the last 30 years has clearly been upward, but this does not mean hospitalization solely in small-town hospitals. Transportation improvements have been a major factor, and many rural patients—especially those of higher incomes—bypass the nearby community hospital to seek more specialized care in a distant urban institution (40).

The actions taken in particular states to improve the supply and operation of hospitals serving rural people are too numerous to review. Many of the state health departments responsible for the Hill-Burton program and for implementation of the hospital licensure laws have given special consultations to upgrade rural hospitals. Some of the state hospital associations have done likewise. In the Appalachian states, with special federal assistance under the Appalachian Regional Development Act, hospitals and health centers have been expanded particularly to meet the needs of the low-income mountain people (59). Perhaps because of the drama of serious illness, the hospital sector of rural health needs has shown striking improvement, and other sectors are now drawing greater attention.

PROGRAMS FOR SPECIAL POPULATIONS. The United States Department of Agriculture and its cooperating state agencies have long operated programs focused on the welfare of farm families. The agricultural extension services, along with advice to farmers on livestock and crop practices, have had their various home demonstration programs which include education on nutrition, sanitation, and hygienic habits.

Probably the most remarkable health service program specifically for farm families of low income was that of the federal Farm Security Administration (FSA) in the 1930s and 1940s (28, pp. 389–431). As part of a generalized effort to rehabilitate low-income and economically marginal farm families, the FSA gave low-interest loans for various agricultural production purposes and also gave assistance on family living. Among the latter were loans (or sometimes grants) for prepaid membership in small local medical care plans providing doctor, hospital, and sometimes dental and drug services. At their peak in 1942 these local health insurance plans served over 600,000 persons in 1,100 rural counties. There were also special experimental rural health programs in six southern counties in which low-income farm families who were not regular FSA-borrowers were invited to join relatively more comprehensive prepayment plans, with government subsidies of premiums on a sliding scale in proportion to family income. Another special program in Taos County, New Mexico, established rural health centers, with salaried doctors and nurses giving general ambulatory care. The overall FSA approach simply accepted the existing private free-choice pattern and heightened access to care through prepayment.

With the retrenchment of federal assistance from the USDA after World War II this program gradually declined, and the health needs of low-income farm families were left to be met by the traditional local welfare departments or through the private sector. The FSA experience, however, doubtless left its mark in a heightened appreciation of the special problems of rural medical care. Some farm organizations, like the Farmers Union and the National Grange, became sensitized to these issues. Enrollment of farm people in Blue Cross and other health insurance plans, the founding of some voluntary rural medical cooperatives, and support for the whole concept of hospital regionalization were among the long-term benefits of this experience.

Another special rural group for which the USDA provided health care were migratory farm workers (27). Originally one sector of the FSA program, this program was shifted during World War II to a special Office of Labor under the War Food Administration. To cope with the special needs of these families who, being nonresident, did not usually qualify for local welfare medical aid, clinics were set up at about 250 locations of seasonal labor concentration around the country. Doctors on part-time salary and full-time nurses with rather broad "standing orders" (shades of the nurse practitioner of the 1970s) staffed these clinics. To cut through bureaucratic impediments in hiring personnel and purchasing supplies, a series of six Agricultural Workers Health and Medical Associations—nonprofit corporations established locally—were organized to take direct responsibility, entirely under federal financial support.

Although this program also died after the war, the plight of migratory families continued and, as happened for American poverty in general, was "rediscovered" around 1962. In that year the Migrant Health Act was passed, reestablishing federal aid for health services to migrant workers and their dependents (66). Instead of direct federal operation or use of quasi-governmental health corportions, this program provided grants from the U.S. Public Health Service to state and local agencies (mostly health departments but sometimes local medical societies, religious missions, or other bodies) for services to migrant families. Family Health Service Clinics, as the law defines them, are the usual modality, although some of the funds have simply been used to strengthen the traditional preventive services of local health departments. Patterns of interstate agricultural migration have obviously changed over the decades; most seasonal farm labor is now evidently drawn from within state borders, simplifying the problems of legal entitlement to welfare medical service. Nevertheless, the federal appropriations of a few million dollars for this program have typically been much less than the congressional authorization and far less than the volume of need.

American Indians are an essentially rural ethnic group which has long been the beneficiary of special federal assistance. Of about 700,000 Indians in the nation, approximately half are living in or near reservations, entitling them to services from a network of special health centers and hospitals (operated from 1849 to 1955 by the U.S. Department of Interior and since then by the U.S. Public Health Service) (62). Most of these facilities are small, staffed by salaried medical and nursing personnel; there are also contractual arrangements with other local hospitals and doctors. The Indian Health Service offers a comprehensive scope of preventive and curative services, putting special stress on problems like tuberculosis and alcoholism, which have high prevalence in this population. While marked progress in increasing life expectancy has been recorded among Indians, their health status is still substantially lower than that of the general population (69).

A more recent governmental approach to helping special population groups has been that of the U.S. Office of Economic Opportunity (OEO), established in 1964. With respect to health services, the strategy of the OEO has been to concentrate efforts in certain "pockets of poverty," establishing neighborhood health centers which offer comprehensive ambulatory services to all low-income persons (not solely to public assistance recipients) in the immediate area (47). These local centers obviously modify traditional patterns of medical care delivery with their combination of preventive and curative services, a range of salaried medical and surgical specialists, and active outreach efforts through community aides to attract the poor into the center for health attention.

The great majority of OEO-supported health centers have been established in central city slums, often in response to urban riots; a few have been specifically rural, as at King City, California, or Mound Bayou, Mississippi. These two units and many others have been subjects of sharp controversy, associated with local medical opposition and the OEO policy of delegating major administrative responsibilities to the poor people themselves (8). In spite of these difficulties, the concept of the broad-gauged health service center for ambulatory care has been spreading throughout the nation under the sponsorship of the U.S. Department of Health, Education and Welfare (HEW) as well as the OEO. In 1973 and 1974 all the OEO-sponsored neighborhood health centers were transferred to HEW.

Not all health actions for special rural population groups stem from governmental initiative. The organized efforts of the Welfare and Retirement Fund for coal miners and their families throughout the United States is one of the best examples of voluntary action. While fringe benefit health programs negotiated between labor and management are typically thought of as urban affairs, the mining industry is primarily in rural regions; thus these efforts obviously improve rural health service.

For a century or so health services in mining and other isolated industries (like lumbering or railroading) were developed separately by each local employer (70). In 1950, after extensive negotiations, the United Mine Workers of America Welfare and Retirement Fund was established through an industrywide agreement between bituminous coal operators and the union. A wide range of welfare benefits is offered to coal-mining families, including specialist, hospital, and some high-cost pharmaceutical or long-term services (56). The general strategy of the fund has been to pay for approved services rendered by local doctors and other providers who have been found to meet quality standards. In a number of locations in the coal-mining districts of Appalachia (but also in Pennsylvania, Ohio, and elsewhere), the local medical care resources were very deficient; the fund stimulated the organization of several new group practice clinics, with well-qualified specialists. These clinics then served eligible mining families as well as other people in the area. In the late 1950s the fund also used its resources to build a network of ten new, well-staffed general hospitals in the Appalachian states where local resources were especially weak (31). Financial pressures compelled transfer of these in the 1960s to other sponsorship, but all ten hospitals—with relatively strong staffs of full-time specialists—are still in operation serving these rural people.

QUALITY PROMOTION. Several of the organized health efforts already discussed have stimulated an improved quality of rural health care, but certain actions—both governmental and voluntary—have specifically focused on this objective. The most important of these have been the movements usually epitomized as "regionalization" and "group practice," supplemented by a variety of "regulatory" programs.

The regionalization concept has been mainly directed to assuring rural people the same quality of medical care as is available to people in the cities where highly specialized resources exist. The first systematic program to apply the idea was in Maine in the 1930s, where the Bingham Associates Fund established a series of professional connections between hospitals in the small towns of that state and a large medical center in Boston (45). There were regular consultation services in pathology, radiology, and other fields, through the mail as well as by visits. The Maine doctors were invited to Boston for postgraduate education, and rural patients with difficult cases were referred to Boston for diagnostic workups or complex therapy. The same concept was implemented in the 1940s in several rural counties around Rochester, New York, also with foundation support.

The Hill-Burton act contemplated cooperative activities among the several echelons of hospitals in a state, following their construction under a regionalized master plan. In practice, however, these interhospital ties did not develop very successfully (25). The autonomy of both private doctors and sovereign hospitals presented obstacles. Instead of a theoretical two-way flow of patients and consultation services, the most viable programs simply offered educational services from a teaching medical center outward to small community hospitals. After World War II several medical schools undertook such programs (7).

It took the enactment of medicare in 1965 to give a substantial boost to the regionalization idea; with all this money being put into paying for sevices to old people, it was argued, something should be done to underpin the quality of those services. The legislative strategy was to focus attention on the three leading causes of death in the nation, especially among the aged—heart disease, cancer, and stroke. In late 1965, therefore, a federal law was enacted to provide grants for regional medical programs (RMP) to deal with the three top killing diseases (23). Gradually the scope of diseases and also of service modalities under the RMP legislation has widened, and its objectives have evolved toward upgrading the quality of medical care for all conditions in the population living outside the metropolitan centers. In the 1970s special priority is being given to improving the quality of services for the poor, both in large cities and rural districts.

One can argue about how well the RMP program has promoted the classical concept of regionalization (3). Its impact has been primarily educational, and it has done relatively little to encourage regionalized flow of patients or true coordination in the management of hospitals. Still it has stimulated a number of new services in the smaller hospitals—coronary care units, stroke rehabilitation centers, or cancer screening programs. The establishment of various RMP district committees, with both providers and consumers of health care as members, has created an additional ferment in the American health service system which has long-term implications for rural health care. A recently reported personnel exchange program between rural and urban hospitals in the state of Washington is one illustrative outgrowth of RMP stimulation (46).

The group practice idea was pioneered in a rural setting, with the initiative of the Mayo brothers in the small town of Rochester,

Minnesota, in the 1880s. However, opposition to the teaming-up of doctors in private clinics was substantial in the urban centers; solo practitioners through the local medical societies looked upon this as unfair competition and often branded it as unethical. As a result, group medical practice has actually developed more extensively in small towns, where the opposition is weaker, than in large cities. A study in 1959 found 8.2 physicians in group practice clinics per 100,000 population in isolated rural counties, compared with 5.0 per 100,000 in metropolitan counties (63).

There are many definitions and forms of group medical practice, but its major import is that a number of physicians and allied health personnel work together and bring to bear many skills on the care of the patient (18). Since about 1965 the growth of group practice in the nation has accelerated; with the generally high demand for medical care in the population, opposition from solo practitioners has declined. Hospitals have always offered an organized setting in which specialists and allied personnel could work, but the group practice clinic makes this teamwork feasible for the ambulatory patient and also provides a reasonable economic base for specialists in small towns where they might not make a satisfactory income working alone.

A few private group practices have taken special initiative to get primary health services to very isolated rural people. The Rip Van Winkle Clinic in Hudson, New York, operated three satellite health stations in outlying villages during the 1950s. The Daniel Boone Clinic in Harlan, Kentucky, has two major and three small satellite stations within a 40-mile radius in this depressed mountain area. The Dickenson-Wise Clinic in Wise, Virginia, is another rural ambulatory care center with five peripheral branches. Other group practice clinics of distinction, serving mainly rural populations, number in the hundreds and provide centers of quality care for miles around. While the vast majority of these are private and not linked to any prepayment plan, they provide a nucleus for what may later evolve as "health maintenance organizations." Group practices are also a natural vehicle for attracting new doctors into an area, since there are no problems of establishing a practice; from the first day the young physician can be busy and useful.

A third stream of quality promotion affecting rural health service includes all the regulatory activities emanating usually from a state or higher political level. These are both governmental and voluntary. Beyond the hospital licensure laws there is the Joint Commission on Accreditation of Hospitals, founded in 1950 (52), whose inspections and approvals may have more influence on hospitals in rural districts than in cities, since these hospitals are subject to fewer general outside contacts. The Specialty Boards in Medicine, starting with ophthalmology in 1916, have steadily increased their impact. The various professional societies in medicine, dentistry, and nursing exert an influence through continuing education. The American Academy of General Practice requires a certain amount of postgraduate study each year for continued membership of general practitioners, who are relatively more numerous in rural areas than in the cities. The most recently established Specialty Board in Family Practice (1969) should help to elevate the status of the GP, which ought to bring long-term rural benefits.

Under medicare every participating hospital must have a "utilization review" process, which induces a certain group discipline in hospital staffs beyond the usual medical staff rules. In late 1972 federal amendments to the Social Security Act mandated the establishment of Professional Standards Review Organizations (PSRO) to blanket the nation with medical bodies that would exercise peer review of all hospital cases under medicare and medicaid. These PSROs, when they become fully implemented, should have special significance for monitoring the quality of inpatient work done by the more frequently isolated rural doctor. Another new development is the recently authorized network of Area Health Education Centers (AHEC), designed to provide continuing education for all sorts of health manpower in isolated or low-income regions—evidently to either supplement or replace the RMP activities.

STRENGTHENED ECONOMIC SUPPORT. A root problem in attaining good medical care everywhere has always been getting the necessary economic support. For the wealthy this has seldom been a problem. But per capita incomes have long been lower in rural areas, and charity—which has historically helped the poor—is scantier in rural areas. Voluntary health agencies supported by private donations are weaker in the more rural states, as reflected in 1966 data from the American Heart Association and the American Cancer Society (41). The Frontier Nursing Service of Kentucky, supported originally by private philanthropy in the 1920s, is now dependent mainly on governmental grants. Church missions in the Southwest and elsewhere still offer some hospital services, but most of their support comes from noncharitable sources.

Much more important than charity since the 1930s have been the various programs of public assistance that include support for medical care. Before the Social Security Act of 1935 the welfare programs in rural counties were extremely meager, but the inauguration of federal grants to the states brought definite improvements (41). Federal assistance is dependent on demographic categories, the largest of which is the program for Aid to Families with Dependent Children (AFDC);

since children are more numerous in rural families (and in low-income families generally), this program has special value for rural populations. Over the years the Social Security Act has been amended, widening its medical benefits for the poor. The actual amounts of financial aid, however, are dependent on matching state funds; thus the net support per case is typically lower in the more rural than the more urbanized states.

After 30 years of experience the Social Security Act was amended in 1965 with Title XIX or medicaid, which put much larger sums into support of medical care for the poor. To qualify for federal grants, states had to assure a relatively wide scope of physician, laboratory, hospital, and extended care services for categorical cash-grant recipients and also (with limitations) to "medically needy" persons who were categorically linked but not getting cash grants (34). The various amendments and regulations under the medicaid programs are too complex to summarize here, but two points should be made: (1) Under the program the rural poor have received more medical care than they got before. (2) They still get less care than the urban poor. The reason is not simply the lesser per-person expenditures but the lower supply of rural doctors and the relative scarcity of hospital outpatient departments which play such a large part in meeting demands of the urban poor.

The rapidly rising general prices and costs of medical care in the nation since 1965 have created obvious pressures on state governments which must finance about half of medicaid costs. This has led to retrenchments of the program in many states, especially with respect to the medically needy or the near-poor. A special investigating commission in 1970 recommended federalization of the whole structure of medical care for the poor and using public funds for enrolling them in existing health insurance plans serving the general population (65). Some states are now doing this on a limited basis.

In even the most generous state jurisdictions only a small percentage of the total population (well under 10 percent) qualifies for formal public assistance; the great majority of people must rely on other forms of economic support for medical care. Voluntary health insurance has provided an increasing share of this support over the last 50 years. The early application of the insurance mechanism in isolated industries and the subsidized FSA programs for low-income farm families have been mentioned; the big national push began with the rise on a community basis of general hospital insurance in 1929, later acquiring the Blue Cross emblem. This was supported by the hospitals themselves, and around 1939 state medical societies began to sponsor parallel insurance (Blue Shield) mainly for doctors' services in hospitalized cases. In the 1940s the commercial insurance companies, which had previously offered limited indemnity policies for loss of earnings or some medical expenses due to accidents or sickness, also began to sell this type of insurance in a big way (53).

The health insurance movement is well known, but it should be noted that its impact on rural populations has been much less than on urban. The rapid growth of insurance coverage has been due mainly to enrollment of employed groups, found mainly in urban industries. Individul farm families or people in small rural trade centers are not so easily enrolled, even if they can afford it. In 1963 about 75 percent of urban people had some form of insurance protection (usually for hospitalization); this applied to 64 percent of rural nonfarm people and to only 51 percent of rural farm people (60). Moreover, the type of insurance held by rural people is more often the individual enrollment type of indemnity policy sold by commercial carriers, which tends to have higher premiums and more restricted benefits (with various exclusions, deductibles, etc.) (36).

Here and there rural cooperatives that had been organized for agricultural purposes applied the same mechanism to insurance for medical care. One of the first and most illustrious of these efforts was at Elk City, Oklahoma, where the local Farmers Union set up the Farmers Cooperative Health Association in 1929. The struggles of Dr. Michael Shadid to keep this consumer-sponsored program afloat against intense opposition from state and local medical societies is one of the sagas of hard-won progress in the rural health field (49). This program, like one developed later at Two Harbors, Minnesota, was associated with salaried group practice and helped to pioneer the principle now heralded nationally as the Health Maintenance Organization (HMO) concept. Most such organizations, however, are confined to city families, particularly the two largest—the Kaiser-Permanente Health Plan and the Health Insurance Plan of Greater New York. This movement has now come to be spearheaded by the Group Health Association of America, but it still reaches only about 5 percent of the total population and a smaller percentage of the rural.

Aside from deficiencies in rural health insurance coverage, the prominent gap in the 1950s was the weak insurance protection of aged persons, since after 65 years of age most people are retired from employment. Moreover, most private insurance companies had specifically excluded older persons from coverage because they are high risks (that is, have greater needs for medical care), or else such persons were enrolled only with higher premiums and numerous benefit restrictions. In 1957 the first federal legislation was proposed to apply social insurance to medical care of the aged, making hospitalization a supplementary benefit along with old-age pensions under the Social Security Act. This proposal by Representative Aimes Forand generated two responses: an intensive campaign of opposition by the American Medical Association, the insurance industry, and others

—reminiscent of the bitter invectives against the first national health bills 15 years earlier; and expansion of benefits for old people by most of the voluntary insurance plans—some even mandated by state laws (16).

Eight years of contention followed before Title XVIII, medicare, was added to the Social Security Act in 1965. Workmen's compensation providing medical care for industrial injuries (usually excluding agricultural work, incidentally) had started on a state-by-state basis in 1910, and unsuccessful proposals for state laws to meet the costs of general nonoccupational illness had been debated from 1915 to 1920. Now at last a social insurance law for hospital, physician, and other services—although confined to old people—was enacted for the whole United States. To secure congressional passage, numerous compromises were made involving restrictions on benefits associated with commercial insurance practice and day-to-day administration by non-governmental health plans designated as "fiscal intermediaries" (11). Administrative procedures also restricted entitlement of people to hospital and extended care facility services compared with the services of physicians.

Aged people in rural areas have probably enjoyed the greatest relative improvement from the medicare law, since their previous insurance coverage was so poor and their socioeconomic status generally so low. One may conjecture that this flow of assured fees also has added appreciably to the income of rural doctors and small-town hospitals. Since aged persons when hospitalized have relatively long periods of stay, and since their frequency of illness is higher, medicare payments now account for about 40 percent of general hospital income and very likely an even higher proportion for hospitals in small towns (67). Payments into the Social Security Trust Fund from rural populations have been lower than from urban; this program has therefore yielded some redistribution of national wealth toward strengthening rural health care resources.

Medicare has also had another important effect of potentially great importance for rural areas. Since many billions of new dollars were injected into the health services without any significant change in delivery patterns, medical prices rose steeply. Demands for care continued to mount, and people of all social classes—especially the poor—found service increasingly difficult to get. In July 1969 the White House was led to issue a statement saying:

> This nation is faced with a breakdown in the delivery of health care unless immediate concerted action is taken by the government and the private sector. Expansion of private and public financing has created a demand for services far in excess of the capacity of our health system to respond.

With widespread talk of a national crisis in health care, a whole series of new legislative proposals were made to extend the social insurance principle to the whole national population. These proposals varied from government subsidy of membership for low-income people in voluntary health insurance plans to mandatory enrollment of all working people in existing plans to universal coverage of the entire national population (10). Most remarkable was the fact that a Republican national administration, long opposed to any compulsion in paying health insurance premiums, now favored such action by all employers in the nation—albeit with various deductibles and cost-sharing features for the patient. Also remarkable was the advocacy of legislative incentives to modify traditional delivery patterns—that is, private solo practice and fee-for-service remuneration—by both major political parties.

All of the recently proposed national health insurance bills would bring some new benefits for rural people, but the greatest would undoubtedly come from legislation that would achieve a centralized flow of social insurance funds which could then be reallocated to local areas in some reasonable relationship to their health needs. Only a program on the classical social security model of our present OASDI system (like the Health Security Bill of 1972) would do this. As of this writing the outcome of these debates is quite uncertain and will obviously depend on larger political events. One can be quite certain, however, that some new legislation will soon be enacted to provide stronger economic support for general medical care, and that such action will have particular value for rural populations.

HEALTH PLANNING. Most of the movements for improvement in rural health service imply a type of social planning. When the American Medical Association set out to "grade" medical schools after the Flexner report of 1910, that constituted health manpower planning. When Titles V and VI of the Social Security Act of 1935 called for state plans in the maternal and child health and general public health fields as a condition for federal grants, that was health service planning. The state master plans for hospital construction under the Hill-Burton act of 1946 compelled facility planning even more obviously. During World War II there was extensive activity on postwar planning, including commissions in every state, stimulated by the agricultural extension service for rural health service improvements (57).

In 1966, soon after medicare, the first federal legislation specifically in support of comprehensive health planning at the state and local (or areawide) levels was enacted (55). This was largely stimulated by the multiplicity of federal grant-in-aid programs for categorical health purposes which had accumulated over the years, each requiring its own special administrative review. The new law consolidated most (though not all) of these into one block health grant to a single health agency, at which point decisions would be made on allocations of the money for different purposes. To make these decisions, there were to be set up state Comprehensive Health Planning councils on which consumers must constitute a majority. Corresponding CHP boards were also financed in local areas, into which each state had to be divided, but the functions of these local boards have not been so explicit. New funds were also made available for "innovative" health service programs in local communities (Public Health Service Act, Section 314-e), not within the scope of the "formula grant" for overall health purposes received by each state (4).

The CHP legislation calls for planning of "health manpower, facilities, and services"—a broad enough scope but without mandatory authority, except as it has been or will be established by subsequent legislation. The most active role of CHP boards has probably been with regard to planning the construction of facilities, and the staffing of many of these boards has been derived from the earlier councils devoted exclusively to hospital planning. Some 20 states have now passed legislation requiring "certificates of need," approved by a CHP agency, for any new hospital construction, regardless of whether governmental subsidy is received or not (1).

The CHP movement has special meaning for rural areas because the free market determination of the allocation of resources, especially in health manpower, has obviously not been adequately responsive to human needs. Only where market mechanisms have been modified—as in the Hill-Burton, the OEO, or the medicare-medicaid programs—have rural areas seen solid health care improvements. At some future time, when overall funds for health service are more systematically allocated, one may expect that the CHP movement will acquire real force. In 1974 the National Health Planning and Resources Development Act (P.L. 93–641) became the latest chapter in this evolutionary process.

A major impetus to health planning in recent years, aside from the earmarked legislative support, has obviously been the rising costs of medical care. This has been going on for many decades, but until about 1950 the rise in our gross national productivity and national income went along at a corresponding pace, so that health costs remained at 3.5–4.5 percent of our GNP (38). Since 1950 health costs have been rising at a noticeably greater rate than the GNP, and today they exceed 8 percent. This has been due to rises in both rates of utilization and prices per unit of service. These cost pressures have stimulated much of the concern for training new types of allied health personnel and for achieving greater efficiency in the operation of hospitals, which remain the most expensive component of health care (35).

Another important outcome of the cost pressures, with special meaning for rural populations, has been the new official national promotion of Health Maintenance Organizations. In a "health strategy" message of February 1971, President Nixon called for nationwide promotion of HMOs as one of the soundest approaches to cost-containment along with quality controls (19). The idea of providing persons a relatively comprehensive range of physician, hospital, and related services for a fixed annual premium is not new; what is new is its promotion by government. Patterns of delivery of service under HMOs may still involve private solo medical practice and fee payments by medical foundations; the commonest interpretation has assumed the more organized framework of group practice clinics, where systematic preventive and curative services as well as quality assurance can be better arranged. There are various hazards of underservicing in the HMO concept, which will require careful governmental surveillance if the pattern becomes widespread through public financial support. After extended debate the Health Maintenance Organization Act (P.L. 93-222) was enacted in December 1973; it authorizes $375 million over a five-year period for stimulating and assisting establishment of new HMOs, with special priorities assigned to covering populations in nonmetropolitan areas.

For rural populations the HMO pattern could have the special advantage of mobilizing many different types of health resources in isolated areas. The patient would not have to wend his way through a dispersed pluralistic maze to get integrated health care. In a sense the HMO idea, if backed up by adequate financial support, would constitute a characteristically American approach to the planning of total health services, with the initiative coming from many local communities instead of being mandated by a central power. Furthermore, opportunities for strong consumer input into the methods by which health needs are met would be greater than ever before.

TRENDS. From early attention focused on disease prevention, the health movement has widened to social concern for comprehensive health service. While the preventive focus was understandably warranted in a period of dramatic new discoveries in community hygiene, the technical inseparability of prevention and treatment and the greater social effectiveness of their combination has become increasingly appreciated.

The interdependence of actions in the several sectors of health service has become recognized as necessary for rural improvements.

Programs for facility construction, manpower expansion, economic support, and quality promotion are all obviously intertwined. These actions in turn are all interdependent with general social changes in agriculture, employment, transportation, education, social security, and other spheres. Reaching goals in any one of these sectors usually depends on parallel actions in several of the others.

It has become clear that health service improvements cannot be left to the initiative of doctors and other health professionals alone. Progress has come largely from the initative of consumers, expressing their will through various citizen organizations and ultimately through elected representatives in government. In fact, much of the progress has been achieved over the opposition of leaders of the private medical profession. This does not mean that consumers could work effectively without sound technical advice, but such advice has been available from many sources.

Because of the complexities and rising costs of health service, improvement has become increasingly dependent on collective economic efforts. The mechanisms of private spending and charity have become gradually replaced by insurance and tax support. Along with this, people have naturally become more concerned with how wisely the collectively raised monies are spent for health service.

As public knowledge of the health sciences has widened, professional discipline has heightened and greater social controls over the quality of services have been developed. These have emanated from both governmental and private sources, but all of them have meant greater social organization of resources.

Significant rural health improvements cannot be expected within the boundaries of rural communities by themselves. Cooperation is needed from the cities, along both economic and technical lines. As the instrumentality for linking rural and urban resources, government has had to play an increasing role. This means government at all levels, but the main thrust has come from state and national rather than town and county levels. National and state taxing powers have been the major vehicles for redistribution of resources toward achieving greater equity for rural people.

At present marked deficiencies still characterize rural health service compared with levels that have been shown to be reachable in the cities. This is seen in wealthy America as much or more than it is seen in many other countries of lesser wealth. The main lesson of history would seem to be that future reduction of rural deficiencies in health resources and services will depend largely on deliberate social actions by the national government.

CHAPTER TWO

DIVERSITY OF RURAL SOCIETY AND HEALTH NEEDS

JAMES H. COPP

RURAL HEALTH has traditionally been viewed as a special problem because of rural people's relative inaccessibility to professional medical care and their greater exposure to socioeconomic conditions conducive to neglect of health problems. The inaccessibility of people living in small towns and widely dispersed homesteads in the open country is obvious and is inherent in the notion of rural, which means beyond the city. The inferior socioeconomic conditions of rural people compared with urban people—as measured by income, education, and quality of housing—are equally obvious. Thus the presumption that rural health continues to be a serious problem in our society appears to be well justified. Earlier studies of rural health have provided ample grounds for the presumption (9).

However, a careful examination of recent data as well as of the conditions of rural life today suggests that the conclusion is not as clear as we might expect and that the identification of population groups with serious health problems is much more involved than the simple blanket designation of rural areas. There are grave health problems in many rural areas, but the inferior status of rural health in general may not be easily demonstrable.

DEFINITIONS OF RURALITY. The U.S. Census of Population makes the designation of rural people deceptively simple: rural people are those who live in places with fewer than 2,500 people or in the open country. But the social conditions of living have changed, and this rural-urban distinction is less discriminating than in

JAMES H. COPP is Professor and Head, Department of Rural Sociology and Department of Sociology and Anthropology, Texas A & M University.

the past. Urban influences on life styles have progressed beyond the city limits. Rural no longer implies farm or agricultural; less than 15 percent of our rural population live on farms. Among those who live on farms, more income is obtained from nonagricultural sources than from agricultural sources. Suburbanites, exurbanites, and commuters are widely scattered over the rural landscape. Putting it briefly, our rural population in the United States is not at all homogeneous and is not primarily identified with agriculture (21, pp. 110–14).

The only thing shared by rural people is location outside a place of 2,500 or more people. Even this characteristic is far from uniform in meaning: 30 percent of our rural people live in metropolitan counties (counties or sets of counties with centers of 50,000 or more people) (20, Table 17), and another 25 percent live in counties immediately adjacent to a metropolitan county. Given the speed of movement by automobile on interstate and limited-access highways, being rural does not necessarily mean being inaccessible. However, isolation from large urban centers remains a serious problem for a great many rural people.

On the other hand, many so-called urban places have become more rural in character. Small cities have become less complete service centers, giving up many of their economic functions to nearby larger places, and have less in common with those centers of 50,000, a million, or more population.

Since the distinction between rural and urban has become less useful than it was in the past, the growing tendency is to distinguish between metropolitan areas (counties or sets of counties with a central city of 50,000 or more population) and nonmetropolitan areas. For many purposes even 50,000 population appears to be too small; 250,000 population might be a better cutting point for distinguishing extensive, dense agglomerations of people from less concentrated settlement. There never will be a perfect cutting point for distinguishing densely settled from widely dispersed populations; for conditions of life in our society, the rural and urban criteria are very imperfect.

Despite the recognized deficiencies of the distinction, rural and urban categories, sanctified by traditions of discourse, will probably continue to be used by policymakers. We should keep in mind that "rural" is too inclusive—comprising both those who are definitely isolated and those who are not—and that rural people are not homogeneous according to occupation, income, or education. "Rural" denotes nothing but location, and even that denotation is highly imprecise.

If "rural" is such a crude category, why do we often find differences in social indicators when we categorize on a rural-urban basis? The answer lies in some modal tendencies in this residual group. Although the rural population is not principally agricultural, the agricultural population is found principally within it. Although rural incomes vary widely, a disproportionate share of low-income families live in rural areas. Although rural educational attainment varies, a disproportionate share of people with the lowest educational attainment live in rural areas. Although rural housing varies widely, a disproportionate share of substandard housing is found in rural areas. Likewise, rural areas are characterized by having a disproportionate share of the elderly (3).

Furthermore, rural areas are characterized by what we may term residual stability. Historically, more people have migrated *from* rural areas than *to* rural areas. Thus whatever rural people tend to have been in the past persists into the present, undiluted by infusions of different stock with sharply divergent demographic or cultural traits. The rural population may be seen as a residual reservoir that changes slowly through the attrition of outmigration and time rather than by the sudden admixture of new populations with divergent life styles (residential suburbs in rural areas would be the striking exceptions).

When we find differences in social indicators between rural and urban categories, what are we to conclude? Is it a difference attributable to the ecology of spatial location, of occupation, of some other demographic characteristic, or of tradition? Rural-urban differences do not tell us much if we cannot specify what it is about rurality that causes the differences. Likewise the deficiencies and handicaps of some subpopulations in rural areas may be masked or offset by the strengths and advantages of other rural subpopulations. Our analytical lines of cleavage for specifying critical subpopulations in our society must be more incisive; "rural" and "urban" are too blunt and crude for exact analysis, yielding shadowy results we cannot confidently interpret when found. We see, but we do not know what we have seen. The increasingly popular metropolitan-nonmetropolitan distinction is subject to the same shortcomings for interpretive purposes.

HEALTH OF RURAL PEOPLE. How healthy are rural people? The truth is that we do not know. If it were possible to conduct physical examinations of large representative samples of various subpopulations, we could make statements with confidence. Such data do not exist, nor is it likely that they will materialize in the near future (if the past record of the National Health Survey in providing physical examination data on *specific conditions* for broad urban and rural categories can be taken as a guide).

Past experience suggests that rural people would not be superior in health to urban residents. At the time of World War II, careful studies of preinduction physical examination data showed that more rural than urban young men were rejected for medical reasons (9, pp.

114–21). Unfortunately, regional variations in those and in more recent data lead one to question uniformity of standards employed by the examining physicians (8). Fairly widespread dental examinations in the population also seem to indicate that rural people obtain less adequate dental care (16). If the physical condition of rural people were greatly superior to that of urban people, such findings would be most unlikely. On the other hand, we do not have good evidence that the health of rural people is decidedly inferior. We can only say the answer is not obvious and that the question is unsettled.

If rural people are physically inferior, as some studies suggest, the fact remains that rural people are affected less by illness than urban people, at least as measured by standard morbidity measures in the National Health Survey. Table 2.1 shows that residents of metropolitan central cities generally have the highest morbidity rates, followed by nonfarm nonmetroplitan people; farm people have the lowest morbidity rates of all. In a number of cases the differences between farm people and the combined nonfarm and metropolitan samples are quite distinct. We do not know if farm people have fewer and less severe illnesses or whether they are less willing to restrict their activity when they are ill.

Given the more or less consistent patterning of the trends in the data from metropolitan or central city to nonfarm to farm, it is tempting to speculate that urban congestion and pollution are taking their toll. Such speculation is premature until we have more refined analyses by density of population and relative pollution of the environment. Who is to say how the dust, exhaust fumes, and agricultural chemicals to which the farm worker is exposed compare with urban smog? Nevertheless, the rather severe air pollution in major metropolitan areas is not easily set aside as an extremely negative health factor.

Taking more extreme measures of health—death rates—the evidence is unfavorable for rural areas. The infant mortality rate has often been taken as the most sensitive measure of the quality of life. On this measure the nonmetropolitan rate of 24.9 deaths per 1,000 live births compares with the metropolitan rate of 22.0. The differential persists for most regions, income, and educational levels, even when considering each race separately (14). The largest differential is by race; infant mortality rates for blacks are twice those for whites in many comparisons. Infant mortality rates for whites in nonmetropolitan areas do not consistently decrease with increases in the income or education of mother or father. Apparently no amount of income or education will counteract nonmetropolitan residence. Although the differentials are small, they suggest that the roots of infant mortality may be quite complex and that infant mortality may be an inexact measure of the quality of life.

With regard to motor vehicle accidental deaths, we find some

Table 2.1. Selected Health Indicators by Metropolitan and Nonmetropolitan Residence

| | Metropolitan | | Nonmetropolitan | |
	Central City	Outside Central City	Nonfarm	Farm
Days of restricted activity per person per year (age adjusted) (12)[a]	15.7	13.7	15.1	11.8
Days of bed disability per person per year (age adjusted) (12)	6.9	5.6	6.1	4.3
Days lost from work per currently employed person per year (age adjusted) (12)	5.9	4.9	5.2	4.2
Limitation of activity due to chronic conditions per 100 persons (age adjusted) (12)	11.5	10.8	12.8	12.2
Days lost from school per school-age child per year (11)	5.4		4.1	4.4
Number of acute conditions per 100 persons per year (age adjusted) (12)	204.1	207.1	199.1	163.1
Infant deaths per 1,000 live births (14)	22.0		24.9	
Motor vehicle accident deaths per 100,000 population (15)	17.1		28.4	
Persons injured per 100 persons (age adjusted) (12)	24.9	26.8	27.6	22.5
Injuries at work, per 1,000 workers, males (17)	87.2		96.8	129.6
Hospital insurance coverage (13)	81.3		74.4	61.9
Surgical insurance coverage (13)	79.6		72.9	59.7
Discharges from short-stay hospitals per 1,000 persons (age adjusted) (12)	129.4	122.8	145.3	107.1
Surgical treatment for discharges per 1,000 persons per year (12)	73.9	70.7	68.3	50.8
Physician visits per person (age adjusted) (12)	4.7	4.6	4.2	3.1
Dental visits per person (age adjusted) (12)	1.6	1.8	1.2	1.1

[a]Numbers in parentheses refer to references at end of book.

interesting differences; nonmetropolitan death rates were two-thirds higher (15). Two factors are probably operating: the high speeds traveled in sparsely populated areas and the greater difficulty in providing fast emergency care. Injuries at work are also higher for farm males—129.6 per 1,000 workers compared with 96.8 for nonfarm male workers and 87.2 for metropolitan male workers (17). Undoubtedly this too is related to the nature of the work in rural areas—more physical and more hazardous. An additional consideration is that the farmer generally lives at his place of work and is not constrained by a 40-hour week, leading to greater exposure to work-related injuries.

Thus it appears that the rural environment is more hostile when it comes to automobile and work accidents. It is curious to note that when very distinct rural-urban differences are found, they are differences peculiar to the nature of rural areas. Since differences in morbidity and infant mortality are patterned but not great, it does not seem reasonable to expect great differences in rural and urban health (if we could get good data on the health of populations classified by degree of rurality).

Despite the lack of supporting evidence for wide rural and urban health differences, a real difference may lie in the extent to which treatment for chronic health problems is sought. The evidence on dental conditions has been cited, and we note that farm people are less likely to let illness restrict their activity. More to the point, four out of every five metropolitan residents have hospital and surgical insurance coverage, compared with three out of every five farm people (13). The pattern of the data in Table 2.1 suggests that the rural person is less likely to have adequate resources available when illness strikes. In such cases treatment is more likely to be avoided or postponed when possible. We suggest that rural people are about as likely as urban people to be ill but less likely to do anything about minor ailments and symptoms. Likewise, farm people suffering from acute conditions experience restricted activity 0.1 of a day longer than SMSA (Standard Metropolitan Statistical Area) and nonfarm categories but spend 0.4 and 0.3 less days in bed (10). Critical examination of this possibility is required, although hospitalization and physician visits show parallel trends in Table 2.1.

However, the major factor differentiating subpopulations is not rural or urban residence. We would do much better in identifying populations with critical health needs if we shifted to other bases of categorization, such as race or income.

SUBPOPULATIONS. Thus far the term "health needs" has been employed rather loosely in an undefined fashion. It would be difficult to be very specific, but certain clarifications can be made. Health needs would be the objective, technically defined need for preventive and treatment measures to improve the physical well-being of people in a medical sense. Health needs are not necessarily recognized by the client public. They are not the same as wants. On the other hand, the public may desire certain measures they believe benefit their health, when these measures do not objectively improve their health (e.g., certain patent medicines). Consequently health needs are not the same thing as the "demand" for medical care.

Health needs also involve the notion of technical determination of priorities. People may demand hospitals when they really require preventive medicine, environmental protection, or improved nutrition. The determination of health needs is a matter of expert technical opinion rather than the expression of the public's conscious desires in health matters. The concept of health needs thus involves the perils of technical arrogance: the technician may make errors in judgment or base his inferences on incomplete or fallacious information. Certainly the medical community is not infallible in its recommendations for health and its judgments of needs, but the medical and health professional *in general* is better able to recognize health needs than the client public. If the qualification of humility can be kept in mind, the concept of health needs can be employed to represent an objective determination, using the best available medical knowledge, of the extent to which positive intervention is required to improve the physical well-being of a population.

A number of subpopulations living in rural areas have been specifically identified as having critical health needs. In identifying a subpopulation there is no assertion that every member or even most members are subject to severe health deprivations. Rather the intent is to suggest that unmet health needs occur disproportionately in that subpopulation. In many cases careful research must be conducted to validate the assertions.

American Indians. The American Indian is the most rural of all our ethnic groups and is also the most economically deprived. He is far from being brought into the mainstream of our economy and society. Infant mortality rates are high and life expectancy is far below the U.S. average (7); other health problems such as alcoholism and tuberculosis are endemic. Because native Americans tend to be located in the most rural and most inaccessible parts of the country, health delivery systems are costly and less effective.

Southern Rural Blacks. Next to the American Indian, the economic condition of the southern rural black is probably lowest. Housing is often as bad as that of the American Indian. Educational attainment, especially among older rural blacks, is low. Persisting patterns of discrimination have meant that the black has had to take second best in medical care. Folk nostrums are common, and a generally inadequate knowledge of health maintenance and preventive medicine prevails. Nutrition has traditionally been poor. Infant mortality is twice as high as for rural whites. Contagious diseases are prevalent. Average expectation of life is significantly lower than for whites. Given high rates of outmigration of the able-bodied young people from the region, physical disability tends to be high among the remaining families (19). The southern rural black, in terms of his numbers and his economic deprivation (2), is one of the most significant subpopulations in the rural United States having critical health needs.

Mexican Americans (Chicanos). A third major rural subpopulation that could be expected to have critical health needs is the Mexican American. Educational attainment is unusually low, families are large, economic deprivation is high, and there is an added barrier —a difference in language and culture. As a result, the Chicano tends to be cut off from modern professional medical care. Folk medicine has been relied upon extensively in rural areas.

The low income position of the Mexican American is compounded by fatalistic views of health. Traditionally illness has been seen as coming from God or even evil spirits—something to be borne rather than avoided. Although there appear to be critical health needs among rural Chicanos, there has been little investigation of health problems. Available data are highly inadequate (5, p. 23).

Appalachian and Ozark Whites. Historically the Appalachians and the Ozarks have been among the more inaccessible and culturally isolated parts of the country. Incomes of residents have been characteristically low, as has been educational attainment. Disability tends to be high in what is a disproportionately aged population (6). Health needs are critical and delivery systems are underdeveloped.

The Aged. Rural aged people constitute one of the least recognized problem segments of our population so far as health is concerned. Incomes are low, chronic illnesses and disability are high. Reluctance to accept public assistance may be a serious barrier to treatment. Transportation to obtain medical care is a problem. Utilization of medicare and other available programs may be low because of misunderstandings about eligibility and confusion over procedures (1). The rural aged, like the urban aged, are a subpopulation with extremely critical health needs (4).

Migrant Workers. Of all the groups with largely unmet critical health needs, the migrant agricultural worker has probably attracted the most attention. As the agricultural industry's demand for workers decreases with mechanization, this group's numbers are rapidly declining. Today probably fewer than 120,000 migrant workers are employed in agriculture for 25 days or more a year, and the number continues to decline (18, p. 6). If family members are included, the total number of people involved is probably about 500,000; thus this is a relatively small and declining group, but one with serious problems.

The migrant worker's annual income is low. His education is low. He lacks the ties of residence to establish his claims for public assistance. He is nobody's problem, and he is everybody's.

Alcoholism and personal instability tend to be high. Exposure to the elements and poor living conditions lead to early and widespread disability, often disqualifying the migrant for further work. The migrant comes to his job economically and socially powerless and very likely jeopardizes his health in the process. Thus far, health delivery systems for the migrant and his family are woefully inadequate.

Illegal Aliens. Even more powerless to obtain health care is the rural worker who has entered this country illegally, most commonly from Mexico. Great numbers of illegal entrants, estimated in the millions, are living and working in urban and rural areas. The rural illegal entrant, working on ranches or construction projects, typically comes from poverty-stricken areas where medical care is generally inadequate; and he must avoid any move that would betray his citizenship status to officials who could immediately deport him. Presently the illegal entrant has no claims to public resources for his health needs and represents the ultimate in limited access to services.

Tourists and Vacationers. Another group of people with occasional special health needs are travelers and vacationers—generally well off economically and in other ways. With accidents and sudden illnesses, getting competent treatment in a strange rural community can be a problem. In some instances the victim is in an extremely isolated area or in rugged terrain. As participation in tourism and outdoor recreation continues, the need for quickly securing competent medical aid persists. In some rural areas the vacation population may be double or triple (or more) the year-round population. The same would hold for any event in a rural community that brings in a great influx of outside people, whether it be a rock festival or a revival.

Environmental Pollution Areas. Until recently, major health needs in communities with noxious industries—smelters, paper mills, refineries—have not been recognized. Only in the past few years have epidemiological studies disclosed community health hazards from dust, radiation, and air pollution. For a long time the need has objectively existed, but the problem has not been acknowledged. The major task in such communities is reduction of hazards; treatment for resulting disabilities is a second priority.

Highly Dispersed Settlement. There is a subpopulation living in rural areas that suffers the classic costs of isolation and sparse settlement to a very high degree. Population density is too low to support a conventional health delivery system, and transportation to a medical center may be a matter of hours. Many areas in the Great Plains, the mountain states, and Alaska are subject to these restrictions. If there is a disadvantage to rural living, people living in such areas exemplify the problem. Fortunately the proportion of the rural population living under such conditions is low, although the aggregate numbers involved are significant.

Metropolitan Hinterland. Within 50 miles of every large city are pockets of low-income people who have not shared in the general affluence of metropolitan growth. Because of this proximity to affluent suburban areas, their existence tends to be masked in the statistics. They have little power or skill in attracting the attention of the authorities. The general body of citizenry cannot believe such conditions exist. Yet such neighborhoods can be found on the back roads in Westchester County, New York; Howard County, Maryland; Prince William County, Virginia; or Harris County, Texas. In other words, some of the most critical health needs in the country can be found in rural areas in the shadows of New York City, Baltimore, Washington, D.C., or Houston. These pockets of poverty are all the more serious because of their invisibility and the hostility and indifference of middle-class suburbanite neighbors.

Communes. The last subpopulation of rural people to be mentioned can easily be overlooked; it is mentioned to illustrate how easily groups with critical health needs can be ignored. These are the young people who have fled to rural areas to live under communal conditions or unconventional circumstances. Income is low, health habits are irregular, sanitary conditions may be poor. Furthermore, there may be strong hatred for these "deviants" among local residents. The number of such youth in rural areas is unknown, but the total for the United States may be around 100,000.

Common Characteristics. This cursory review of several rural subpopulations with critical health needs suggests that they share certain common characteristics. They tend to be low-income; powerless; and despised because of race, culture, or life style. They tend to embody values that are held in low esteem in our society—age, color, rootlessness, poverty, or presumed immorality. They tend to be what we popularly call losers. They are people who have been exploited or bypassed in the name of progress or economic development. We have tended to overlook the plight of residents of the community with a noxious industry; Indians, blacks, Chicanos, and hillbillies have been dismissed as backward; the migrant worker and the metropolitan hinterland poor are invisible; and the illegal entrant is not our responsibility at all. Most of these subpopulations cannot be found with the aid of present statistical information; yet their health needs far exceed what would be expected from statistics on the rural population. We need to examine our population along new analytical lines of cleavage if we are to identify those with the greatest need; our present demographic breakdowns can be next to useless, even deceptively reassuring, as the preceding data from the National Health Survey have shown.

RECOMMENDATIONS FOR RESEARCH. The foregoing discussion has made one point abundantly clear: useful data on rural health needs are almost totally lacking. Only the data from the National Health Survey give any hint of the situation, and even then the data reported on a metropolitan-nonmetropolitan, farm-nonfarm basis are rather limited. Not only are present data sparse, but the rural-urban categories employed are not very diagnostic in locating the problems because they confound affluent and impoverished rural subpopulations.

Much better assessment of rural health needs could be made if the National Health Survey were to include additional questions that would make it possible to clearly identify subpopulations by ethnicity (Negro, Mexican-American, Indian, Eskimo), by age, by income level, by degree of accessibility to medical centers, and by cultural barriers (language and cultural traits, including countercultural). The survey samples would have to be substantially increased, but until data can be provided on high-exposure subpopulations, they will not be of much programmatic use anyway, except for giving a broad national picture.

Moreover, the data obtainable from an interview survey (such as the National Health Interview Survey) are imprecise, based on self-reports and recall. Self-judgments of morbidity and chronic disability will vary from person to person. The survey does not tell us much about the individual's objective impairment. People tell us they have been ill or incapacitated, but we do not know anything about their physical condition. Neither can the Health Survey tell us about health problems of which the respondent is not aware.

If we want to know something about the health and health needs of rural people, we will have to perform physical examinations on substantial samples of the different rural subpopulations. Objective determinations will have to be made of accessibility to medical care and of exposure to noxious environmental influences. Now here is a problem: If the comparability of preinduction physical examinations among races, education levels, and regions of the country is suspect (8, pp. 20–24), would physical exams accurately portray the health conditions of rural Americans? Can we assume that physical examinations have high reliability? Evaluations of health by physicians are judgmental. What is a critical health problem in one physician's eyes might be a tolerable condition in another's judgment. The manifold physical measures will have to be standardized, and the integration and interpretation of the resulting great number of specific measures will have to be done impersonally—perhaps by computers. Given the present state of the art, physical exams may be no more reliable than self-reports by respondents. National Health Survey physical examination data are reported in terms of specific measures rather than in terms of summary interpretations of physical condition. So far no publication from the Health Survey integrates the physical examination data in summary fashion for individuals. We are not told anywhere about the state of health in the nation. Apparently the more carefully we measure health indicators, the less able we are to talk about health.

In the above discussion, nothing has even been said about clarifying the concept of health. What is health? Is normal aging health? Is a certain amount of morbidity healthy, say, in building up resistance? What indicators shall we use to measure health? It has been suggested that indicators used in the National Health Survey or in physical examinations may not be valid, reliable, or interpretable in a policy sense. Thus a tremendous amount of work needs to be done on the methodology of assessing health.

Once we have improved measures and applied them to strategic subpopulations, we will be prepared for some basic research on the relative influence of various classes of background factors on health. Furthermore, we will be able to study the changes in the values of measurements over time to ascertain the relative efficacies of health programs and what effects environmental changes are having on health. Today we can only identify those environmental influences that have obvious gross effects. A great deal of work on the methodology of assessing health must be done before we can speak authoritatively about health needs in rural areas.

CHAPTER THREE

RISK OF ILLNESS AND DEATH IN METROPOLITAN AND NONMETROPOLITAN AREAS

HERBERT I. SAUER

GOOD HEALTH is an exceedingly difficult quality to measure with reasonable objectivity. Illness and disease provide a more tangible approach for measurement (23). Five levels of evaluation of poor health are suggested: dissatisfaction, discomfort, disease, disability, and death (22). Dissatisfaction is as difficult to measure as good health, and questions may be raised as to whether the absence of dissatisfaction is either necessarily related to health or desirable. Discomfort is also somewhat difficult to measure objectively. Therefore, attention is focused on the latter three levels of evaluation, and patterns of illness are compared for both rural and urban areas.

RATES OF ILLNESS AND DEATH. Various measures or indices of illness may be obtained from interviewing large samples of the population of the United States, focusing on degrees of disability and disease. Such information has been obtained by the National Health Survey, the latest report being for the years 1969 and 1970 (7).

Four measures of the prevalence of disability or illness are presented in Table 3.1: restricted activity days, bed disability days, workloss days, and percent of the population with limitation of activities due to chronic conditions. On the average, persons living on farms reported the fewest days per year of either restricted activity or bed disability. Data (not in Table 3.1) also indicate that the average number

HERBERT I. SAUER is Assistant Professor, Department of Community Health and Medical Practice, University of Missouri.

This work was supported in part by designated research grants from the University of Missouri-Columbia Development Fund and the Office of Creative Ministries, Missouri Area United Methodist Church.

Table 3.1.   Prevalence of Illness by Place of Residence, United States, 1969–70

| Index of Illness | Nonmetropolitan Areas | | | Standard Metropolitan Statistical Areas |
	Total	Nonfarm	Living on farms	
Restricted activity, days per year	14.9	15.2	12.6	14.5
Days of bed disability per year	6.0	6.2	4.5	6.2
Work-loss days per currently employed person (17+ years) per year	5.1	5.2	4.7	5.3
Percent of population with limitation of activity due to chronic conditions	13.1	13.0	13.9	10.9

Source: Namey and Wilson (7, Table O, p. 12).

of days per person per year of both restricted activity and bed disability increases moderately with age, for age 65+ being roughly three times as great as for those under 45. But for each of four broad age groups (under 17, 17–44, 45–64, 65 and over), those living on farms had fewer average days reported than did those in metropolitan areas.

Families living in the open country but not on farms and those living in villages, towns, and small cities constitute the nonfarm group living in nonmetropolitan areas. Their average number of days of limited activity and bed disability tended to be similar to the averages for those living in metropolitan areas. Additional data (not in Table 3.1) indicate that for the two age groups under age 45 (under 17 and 17–44), the averages for the nonfarm group tended to be less than those for the metropolitan areas; for the groups age 45–64 and 65+, they were higher for the nonfarm group than for the metropolitan group.

There may well be a difference in health and health care needs for the two groups, even though the difference may be partly due to the way in which human beings move about and arrange for care. For example, it has been customary for decades for farmers to retire from their farms because of age and failing health. In the process they often become part of the normal nonfarm population. Further, the data are derived from a probability sample of the civilian noninstitutional population. If there are differences among different segments of the population in utilizing nursing homes or other resident institutions for the delivery of health care, the indices based on those at home will also be affected.

The average annual number of days of work lost per currently employed person is likewise less for those on farms than for others, but this differential is less than for the restricted activity and bed disability indices of illness (Table 3.1). Data (not in Table 3.1) reveal that for age group 45–64 and particularly for age group 17–44, those on farms average fewer days of work lost than do those in metropolitan areas. However, for those 65 and over, the number of days of work lost is greater for those on farms than for those in metropolitan areas. This might mean that farmers with borderline health could continue working, whereas factory and white-collar workers would be more likely to be retired for disability. If so, then one might expect middle-aged and older farm residents to have a higher percentage "with limitations of activity due to chronic conditions" then do those living in metropolitan areas. The data are consistent with this line of thought, even though for those under 45 years of age, farm residents have the lower percentage "with limitations of activity due to chronic conditions":

	Nonmetropolitan Areas (farm residents)	Metropolitan Areas
Under age 45	4.7%	5.2%
Age 45–64	21.5%	17.8%
Age 65+	46.7%	39.8%

These percentages also make clear a close association between the prevalence of chronic conditions and age. Thus, even if age-specific percentages are fairly low for a given area compared with other areas, the overall percentage for such an area may be high if the area's population is largely in the older age groups.

The average annual incidence of acute conditions per 100 persons per year is lower for those living on farms than for those living in metropolitan areas (Table 3.2). (This trend applies for age-specific rates as well, even though individuals under age 17 have the highest rates and those age 45+ have the lowest rates.) Since these are defined as acute conditions that are medically attended, it is not possible (with these data) to separate completely the incidence of disease from the delivery of health care. Indices of delivery of health care—such as "short-stay hospital discharges per 1,000 persons per year" and "percent of population with 1+ physician visits within a year"—are thus to some extent measuring the incidence of illness for which health care is needed, along with the extent to which health care is delivered.

The several indices of illness together do not present a sharp contrast in the level of health of people in nonmetropolitan United States compared with those in metropolitan areas. For those living on farms, however, the various indices of illness rather consistently

Table 3.2. Incidence of Illness and Delivery of Health Care by Place of Residence, United States, 1969–70

| | Nonmetropolitan Areas | | | Standard Metropolitan Statistical Areas |
Index of Illness	Total	Nonfarm	Living on farms	
Acute conditions per 100 persons per year	195.1	200.0	159.6	205.8
Short-stay hospital discharges per 1,000 persons per year	141.0	145.4	108.7	125.7
Percent of population with 1+ physician visits within a year	68.5	69.4	62.4	71.8

Source: Namey and Wilson (7, Table O, p. 12).

tend to be lower than for those in metropolitan areas, with one major exception: of the farm population who are middle-aged or older, a higher percentage report limitation of activity due to chronic conditions compared with the corresponding individuals in metropolitan areas. Less clear-cut differences, as well as this difference, may very well be worth further study.

Rural areas generally tend to have lower death rates in middle-age populations than do urban areas, although this difference seems to be decreasing. In 1940 white death rates for ages 35–44, 45–54, 55–64, and 65–74 for rural United States were only about three-fourths as high as for cities 100,000 and over; under age 35 the various rates were as high or higher in rural areas (5). Cities of 2,500–10,000 and 10,000–100,000 populations had varying death rates, generally intermediate between the rural and large-city rates.

In 1950 the nonmetropolitan areas had rates for middle-aged whites about 14 percent less than metropolitan areas; in 1960 this difference was 9 percent (3). The rates per 1,000 for whites, both sexes, age 35–74 (age-adjusted by direct method by ten-year age groups to the total U.S. population in 1950) were as follows:

	U.S.	Metropolitan Counties	Nonmetropolitan Counties
1950	12.9	13.6	11.7
1960	11.7	12.1	11.0

In both these time periods the nonmetropolitan areas had higher rates for each age group under 35.

Since the various rates under age 35 are less favorable for the rural or nonmetropolitan areas and the rates for age groups 45–84 are more favorable for nonmetropolitan areas, a single all-ages rate tends to minimize the differences between nonmetropolitan and metropolitan areas. Further, the amount and direction of the differences will be determined by the population used as the standard. In spite of such limitations, the usual procedure in vital statistics analyses is to present the all-ages rates, age-adjusted by the direct method. Using the total U.S. population in 1940 as the standard population, in compliance with convention, the usual death rates per 1,000 population for all ages, age-adjusted, are presented as follows:

	U.S.	Nonmetropolitan Counties
1950	8.0	7.7
1960	7.3	7.1
1969–71	6.7	6.8

In the past for the United States as a whole, death rates for all ages, age-adjusted, have been somewhat lower for nonmetropolitan than for metropolitan counties. In recent years, however, rates for metropolitan counties have declined more, so there is uncertainty as to the magnitude and direction of this difference at present. Detailed analyses of Missouri mortality by counties now being made for the 1968–72 period compared with the 1950–59 period also show a greater average decline for metropolitan than for the nonmetropolitan counties (13, 16, 17).

Many other similarities between various groups in the risk of death may also be identified. Of even greater interest and importance are the differences in death rates between specific areas. The focus of our study is on geographic differences in the risk of death due to chronic diseases in middle age, broadly defined. External causes—specifically motor vehicle accidents, other accidents, suicide, and homicide—are of concern to those involved in the delivery of health care regardless of age. However, for those age 35 and over, particularly those 45 and over, external causes as a group are responsible for a very small portion of total deaths. Further, deaths from external causes tend to vary by geographic area independently of chronic disease deaths. Communicable diseases are of even less importance in the number of deaths in these age groups. Thus, for those of middle age and older, the age-specific death rates for all causes of death combined constitute an excellent measure of the risk of death due to chronic diseases.

RISK FACTORS AND GEOGRAPHY. The exact causes of the various chronic diseases generally are not known, but various risk factors have been identified, some of which may be causal in nature. For example, cigarette smoking, obesity, high caloric and saturated fat intake, and lack of exercise are all associated with a high risk for one or several chronic diseases. Various cultural and socio-economic variables have been identified as being either actual or possible risk factors.

Age, sex, and race or major ethnic group have geen recognized as major risk factors for which information is generally available by geographic area. However, chronological age cannot be assumed to be a precise measure of aging. For example, the 60-year-old who has exposed himself to heavy cigarette smoking, overeating, and lack of exercise for 40 years may be assumed to be at a much greater risk of attack from a chronic disease than the 25-year-old who has exposed himself to such factors for only 5 years—even if aging did not exist. In early adult life the risk of death due to chronic diseases is very low, but this risk doubles every 7 or 8 years. This steep rise in risk with age and geographic variations in this rise may be studied without assuming that the cause of this increase is known.

Differences by sex and race, even though much less marked, may be approached in a similar manner. In recent years the middle-aged white male is very clearly the weaker sex, with much higher risk of death than the white female of the same age. More specifically, white men age 45–54 have cardiovascular disease death rates about three times as high as do white women of the same age, even though around 1920 there was no difference in the rates. Thus anyone who wishes to propose the hypothesis that sex differences in risk are due solely to physiological factors (hormonal or other) has the challenging task of explaining how sex differences in physiology could change so dramatically in the short span of half a century. Therefore, it seems necessary to concur with the view that risk factors such as sex and race may in some instances be identifiers of relative risk; the underlying causes may in some way be due to differences in the environment—physical, biological, or cultural—and their interactions.

The conventional epidemiological approach of using age-, sex-, and race-specific rates seems to be necessary and appropriate; these should be considered only as three important risk factors which are brought under statistical control so that the search for other risk factors may continue.

State Economic Areas (SEAs). The National Center for Health Statistics has made available the number of deaths by age, sex, and race for each county and county equivalent in the United States for each year 1959–69 inclusive. In Tables 3.3–3.9 we have summed these deaths and calculated conventional average annual death rates per 1,000 population, with the estimated population at risk being the arithmetic interpolation of counts from the Bureau of the Census for 1960 and 1970 (18, 20).

To minimize the role of chance fluctuation without appreciably minimizing differences in risk, attention is focused on death rates for white males age 35–74, age-adjusted by ten-year age groups by the direct method to the total U.S. population in those age groups in 1950 (5).

Rates have been calculated for each of approximately 3,100 counties and county equivalents in the United States. However, for many of these counties the population at risk is so small, even using the experience of the 11-year period 1959–69, that chance fluctuation or standard error is substantial. Two simple approaches are used to minimize the effect of chance fluctuation:

1. Data are presented by state economic areas (SEAs) as defined by Bogue and Beale (1). Metropolitan SEAs are either similar or identical to Standard Metropolitan Statistical Areas (SMSAs) with a few exceptions and consist of one or more metropolitan counties. Nonmetropolitan SEAs usually consist of about 6–20 contiguous counties which are relatively homogenous in occupational and related activities. There are 206 metropolitan SEAs and 303 nonmetropolitan SEAs, a total of 509. More details of the specifications for SEAs and the names of the counties in each SEA have been published by the Bureau of the Census (19, 21).

2. Large counties have been defined as those which in the 1960 census had either 30,000 or more total population or 1,000 or more white males age 55–64 and also 200 or more deaths in 1959–61 among whites, both sexes, age 35–74. A total of 1,205 counties thus defined as large provide more stable rates than do counties with very small populations (14).

LOWEST-RATE AREAS. The lowest 5 percent of the SEAs (the 25 with the lowest rates) for white males age 35–74 are presented in Table 3.3.

Nonmetropolitan SEAs are designated by numbers, metropolitan SEAs by letters.

Chance fluctuation has been brought under reasonable control through the use of (1) 11 years of mortality experience, (2) four 10-year age groups, and (3) state economic areas, which are much larger than counties. In this lowest-rate group the average standard error is slightly less than 0.2; the largest standard error is 0.3.

Three of the lowest-rate SEAs are small metropolitan areas, and 22 are nonmetropolitan. Twenty of these are contiguous to each other, scattered from west central Wisconsin to Colorado (Fig. 3.1). All are west of the Mississippi River except for the two Wisconsin

Table 3.3. All-Causes Death Rates by Sex, Whites Age 35–74 (age-adjusted), 25 State Economic Areas with Lowest Male Rates in Rank Order, 1959–69

State Economic Area				Male	Female	Ratio, Male to Female
	UNITED	STATES		15.41	7.96	1.94
Nebr.	SEA	4	(South central, west)	11.66	6.31	1.85
Kans.	SEA	4	(North central)	11.69	6.24	1.88
N.Dak.	SEA	5	(Southeast)	11.73	6.14	1.91
Utah	SEA	2	(Central)	11.76	6.73	1.75
Nebr.	SEA	5	(South central, east)	11.82	6.48	1.82
Minn.	SEA	6	(East central, south)	11.99	6.51	1.84
Minn.	SEA	5	(West central)	12.07	6.52	1.85
Colo.	SEA	4	(East central)	12.07	6.81	1.77
Minn.	SEA	8	(Southwest)	12.08	6.36	1.90
Minn.	SEA	3	(West central, north)	12.10	6.50	1.86
Utah	SEA	1	(North)	12.11	6.62	1.83
Nebr.	SEA	6	(South central, east)	12.18	6.50	1.87
S.Dak.	SEA	4	(Northeast)	12.26	6.44	1.90
Minn.	SEA	4	(East central, north)	12.28	7.26	1.69
Colo.	SEA	D	Boulder	12.43	6.23	2.00
Minn.	SEA	7	(Southeast)	12.43	6.50	1.91
Ark.	SEA	9	(North central)	12.47	5.93	2.10
Wis.	SEA	2	(West central)	12.48	7.13	1.75
Colo.	SEA	3	(North)	12.56	6.30	1.99
Colo.	SEA	B	Colo. Spgs.	12.59	6.82	1.85
Wis.	SEA	4	(North central)	12.60	7.07	1.78
Oreg.	SEA	B	Eugene	12.66	6.30	2.01
Kans.	SEA	7	(East central)	12.68	6.55	1.94
Iowa	SEA	1	(West)	12.68	6.53	1.94
Nebr.	SEA	7	(Southeast)	12.72	6.70	1.90

Source: Compiled from Refs. 18 and 20 and unpublished data from the National Center for Health Statistics.

areas. The only lowest-rate area in the South is Arkansas SEA 9, a group of rural Ozark counties along the Missouri border.

Of the 25 SEAs with the next lowest rates, 17 are contiguous to lowest-rate areas, providing further evidence of a consistent pattern of low-rate areas. Of the eight noncontiguous areas, two are in northern Washington, four are in Oklahoma and Texas, and one (with a small population) is in northern Illinois. While Ft. Lauderdale-Broward County (Florida) is in this next-lowest group, evidence from a prior study (1959–61) suggests that this is very likely due to selective migration from the North (11). However, both this 1959–61 study and an earlier study for 1950 present evidence that geographic

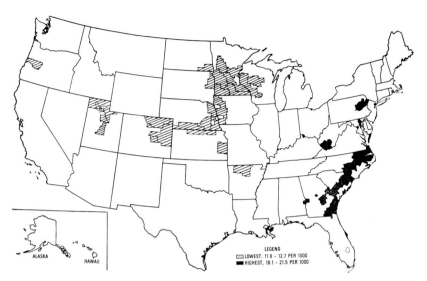

FIG. 3.1. All-causes death rates for white males age 35–74, 25 lowest and 25 highest rate state economic areas, 1959–69. (Computed from Refs. 18 and 20 and unpublished data from the National Center for Health Statistics)

differences generally are not to an appreciable extent the result of selective migration (8, 11).

The task of identifying the lowest-rate counties is much more difficult than identifying the lowest-rate SEAs, mostly because of larger standard errors. About 170 counties have lower rates than do any of the SEAs, and about 500 counties fall in the range of the lowest-rate SEAs, with rates less than 12.72 deaths per 1,000 population. Of the 100 lowest-rate counties (rates less than 11.31) 96 are west of the Mississippi River, two are in the lowest-rate SEAs in Wisconsin, and two are in other states bordering the Mississippi River; only one is in a metropolitan area. Eight of the 100 counties had sufficient population to be included in the study of 1,205 "large" counties, and seven of these were classified among the 25 lowest-rate counties in 1959–61 (14).

Nebraska has 92 counties, of which 26 were among the 100 lowest-rate counties of the United States. About three fourths of the lowest-rate counties were either in the western north central states or in Colorado or Utah. Clearly then, even for small or sparsely settled rural units, the geographic patterns appear to have epidemiological meaning; further study is needed to analyze the role chance fluctuation may be playing. These county rates lend support to the generalization from the SEA data that the lowest-rate areas are mostly non-metropolitan, often very rural, and nearly always located west of the Mississippi River.

HIGHEST-RATE AREAS. The 25 SEAs with the highest rates generally have rates more than 1.5 times those of the lowest-rate areas (Table 3.4). All are located east of the Mississippi River and fall into one or more of three categories: 16 are located in the Southeast (Fig. 3.1), four are areas with a history of mining, five are scattered metropolitan areas. Nine areas in the first two groups are also metropolitan, making a total of 14 metropolitan SEAs in the highest-rate group. Large metropolitan areas tend to have high rates, but there are also several small metropolitan areas along with 11 nonmetropolitan areas in this highest-rate group. Of the 25 SEAs with the next highest rates,

Table 3.4. All-Causes Death Rates by Sex, Whites Age 35–74 (age-adjusted), 25 State Economic Areas with Highest Male Rates in Rank Order, 1959–69

State Economic Area			Male	Female	Ratio, Male to Female
UNITED STATES			15.41	7.96	1.94
Ala.	SEA	B	Russell Co.	21.54	9.46	2.28
Pa.	SEA	G	Wilkes-Barre	20.33	10.29	1.98
Pa.	SEA	C	Scranton	20.15	10.88	1.85
La.	SEA	B	New Orleans	19.72	8.98	2.20
Ga.	SEA	D	Augusta	19.72	8.40	2.35
S.C.	SEA	7	(Northeast)	19.57	8.72	2.24
S.C.	SEA	6	(East central)	19.53	8.58	2.28
N.J.	SEA	H	Jersey City	19.35	10.46	1.85
Ga.	SEA	F	Macon	19.34	7.68	2.52
Ga.	SEA	F	Savannah	19.25	8.51	2.26
N.C.	SEA	8	(East central)	19.19	8.50	2.26
Va.	SEA	9	(East)	19.15	7.91	2.42
S.C.	SEA	C	Charleston	19.14	8.72	2.20
Pa.	SEA	6	(East central)	19.13	10.36	1.85
D.C.	SEA	A	Washington, D.C.	19.09	7.75	2.18
Ga.	SEA	C	Columbus	18.93	8.00	2.37
W.Va.	SEA	4	(South)	18.88	9.06	2.08
Ga.	SEA	6	(Central, south)	18.79	7.42	2.53
N.C.	SEA	9	(South Central)	18.67	8.34	2.24
N.C.	SEA	6	(Central)	18.65	7.86	2.37
Va.	SEA	D	Norfolk-Portsmouth	18.26	8.53	2.14
N.C.	SEA	10	(Northeast)	18.22	7.64	2.38
Ky.	SEA	B	Covington	18.07	9.24	1.96
Md.	SEA	A	Baltimore	18.06	9.19	1.97
Ga.	SEA	9	(Southeast)	18.06	7.95	2.27

Source: Compiled from Refs. 18 and 20 and unpublished data from the National Center for Health Statistics.

about two thirds are contiguous with or near one or more of the highest-rate areas. From these two groups the Southeast high-rate area might be defined somewhat arbitrarily as extending from the Virginia portion of the Delmarva peninsula north of Norfolk to Montgomery, Alabama, including counties adjacent to or below the fall line.

The 100 highest-rate counties include a few with very small populations, thus introducing uncertainty as to whether they would be very high in any future study. In general the highest-rate counties tend to be rather populous counties; in fact, of the 100, 46 were included in the 1,205 large counties in a prior study, seven more than one would have expected by chance alone. Of these 46 large counties, 19 were included in the 25 highest-rate counties in that study.

The 100 highest-rate counties on the average had rates approximately 84 percent higher than did the lowest-rate counties. In general they may be characterized in the same way as the highest-rate SEAs. Even though the Southeast as defined above contains less than one tenth of the counties of the United States, more than half of the highest-rate counties fall in this area.

LOWEST VERSUS HIGHEST. The SEAs with the lowest and highest death rates for white males, age 35–74, 1959–61, also had the extreme death rates for the 11-year period 1959–69 (Table 3.5). Nebraska SEAs 4 and 5 together are made up of 24 counties in the Republican River valley area west of Lincoln and extending south to the Kansas state line. In 1959–61 the eastern half of this area (SEA 5) had the lowest rate for white males age 45–64; the western half of this area (SEA 4) had the lowest rate for age 35–74, but with differences in rates so slight as to have neither epidemiological nor statistical significance. The lowest-rate areas are so closely grouped together that there is a different lowest-rate area for each age-specific group. The highest-rate SEA, Alabama SEA B, Russell County, is a metropolitan county and a part of the Columbus (Georgia) SMSA; for ages 45–54 and 55–64 it very clearly has the highest rate of any SEA in the nation, and for ages 35–44 and 65–74 it has very high rates, ranking third in each instance. For ages 35–64 the rates for Russell County are roughly double those for Nebraska SEA 4. The amount of the difference in rates between the areas increases with age for both males and females, even though the percentage difference declines after age 45–54. Age 85+ is omitted because it is an open-ended age group, roughly equivalent to a crude death rate. At present we do not have the data needed for appropriate age adjustment for this group, even though the need for such adjustment became apparent in another study (15).

The counties with the lowest and highest rates for white males

Table 3.5. Death Rates for State Economic Areas with Lowest and Highest Male Rates, Whites by Age and Sex, 1959–69

Sex and Age	United States	Highest: Russell Co., Ala. SEA B	Lowest: Nebr. SEA 4	Differ- ence	Percent Differ- ence
Male:					
All ages (age-adj.)	9.08	11.89	7.58	4.31	56.8
35–74 (age-adj.)	15.41	21.54	11.66	9.88	84.8
25–34	1.61	2.32	1.86	0.46	24.8
35–44	3.43	5.31	2.49	2.82	113.8
45–54	9.11	14.45	6.60	7.85	118.8
55–64	22.07	31.06	16.67	14.39	86.4
65–74	48.42	62.46	37.53	24.93	66.4
75–84	103.48	118.21	91.22	26.99	29.6
Female:					
All ages (age-adj.)	5.29	6.14	4.54	1.60	35.3
35–74 (age-adj.)	7.96	9.46	6.31	3.15	49.9
25–34	0.82	1.10	0.75	0.35	47.3
35–44	1.96	2.60	1.90	0.70	37.1
45–54	4.61	5.47	3.11	2.36	76.2
55–64	10.28	12.92	8.51	4.41	51.8
65–74	26.46	29.73	20.73	9.00	43.4
75–84	72.32	80.82	63.18	17.64	27.9

Source: Compiled from Refs. 18 and 20 and unpublished data from the National Center for Health Statistics.

35–74 among the 1,205 largest counties in 1959–61—Richland, North Dakota, and Silver Bow, Montana—were identified in a prior study (14). Richland County, in extreme southeastern North Dakota, also had a low rate in the 11-year period 1959–69 but did not quite qualify as one of the 100 lowest-rate counties. Silver Bow County, in southwestern Montana, ranked fourth highest among all counties in the United States, 1959–69; the three counties with higher rates were counties with very few inhabitants. The contrast in rates for these two counties is substantially greater than the contrast for the SEAs with extreme rates (Table 3.6). Silver Bow rates for both males and females age 35–54 and also for males 55–64 were more than double the Richland rates, with pronounced differences for other age groups as well. In fact, the amount of the difference in rates increased with age. If the large county with the lowest rates for the entire 11-year period—Cache County, Utah—were chosen for comparison, the contrasts would be even greater.

Table 3.6.   Death Rates for Counties with Lowest[a] and Highest[a] Rates, White
             Males by Age, 1959–69.

Age	Highest: Silver Bow, Mont.	Lowest: Richland, N.Dak.	Differ-ence	Percent Differ-ence
Male:				
All ages (age-adj.)	12.87	7.21	5.66	78.5
35–74 (age-adj.)	22.49	11.38	11.11	97.6
25–34	2.53	1.41	1.12	79.4
35–44	5.79	2.28	3.51	153.9
45–54	14.84	6.62	8.22	124.2
55–64	32.35	14.27	18.08	126.7
65–74	65.24	39.80	25.44	63.9
75–84	135.00	94.78	40.22	42.4
Female:				
All ages (age-adj.)	6.84	4.41	2.43	55.1
35–74 (age-adj.)	10.83	6.13	4.70	76.1
25–34	1.29	0.75	0.54	72.0
35–44	2.99	1.08	1.91	176.9
45–54	7.24	3.32	3.92	118.1
55–64	13.20	8.65	4.55	52.6
65–74	34.51	20.80	13.71	65.9
75–84	82.94	63.70	19.24	30.2

[a]Counties with highest and lowest rates in 1959–61, selected from 1,205 largest
counties (11).

Areas may also be chosen on the basis of having extreme rates for
white females age 35–74 (Table 3.7). Arkansas SEA 9, consisting of a
group of Ozark counties northeast of Fayetteville, was part of a lowest-rate area in 1949–51 as well as having the lowest rate in more recent years. (The analytic work necessary to identify the county that
might with reasonable confidence be labeled the lowest-rate county
has not yet been completed.) Schuylkill County, Pennsylvania, was
selected as a highest-rate area because (1) its rate is substantially higher than that for any SEA, (2) its population is substantially greater
than that of many SEAs, thus holding chance fluctuation under control, and (3) it is part of the economic subregion that had the highest
rate in 1949–51. The contrasts are substantial but greatest for age
65–74. The amount of the difference in rates increases substantially
with age and is greater for males than for females, even though the
areas were chosen because of the large percentage difference in rates
for females.

Table 3.7.   Death Rates for Areas with Lowest and Highest Female Rates, Whites by Age and Sex, 1959–69

Sex and Age	Highest: Schuylkill Co., Pa.	Lowest: Ark. SEA 9	Differ- ence	Percent Differ- ence
Males:				
All ages (age-adj.)	11.99	7.89	4.10	52.0
35–74 (age-adj.)	21.20	12.47	8.73	70.0
25–34	2.19	2.19	0.0	0.0
35–44	4.48	3.77	0.71	18.8
45–54	12.63	7.71	4.92	63.8
55–64	30.62	17.61	13.01	73.9
65–74	66.63	36.38	30.25	83.2
75–84	135.44	84.88	50.56	59.6
Female:				
All ages (age-adj.)	7.01	4.47	2.54	56.8
35–74 (age-adj.)	11.45	5.93	5.52	93.1
25–34	0.78	0.92	—0.14	—15.2
35–44	2.33	1.51	0.82	54.3
45–54	5.91	3.53	2.38	67.4
55–64	14.90	8.01	6.89	86.0
65–74	40.65	18.86	21.79	115.5
75–84	96.21	61.58	34.63	56.2

Source: Compiled from Refs. 18 and 20 and unpublished data from the National Center for Health Statistics.

For all of these geographic comparisons (Tables 3.5, 3.6, and 3.7) the amount of the difference in rates increases with age through age 75–84, even though the percentage difference declines with age. The contrasts are marked for each sex, even though the areas were chosen on the basis of rates for one sex only.

Sex Contrasts. Male death rates are consistently higher than female death rates, not only for the United States as a whole but also for those areas with extreme rates. Table 3.8 shows the differences in rates by sex for each of the areas presented in Tables 3.6 and 3.7. The amount of the differences in rates between the sexes increases with age, even though the percentage difference declines with age. Patterns in both trend and amount are similar to those presented for geographic contrasts.

Thus far we have not identified any areas or counties with male rates lower than those for females of the same age except for a very

Table 3.8. Sex Difference and Percent Difference in Rates, Whites by Age, Areas with Extreme Rates, 1959–69

Age	Richland Co., N. Dak.	Silver Bow Co., Mont.	Ark. SEA 9	Schuyl- kill Co., Pa.
Difference in Rate				
All ages				
(age-adj.)	2.80	6.03	3.42	4.98
35–74				
(age-adj.)	5.25	11.66	6.54	14.19
25–34	0.66	1.24	1.27	1.41
35–44	1.20	2.80	2.26	2.15
45–54	3.30	7.60	4.18	6.72
55–64	5.62	19.15	9.60	15.72
65–74	19.00	30.73	17.52	25.98
75–84	31.08	52.06	23.30	39.23
Percent Difference				
All ages				
(age-adj.)	63.5	88.2	76.5	71.0
35–74				
(age.-adj.)	85.6	107.7	110.3	123.9
25–34	88.0	96.1	138.0	180.8
35–44	111.1	93.6	149.7	92.3
45–54	99.4	105.0	118.4	113.7
55–64	65.0	145.1	119.9	105.5
65–74	91.3	89.0	92.9	63.9
75–84	48.8	62.8	37.8	40.8

Source: Compiled from Refs. 18 and 20 and unpublished data from the National Center for Health Statistics.

few counties with such a small white population and such erratic age-specific rates that they obviously lack any statistical significance. Thus the generalization holds: When in the same geographic environment in the United States, the white male has a greater risk of dying than the white female of the same age. Generally males in low-rate areas have rates equal to or higher than females in high-rate areas. Two exceptions may be noted: the males of Richland County (N.Dak.) have age-specific rates nominally lower than the females of Schuylkill County (Pa.). Cache County (Utah) has even lower rates for males and thus presents a pattern of lower age-specific rates than the female rates of Schuylkill County (Table 3.9).

Relevant Factors. What factors are causing these geographic differences in age-specific rates? Since deaths in middle age and beyond are primarily due to chronic diseases, with causes not clearly recognized for the most part, it is obviously not realistic to expect an

Table 3.9. Comparison of Lowest Male and Highest Female Rates, Whites by Age, 1959–69

Age	Lowest Male Rates: Cache Co., Utah	Highest Female Rates: Schuyl-kill Co., Pa.	Differ-ence	Percent Differ-ence
All ages				
(age-adj.)	6.71	7.01	—0.30	—4.3
35–74				
(age-adj.)	10.64	11.45	—0.81	—7.1
25–34	1.18	.78	.40	51.3
35–44	2.28	2.33	—.05	—2.1
45–54	6.50	5.91	.59	10.0
55–64	13.85	14.90	—1.05	—7.0
65–74	35.41	40.65	—5.24	—12.9
75–84	87.91	96.21	—8.30	—8.6

Source: Compiled from Refs. 18 and 20 and unpublished data from the National Center for Health Statistics.

answer to this question. However, some associations may be relevant for consideration as possible risk factors.

More than 100 possible risk factors have been studied, selected from various measures of weather characteristics, content of the drinking water, geography, and socioeconomic indices. The 36 factors with the highest correlations with death rates were entered in multiple regression matrices; the variable that consistently turned up in the computer program as first or second in importance was the percentage of employed males engaged in farming, professional, or managerial occupations (10). This and other socioeconomic associations were consistently stronger than the often-cited association of hardness of the drinking water with low death rates. All of the low-rate areas presented in Tables 3.5–3.9 are farming areas. The lowest-rate county (Cache) is in Utah, the state that has the lowest per capita sale of cigarettes (2). Two of the high-rate counties have a history of mining.

Efforts are being made to define with more precision the socioeconomic indices and other variables, particularly the essential characteristics of a specified variable most likely to be related to the risk of dying. One example is population density. The population per square mile is on the average greater in the high-rate areas than in the low-rate areas, just as it was in a prior study of low- and high-rate counties (p < .001) (14). However, there are some very sparsely settled rural counties in the high-rate areas of the Southeast. Further, one may raise questions about the appropriate measure of population density. If most of the population is concentrated in the county seat, is it relevant to calculate the density based on the number of square miles in the entire county? McDowell County in the West Virginia high-rate area presents another aspect: the county's population is scattered in small communities in valleys, with houses on tiny lots, simply because there is not enough level space for larger lots. It therefore seems desirable to explore other measures of population density as part of the task of studying the relationship of this variable to the risk of dying.

Elevation above sea level also continues to show a statistically significant association with the risk of dying. Studies have indicated that the higher the elevation, the lower the risk (8). However, in 1959–61 the entire country of the Netherlands had a lower rate than did any of the 509 SEAs of the United States (12). The province in the Netherlands with the lowest rate is Zeeland, which is southwest of The Hague and below sea level. This observation suggests the strong possibility that in the United States elevation is an indicator or measure of presently unrecognized risk factors and not of itself a causal agent.

While race or major ethnic group is an important factor, the various ethnic groups in the United States of European origin appear to have rather moderate variations in risk—less than the differences between those same countries in Europe (6, 8). Among whites only the Spanish-American group appears to have special characteristics which deserve high priority for study. "All other races" consists of a rather heterogeneous group as regards the risk of dying. Many areas have a small population in this category with a resulting random error so large as to make their rates of little value; further, age is frequently not reliable (4). Because of special problems of this type, our analyses of rates for "all other races" are still very incomplete.

Age-specific male rates are consistently higher than those for females of the same age. However, because of the substantial increasing risk with increasing age, female rates are higher than the rates for males ten years younger; specifically, white women age 55–64 have higher rates than do white men age 45–54. A similar generalization may be made in comparing geographic areas with extreme differences in rates. The risk of death at age 60 in a low-rate area is comparable to the risk of a 50–55-year-old in a high-rate area, just as the risk of death for a 60-year-old white female is similar to that of the 50–55-year-old white male.

Many other factors in the environment—physical, biological, and cultural—are being explored. At present there is a plethora of such statistically significant factors; many of the factors are not independent of each other, making it difficult to separate the coincidental associations from risk factors that may be causal.

RECOMMENDATIONS FOR RESEARCH. Geographically the various chronic diseases are not randomly distributed. Areas with high rates for coronary heart disease specifically, and for the broader category cardiovascular-renal diseases, show a persistent tendency to have high rates for malignant neoplasms (9). This generalization applies for lung cancer, but it also applies to malignant neoplasms other than lung cancer—the correlations usually being in the vicinity of +.50 to +.55. (In this study of SEAs with $n = 509$, any correlation in excess of .11 would, according to conventional standards, be considered statistically significant at the .01 level.)

In order to facilitate the search for persistent, substantial associations that may be causal, emphasis is being placed on the disease-specific approach as well as on all causes of death. Even if complete prevention of a specific chronic disease is not possible, a postponement by a decade or more in the age at onset would be of decided benefit.

The study of geographic patterns in the risk of death also has potential value to those concerned with the delivery of health care after onset of disease. In rural areas of Iowa, Missouri, Nebraska, and Kansas the proportion of the population age 65 and over tends to be high, often in excess of 20 percent. Because of this age distribution, the prevalence of chronic diseases and death rates is almost certain to be high, even though this area tends to have very low age-specific rates for the cardiovascular diseases and malignant neoplasms as well as for all causes of death. It therefore seems reasonable to hypothesize that this area will need higher levels of staffing for delivery of health care than will areas with very few elderly people.

Parts of the Southeast and other areas with high age-specific rates may be hypothesized to need to a greater extent than other areas any preventive health services that seem to offer promise of either preventing or postponing the onset of specified chronic diseases. In areas of high death rate the chronic illnesses strike individuals either earlier or harder or both than they do in low-rate areas. It therefore seems reasonable to suggest that in such areas the patients in need of delivery of health care will tend to be younger than those in low-rate areas. Thus age-specific death rates would appear to be part of the body of information needed by comprehensive health planning groups.

As programs designed to reduce the incidence and lethality of various chronic diseases develop, there will be a need for evaluating the extent to which age-specific death rates are reduced. Death rates of the type presented in Tables 3.5–3.7 provide baseline data necessary for measuring the extent of progress being made toward such reduction.

CHAPTER FOUR

DISTRIBUTION OF PHYSICIAN MANPOWER

SAM M. CORDES

ANY SERIOUS discussion of medical care delivery—whether the focus is on rural-urban differences or another taxonomy—invariably involves a careful analysis of at least some facet of physician manpower. The rationale for such an analysis stems from the central role of the physician in the delivery of medical care. In examining this role, Dr. John Knowles, director of Massachusetts General Hospital and an astute observer of the American medical scene, notes:

> It is through [the physician] that the "consumer" gains entry to our health system. It is he who determines the need for and utilization of other health workers. It is he who controls the organization, distribution, and utilization of health services. It is he who ultimately controls and determines health expenditures and the cost of medical services, be they drugs, hospitals, laboratories, or office visits. Finally, it is he who controls the numbers recruited, produced, and retained in the profession, largely through his membership in medical school faculty, teaching hospital staff, the American Medical Association, the Association of American Medical Colleges, specialty boards, or special public or private commissions (41, pp. 81–82).

Six major aspects of physician manpower are considered:

1. Physician manpower from a national perspective
2. Physician manpower in rural areas
3. Shortages of physician services in rural areas

SAM M. CORDES is Assistant Professor of Agricultural Economics, Pennsylvania State University.

The excellent comments and suggestions of Charles Crawford, Frank Goode, J. Patrick Madden, and Michael Miller of the Department of Agricultural Economics and Rural Sociology, Pennsylvania State University, and Richard Lee of the Health Services Administration, Department of Health, Education and Welfare, are gratefully acknowledged. Errors of omission and commission are solely the responsibility of the author.

4. Limitations of and alternatives to physician-population ratios
5. Locational decisions of physicians
6. Future research needs

The term "physician services" is used comprehensively to include all medical care produced by the physician or under his supervision regardless of whether the delivery takes place in the physician's office, a hospital or nursing home, or the patient's home.

PHYSICIAN MANPOWER FROM A NATIONAL PERSPEC-TIVE. Tables 4.1 and 4.2 include data on physician-population ratios for selected years beginning in 1931.[1] Definition changes preclude comparisons of the numerical values for all years; however, yearly comparisons can be made for the intervals 1931–57, 1963–67, and 1968–72.[2] This allows for the examination of trends within each of these three intervals. From this information certain inferences can be made for the entire time period 1931–72. Physicians who are retired or inactive have been excluded from the analysis.

The growth since 1931 in the total number of physicians as well as nonfederal physicians is quite evident, being particularly rapid since 1963. Many of the factors underlying this growth are reflected in Table 4.3. For example, 27 new U.S. medical schools were opened between the academic years 1930–31 and 1970–71, with well over half of these opening since 1962–63.[3] Concomitantly the absolute number of medical students and graduates increased significantly, with the growth rate accelerating since 1962–63.

Another significant factor underlying the growth in physician numbers has been the influx of graduates from foreign medical schools. In 1966–67 for the first time ever, the number of foreign graduates entering the country exceeded the number graduating from U.S. medical schools. Not all of these 8,540 foreign graduates represent permanent additions to the nation's physician manpower; about 60 percent of them are on temporary visas, and many of these will return

1. Unless stated otherwise, it will be assumed throughout this chapter that the number of physicians and changes in the number of physicians refer to the number of physicians per 100,000 population.
2. The definitional changes causing problems of comparability between the 1968–72 data and prior years had substantial impact. If the 1963–67 definitions had remained in effect, the 1968–72 data would have shown significantly more physicians in (1) patient-care activities, (2) office-based practice, and (3) hospital-based practice. In addition, more physicians would have been included as general practitioners and fewer would have been considered "inactive" and involved in "other professional activities" (37, pp. 12–13).
3. A 1973 report indicates 112 medical schools are either in operation or in the developmental stage (69, p. 902).

Table 4.1. Active Federal and Nonfederal Physicians (MDs) by Specialty, U.S., selected years 1931-72

Year	All Physicians /100,000 population (col. 1)	Total		Primary Care Physicians								General Surgeons	
				General Practitioners		Internists		Pediatricians[a]		Obstetricians/ Gynecologists			
		/100,000 pop.	% of col. 1	/100,000 pop.	% of col. 1	/100,000 pop.	% of col. 1	/100,000 pop.	% of col. 1	/100,000 pop.	% of col. 1	/100,000 pop.	% of col. 1
1931	122.8	106.1	86.4	97.0	79.0	3.2	2.6	1.3	1.1	1.1	.9	3.5	2.8
1940	127.7	104.6	81.9	90.9	71.2	4.9	3.8	1.8	1.4	1.9	1.5	5.0	3.9
1949	131.8	94.8	71.9	74.0	56.2	7.8	5.9	2.9	2.2	3.4	2.6	6.7	5.1
1957	131.0	84.7	64.6	56.6	43.2	10.9	8.3	4.4	3.4	4.8	3.7	8.0	6.1
1963	134.8	89.7	66.5	43.3	32.1	17.9	13.3	7.3	5.4	8.1	6.0	13.1	9.7
1967	144.4	91.7	63.5	38.9	26.9	20.8	14.4	8.6	6.0	8.8	6.1	14.6	10.1
1968[b]	148.7	82.3	55.3	30.9	20.8	19.3	13.0	8.8	5.9	9.0	6.0	14.3	9.6
1972[c]	154.7	84.4	54.6	26.7	17.2	23.1	14.9	9.9	6.4	9.7	6.3	14.9	9.6

Source: Health Manpower Source Book (79), pp. 33, 34, 42, 43; Haug et al. (37), pp. 20, 39; and Roback (63), pp. 14, 21.
[a] Includes pediatric allergy and pediatric cardiology.
[b] Population data used for calculations were for 1967. Physician data were for 1968.
[c] Population data used for calculations were for 1971. Physician data were for 1972.

Table 4.2. Active Nonfederal Physicians (MDs and DOs) by Type of Activity, U.S., selected years 1931–72

	MDs						DOs
	Total		Patient Care Activity				
			Total		Hospital Based		
Year	/100,000 pop. (col. 1)	% of all active federal and non-federal MDs	/100,000 pop.	% of col. 1	/100,000 pop.	% of col. 1	/100,000 pop.[a]
1931	118.4	96.4	N.A.[b]	N.A.	N.A.	N.A.	N.A.
1940	121.5	95.1	N.A.	N.A.	N.A.	N.A.	N.A.
1949	120.0	91.0	N.A.	N.A.	N.A.	N.A.	N.A.
1957	116.4	88.9	N.A.	N.A.	N.A.	N.A.	N.A.
1963	123.5	91.6	116.9	94.6	24.5	19.8	5.5
1967	130.8	90.6	122.4	93.6	29.0	22.2	5.5
1968[c]	132.7	89.2	118.7	89.4	28.4	21.4	N.A.
1972[d]	140.0	90.5	128.5	91.8	33.3	23.9	N.A.

Source: *Health Manpower Source Book* (79), pp. 32, 34, 35, 39; Haug et al. (37), and Roback (63), p. 7.

[a] Approximately 98 percent of all active nonfederal osteopathic doctors were in patient care in both 1963 and 1967. The percent hospital based was approximately 9 percent in 1963 and 10 percent in 1967.

[b] N.A.: Not available.

[c] Population data used for calculations were for 1967. Physician data were for 1968.

[d] Population data used for calculations were for 1971. Physician data were for 1972.

to their native lands upon completing advanced training programs in this country (44, p. 75). Nevertheless, in 1967 almost one fourth of the physicians licensed for the first time in the United States were graduates of foreign medical schools (79, p. 69).

The data in Table 4.2 do not give strong justification to the frequently expressed concern that fewer physicians are involved in patient-care activities and more are becoming involved in such activities as teaching, research, and administration. The number of physicians in patient-care activities increased between 1963 and 1967 and again between 1968 and 1972. Although the percentage of physicians in patient-care activities decreased slightly between 1963 and 1967, this percentage increased between 1968 and 1972.

Another concern is the alleged decline in the number of physicians providing primary care. Primary care is often defined as "the type of care most of the people need most of the time" and historically has been the exclusive domain of the general practitioner. However, recent evidence suggests specialists in internal medicine, pediatrics, general surgery, and obstetrics/gynecology are regular sources of primary

Table 4.3. Selected Data on Medical Education and Foreign Medical Graduates (MDs), U.S., selected years 1930–70

Academic Year	No. of Medical Schools	No. of Medical Students	No. of Medical Graduates	No. of Medical School Applicants	Percent of Medical School Applicants Accepted	No. of Graduates of Foreign Schools Entering U.S.
1930–31	76	21,982	4,735	N.A.[a]	N.A.	N.A.
1940–41	77	21,379	5,275	N.A.	N.A.	N.A.
1950–51	79	26,186	6,135	22,279	32.6	N.A.
1955–56	82	28,639	6,845	14,937	53.4	N.A.
1962–63	87	31,491	7,264	15,847	56.5	6,730
1966–67	90	33,449	7,743	18,250	50.0	8,540
1970–71	103	40,487	8,974	24,987	46.0	N.A.

Source: *Health Manpower Source Book* (79), pp. 7, 15; *Health Manpower and Health Facilities, 1972–73* (78), p. 200; Dubé and Johnson (27), p. 850; and Margulies and Bloch (44), p. 75.
[a] N.A.: Not available.

care for many persons (4, p. 16; 29; 82, p. 143). These four groups of primary care specialists as a percentage of all physicians have constantly increased over time (Table 4.1), although the increase has not been sufficient to offset the tremendous decline in the proportion of all physicians involved in general practice. However, on a per 100,000 population basis, the combined total of general practitioners and primary care specialists did increase slightly between 1963 and 1967 and between 1968 and 1972.

Scattered evidence suggests this trend may continue in the future: (1) The percentage of residents training for careers in primary care specialties is greater than the percentage of all specialists currently practicing in these fields (Table 4.4); (2) 30 percent of those entering medical schools in the 1972–73 academic year who expressed a career preference chose general practice (27, p. 867). This figure is significantly greater than the percentage (17.2) of physicians who were general practitioners in 1972 (Table 4.1). Of course some of those who initially express a preference for general practice may subsequently change their minds.

A final trend is the steadily increasing proportion of physicians engaged in hospital-based practice. The percentage of all nonfederal physicians in hospital-based practice increased between 1963 and 1967 and between 1968 and 1972. By 1972 almost one fourth of all nonfederal physicians were hospital based (Table 4.2).

PHYSICIAN MANPOWER IN RURAL AREAS. Tables 4.5 and 4.6 present data on the number of active nonfederal physicians by activity and type of practice in rural and urban counties for the years 1963, 1967, 1968, and 1972. Again the data must be viewed as two sets: 1963–67 and 1968–72.

In all four years a strong negative relationship is evident between total number of physicians and degree of rurality. This relationship

Table 4.4. Type of Specialty Practiced among All Specialists and Residents (MDs), U.S., 1972

Type of Specialty	Percent of All Active Specialists	Percent of All Residents
Internal medicine	18.1	18.9
Pediatrics[a]	7.1	8.0
Obstetrics and gynecology	7.6	6.9
General surgery	11.6	15.6

Source: Seventy-third Annual Report on Medical Education (69), p. 927; Roback (63), p. 21.

[a] Includes pediatric allergy and pediatric cardiology.

Table 4.5. Active Nonfederal Physicians (MDs) by Type of Practice and County Type, U.S., 1963 and 1967

County Type	Number of Physicians per 100,000 Population											
	Total			Office-Based General Practitioners[a]			Hospital-Based Physicians and Office-Based Specialists			Other Types of Practice		
	1963	1967	1967 minus 1963	1963	1967	1967 minus 1963	1963	1967	1967 minus 1963	1963	1967	1967 minus 1963
All counties	125	134	+9	36	32	−4	83	93	+10	6	9	+3
Counties in SMSAs with 1,000,000 or more inhabitants	173	185	+12	38	33	−5	124	138	+14	11	14	+3
Counties in SMSAs with 50,000–999,999 inhabitants	125	131	+6	31	27	−4	87	95	+8	7	9	+2
All other counties	75	76	+1	38	35	−3	35	39	+4	2	2	0

Source: *Health Manpower Source Book* (79), p. 68.
[a] Approximately 90 percent of all general practitioners are office-based.

Number of Physicians per 100,000 Population[a]

County Type	Total			Physicians Not in Patient Care			Physicians in Patient Care								
							Total			Office-Based General Practitioners[b]			Hospital-Based Physicians and Office-Based Specialists[c]		
	1972	1968	1972 minus 1968	1972	1968	1972 minus 1968	1972	1968	1972 minus 1968	1972	1968	1972 minus 1968	1972	1968	1972 minus 1968
All counties	140.0	132.7	+7.3	11.6	14.0	−2.4	128.5	118.7	+9.8	23.5	26.6	−3.1	105.0	92.1	+12.9
SMSA counties															
5,000,000 or more inhabitants	212.9	207.0	+5.9	19.8	24.7	−4.9	193.1	182.3	+10.8	26.0	30.2	−4.2	167.1	152.1	+15.0
1,000,000–4,999,999 inhabitants	180.6	172.2	+8.4	18.0	22.7	−4.7	162.6	149.5	+13.1	21.0	24.1	−3.1	141.6	125.4	+16.2
500,000–999,999 inhabitants	149.4	145.5	+3.9	13.0	15.5	−2.5	136.3	130.0	+6.3	19.8	23.6	−3.8	116.5	106.4	+10.1
50,000–499,999 inhabitants	130.8	117.3	+13.5	9.1	9.7	−.6	121.7	107.6	+14.1	21.2	23.0	−1.8	100.5	84.5	+16.0
Counties considered potential SMSAs	94.2	111.2	−17.0	4.0	9.9	−5.9	90.3	101.4	−11.1	22.1	24.1	−2.0	68.2	77.3	−9.1
Nonmetropolitan counties															
50,000 or more inhabitants	94.2	91.7	+2.5	5.1	6.5	−1.4	89.1	85.2	+3.9	24.4	27.8	−3.4	64.8	57.4	+7.4
25,000–49,999 inhabitants	70.2	68.4	+1.8	2.2	2.9	−.7	68.0	65.5	+2.5	28.6	31.1	−2.5	39.5	34.4	+5.1
10,000–24,999 inhabitants	50.2	51.3	−1.1	1.1	1.5	−.4	49.2	49.9	−.7	31.4	34.0	−2.6	17.7	15.8	+1.9
0–9,999 inhabitants	42.5	42.2	+.3	.6	1.1	−.5	41.9	41.1	+.8	32.1	33.4	−1.3	9.8	7.7	+2.1

Source: Haug et al. (37), p. 20; Roback (63), p. 7.

[a] Population data used for calculating 1968 ratios were for 1967; physician data were for 1968. Population data used for calculating 1972 ratios were for 1971; physician data were for 1972.

[b] Approximately 90 percent of all general practitioners are office-based.

[c] Of all federal and nonfederal physicians in hospital-based patient care activities in 1968 and 1972, 6.9 percent and 5.1 percent respectively were specialists.

Table 4.7. Active Nonfederal Physicians (MDs) by Specialty, Type of Activity, and County
Type, U.S., 1972

| | Type of Activity | | | |
| | All Activities | | Patient-Care Activities | |
Specialty	SMSA Counties[a] (/100,000 pop.)	Non-SMSA Counties (/100,000 pop.)	SMSA Counties[a] (/100,000 pop.)	Non-SMSA Counties (/100,000 pop.)
All physicians:	165.5	74.1	150.6	71.1
All primary care physicians	87.6	52.0	82.4	51.2
General practitioners	23.7	30.6	23.3	30.5
Internists	25.6	6.3	23.1	6.0
Pediatricians[a]	11.3	3.2	10.1	3.1
Obstetricians/ gynecologists	11.2	3.7	10.7	3.6
General surgeons	15.8	8.2	15.2	8.0
All nonprimary care physicians	77.9	22.1	68.2	19.9

Source: Roback (63), Vol. 1, pp. 7, 14; Vol. 2, p. 50.
[a]Includes counties considered potential SMSAs.
[b]Includes pediatric allergy and pediatric cardiology.

also holds for physicians involved only in patient-care activities, those
not in patient-care activities, and for hospital-based physicians and
office-based specialists.[4] The one situation in which the negative relationship between the number of physicians and rurality does not
hold is with office-based general practitioners. The more rural counties
generally have at least as many office-based general practitioners as the
more urban counties. However, if we look at other primary care
physicians—specialists in internal medicine, pediatrics, general surgery,
and obstetrics/gynecology—it is evident that these physicians are more
abundant in urban than in rural counties (Table 4.7). Their relative
abundance is sufficient to give urban counties a decided edge in the
total number of primary care physicians.

Although the previously dicussed aspects of physician distribution
are fairly well known, usually little attention is focused on changes in
this distribution over time. This is an important question and can be
addressed from different perspectives. One perspective is to examine
changes in physician-population ratios for each county group independently of other county groups. Here the data show an increase

4. The 1963 and 1967 data do not make a distinction between patient-care
activities and nonpatient-care activities. Hence reference to changes in these two
categories are only for the interval 1968–72. In addition, the categories of (1)
office-based general practitioners and (2) office-based specialists and hospital-based
physicians are not strictly comparable between the two intervals. In 1963 and
1967 these two categories refer to all physicians; in 1968 and 1972 these categories
are restricted to physicians in patient-care activities.

in total active physicians for all county groups between 1963 and 1967 and for all but two county groups between 1968 and 1972 (Tables 4.5 and 4.6).[5] These two county groups were potential Standard Metropolitan Statistical Area (SMSA) counties and nonmetropolitan counties with 10,000–24,999 inhabitants. The same two county groups also registered a decline in the number of physicians in patient care. Potential SMSA counties were also the only county groups experiencing a decline in the number of hospital-based physicians and office-based specialists. In all county groups the number of office-based general practitioners and physicians not in patient-care activities decreased.

Another approach is to compare changes over time in the size of physician-population ratios among county groups. From this perspective the *net addition* to the total supply of physicians and to the number in patient-care activities was greatest in the more urban counties. A similar widening of the gap between rural and urban physician-population ratios occurred with respect to hospital-based physicians and office-based specialists. On the other hand, the number of office-based general practitioners and physicians not in patient care did not decrease as much in rural counties as in urban counties.

It is difficult to draw a single general conclusion about physician manpower in rural areas. Conclusions will vary depending on type of physician (e.g., general practitioner vs specialist) and type of physician activity (e.g., patient care vs nonpatient care) under study; whether or not the analysis focuses on a single year or changes between years; and whether the interest is in the absolute value of physician-population ratios in rural areas or differences in physician-population ratios between rural and urban areas.

Most policymakers and discussions of rural health care problems tend to focus on physician-population ratios (1) of primary and nonprimary care physicians in patient care, (2) at a single point in time, and (3) in rural areas relative to urban areas. Data indicate that rural areas do not currently have as many primary or nonprimary care physicians in patient-care activities as do urban areas. While this represents a skewed distribution between rural and urban areas, it does not necessarily represent maldistribution. Unfortunately the fact that urban areas have more physicians per 100,000 population is frequently used as prima facie evidence that rural areas have a shortage of physician services. Such a conclusion is predicated on the assumption that fewer physicians in rural than in urban areas is synonymous with a shortage of physicians' services in rural areas. This is an ex-

5. A change in the physician-population ratio does not necessarily mean that the absolute number of physicians has changed in the same direction. For example, if the absolute number of physicians decreases but population decreases at an even faster rate, the physician-population ratio will increase.

tremely questionable approach. A more rigorous approach to the
question of shortage is needed.

SHORTAGES OF PHYSICIAN SERVICES IN RURAL AREAS.

Unfortunately the term shortage—whether used in connection
with health care policy, energy policy, or some other issue—is
commonly used with little discretion. Two very different types of
shortages are possible: one in which the *human* need for a good or
service exceeds the quantity supplied and another in which the
effective demand for a good or service exceeds the quantity supplied.
The first type of shortage can be appropriately labeled a normative
shortage and the second type an economic shortage.[6] The difference
between them is that a normative shortage is concerned with human
need and an economic shortage with effective demand. Effective demand is an economic concept referring to the quantity of a good or
service an individual is willing and able to purchase; human need is
a humanistic concept referring to the quantity of a good or service an
individual needs to achieve some desirable state of affairs. Here the
human need for physician services is defined as the quantity of services
that should be produced and consumed in order to keep an individual
healthy, given existing medical knowledge.[7]

The above definition of human need is fraught with difficulties,
but these difficulties do not diminish the importance of the concept.
The American Medical Association's endorsement of health care as

6. Another type of economic shortage is when the price of a good or service
exceeds its cost of production. This results in "excess" or "monopoly" profits and
frequently happens when a good or service is not produced in a competitive
market. There is considerable evidence that physician manpower fits into this
category in that physicians' incomes are greater than necessary to attract additional
physicians into the profession. The income "necessary" is a proxy for cost of
production, because in order for persons to want to become doctors, this income
must be at least equal to the cost of medical education plus the "opportunity cost"
(income foregone) of not choosing the next preferred occupation. This type of
economic shortage is relevant to the larger question of the *national* supply of
physicians but is irrelevant to the question of whether the present number of
rural physicians is producing and pricing at levels that equate the quantity of
physicians' services supplied to the quantity demanded.

7. This is not to say that health services in general and physician services in
particular are the only inputs or the most important inputs to health. Health is
influenced by countless factors including safer highways and autos, environmental
improvements, changes in life-styles (such as more exercise or less tobacco), and
health services. Anderson has shown that neonatal and postneonatal mortality
decline as health services become more available (5); similarly, Radtke found a
negative relationship between mortality and availability of physicians and paramedics (59). Aside from mortality there is little question that effective utilization
of health services can decrease suffering, illness, and disability; their sheer presence
even when not being used can ease mental anxiety.

a basic human right for all persons, similar pronouncements by recent U.S. presidents, and the fact that national health insurance is almost a foregone conclusion all indicate that an individual's willingness and ability to pay (i.e., effective demand) is fast becoming an unacceptable criterion for determining the quantity of health services that should be produced and consumed.[8]

Given the distinction between a normative and an economic shortage, a relevant question is whether either type of shortage exists in rural areas. This question can be approached by using either direct or indirect evidence or measures of each type of shortage.

Indirect measures try to determine whether or not the effects of either type of shortage are present. A normative shortage is assumed to exist if health could be enhanced by the production and consumption of an additional quantity of physician services. Similarly, an economic shortage is assumed to exist if some of those who are desirous of physician services and able and willing to purchase them are either going without these services or experiencing excessively long waits before seeing a physician.

An abundance of indirect evidence suggests that a significant portion of the rural population faces a normative shortage of physician services. The literature—especially literature dealing with poverty—is replete with "horror stories" and statistical data on the lack of availability and accessibility of physician services to many rural people in need of these services (3; 9; 12; 16; 23; 32; 42, pp. 218–20; 51; 58; 61, pp. 508–30; 74; 75, pp. 458–83; 83). Among those most likely to be in need are migrant workers, native Americans, southern black farm workers, and the mountain people of Appalachia.

Indirect evidence of an economic shortage of physician services in rural areas is extremely scarce. One piece of empirical evidence suggests a substantial economic shortage exists in two of Utah's doctorless rural counties. In this study residents were asked, "Would you visit a doctor more often if one were more readily available?" Over 50 percent of the respondents answered yes. If it is asumed that these potential visits would require an out-of-pocket payment, then an economic shortage of physician services existed. Much smaller economic shortages apparently existed in a rural county with several

8. From a pragmatic viewpoint the reduced emphasis on price rationing as a criterion for access does not mean that all individuals will eventually have equal or free access to all types of health services. For example, to most people—especially the policymaker—the right to health services is not likely to include surgical hair transplants, chamber music in the physician's office, and a personal physician constantly in attendance. Hence the quantity of services required to keep an individual as healthy as possible may never be fully realized. What can be realized is equal access (or at least less inequality in access) to a basic or minimum set of services.

physicians and in urban Salt Lake County. Four percent of respondents in the rural county and 12 percent in Salt Lake County said
they would visit a doctor more often if one were more readily available
(3).

Direct measures of normative and economic shortages typically
rely on the comparison of a "suggested" or "desirable" physician-
population ratio with the existing ratio.[9] Table 4.8 presents several
different suggested ratios based on various studies, surveys, and legislation. Schonfeld, Heston, and Falk estimate the human need for
primary care alone requires 133 primary care physicians in patient-
care activities per 100,000 population. This figure was based on
judgments as to what constituted "good" primary care and data on
the frequency of conditions requiring this type of care (67). Recent
legislation enables the federal government to pay a portion of the
cost of a physician's education if he agrees to practice in an area
having a need for physicians (38, p. 7446). These areas have been
defined as those having fewer than 67 physicians per 100,000 population. In 1972 *Medical Economics* asked medical leaders to estimate
the ideal physician-population ratio needed to bring supply and demand into balance for various specialties. Considering only primary
care physicians, the estimates ranged from 9 per 100,000 population
for obstetricians/gynecologists to 50 per 100,000 population for general and family practitioners (54).

Another useful yardstick is physician-population ratios in prepaid
comprehensive medical groups. The direct cost of using most of the
services in these groups is zero or near zero. Hence their physician-
population ratios can be thought of as a crude measure of the number
of physicians required to satisfy human need when price rationing is
removed as a barrier for utilizing physician services.[10] The average
ratio for six major prepaid medical groups compiled by Mason is presented in Table 4.8.

Three limitations or problems complicate the extrapolation of
physician-population ratios of prepaid medical groups to other populations. First, enrollees in the prepaid groups may be atypical of
other populations with respect to their human need for physician
services. For example, Mason reports that the percentage of enrollees
over age 65 in the six prepaid groups is generally smaller than for
the U.S. population (47). Second, some prepaid groups contract with

9. This approach has been used less extensively in detecting shortages at one
point in time than in projecting or predicting the amount of manpower required
to avoid future shortages. For a review and critique of these predictions see
Fein (31), Klarman (40), and Senior and Smith (68).
10. Nonprice rationing, in the form of long waits to see a physician and
verbally discouraging patients from using the services as often as they would like,
may still exist.

Table 4.8. Suggested Number of Physicians per 100,000 Population

Name of Researcher or Recommending Agency	Criteria Used	Suggested Number
Schonfeld, Heston, and Falk (67)	Provision of "good" primary care on the basis of human need	133 primary care physicians
Department of Health, Education and Welfare (38) (loan forgiveness program for medical education)	Effective demand	67 total physicians
Paxton (54)	Effective demand	50 general and family practitioners 20 internists 10 pediatricians 9 obstetricians/ gynecologists 10 general surgeons 89 primary care physicians
Mason (47)	Average physician-population ratios in six major prepaid medical groups. This ratio represents human need as expressed in the absence of price rationing.	16 family practitioners 23 internists 16 pediatricians 6 obstetricians/ gynecologists 10 general surgeons 71 primary care physicians 94 total physicians
Stevens (72)	Adjusted physician-population ratio in prepaid Kaiser Health Plan (Portland, Ore.). This ratio represents human need as expressed in the absence of price rationing.	71–98 total physicians

nongroup physicians for some highly specialized services. Third, some enrollees of prepaid groups frequently purchase some of their services directly from nongroup physicians. These three factors have the effect of underestimating the number of physicians required if prepaid group practice were the universal mode of practice organization for the entire population. Stevens's research on the prepaid Kaiser Health Plan in Portland, Oregon, is more sophisticated and largely overcomes the above-mentioned problems of comparability and extrapolation (72). Rough calculation based on Stevens's work suggests that 71–98 physicians in patient-care activities per 100,000 population would be required if Kaiser's Oregon plan were emulated nationally.

The disparity between the suggested physician-population ratios in Table 4.8 to the actual ratios in rural counties (Tables 4.6 and 4.7) is indicative of substantial normative and economic shortages of physician services for those living in these counties. For example, the standard of 67 physicians per 100,000 population used in the loan forgiveness program for medical education—the most niggardly standard of all—is still well above the average number of physicians per 100,000 in the nation's two most rural groups of counties. These two county groups have a combined population of almost 21 million persons and represent approximately 60 percent of the nation's counties. In addition, a comparison of the data in Table 4.7 with the suggested number of primary care physicians as determined by *Medical Economics,* Schonfeld, and Mason also suggests rural counties have substantial normative and economic shortages of primary care physicians. This information, combined with the previously discussed indirect evidence on shortages, suggests rather strongly that many and perhaps most rural residents are confronted with both normative and economic shortages of most types of physician services.

PHYSICIAN-POPULATION RATIOS. Physician-population ratios are a crude but important and appropriate standard for drawing general conclusions about large geographical categories, such as "all rural counties." The utility of physician-population ratios was borne out in a recent North Carolina study. Results of the study showed a strong negative correlation between physician-population ratios and the percentage of population in multicounty planning regions that believed a moderate or serious health manpower problem existed (18). Despite the utility of the ratio approach, no single physician-population ratio can be applied universally to determine whether or not any specific small geographical area (such as a particularly rural county) has a shortage of physician services. The following discussion briefly (1) outlines six major limitations of the ratio approach and (2) reports on the development of new measures for detecting shortages of physician services.

1. *Productivity.* Physician-population ratios do not reflect possible differences in productivity among physicians and groups of physicians. Some physicians are naturally more productive than others; even among those with similar talents, productivity will likely be influenced by type of practice (e.g., solo vs group practice) and the quantity and quality of technology, equipment, and supportive personnel employed. Output will also vary depending on the amount of time worked. For example, recent surveys show that most rural physicians work substantially more hours per week (total hours as well as patient-care hours) and see more patients per hour than do

urban physicians (6, pp. 54, 56; 80, pp. 50, 53). The ultimate consequence of these two factors is that primary care physicians in rural areas see anywhere from 13 percent (in the case of obstetricians and gynecologists) to 30 percent (in the case of general surgeons) more patients per week than their urban counterparts (80, p. 59).

2. *Quality.* Physician-population ratios are oblivious to quality considerations. In highlighting this point, Albrecht and Miller refer to a rural county they studied that has only two physicians but such a small population that it has one of the higher physician-population ratios in its state. The problem is that one of the physicians is in his seventies and nearly blind and the other is an alcoholic (2). More generally the quality of physician services in rural areas has been questioned on the basis that rural physicians are older, more frequently overworked, and more isolated than urban doctors (19, pp. 37–39). On the other hand, a survey by Aday and Andersen shows rural people are somewhat more satisfied with the quality of care they receive than are urban people (1).

3. *Population characteristics.* Physician-population ratios typically assume that populations are the same with respect to their human need for physician services and the quantity of physician services demanded. This assumption is often invalid. For example, the rural population is generally older than the urban population; less affluent; less educated; and more frequently engaged in hazardous occupations such as mining, forestry, and farming. These factors increase the human need for physician services. On the other hand, the lower incomes of rural people and their less extensive health insurance coverage decrease their effective demand for physician services (19, pp. 23–33; 21).

4. *Accessibility.* Physician-population ratios are a measure of how many physicians are present or available but say nothing about how easy it is to use the physicians. Potential barriers to accessibility are almost limitless; the more important ones likely include an inability to pay the going price, lack of transportation, traffic congestion, inclement weather, impassable or nonexistent highways, language barriers, racial discrimination, and office hours that do not mesh with the patient's schedule. Aday and Andersen report that rural people—especially the nonfarm population—are more dissatisfied than urban people with respect to length of office waiting time, availability of care after hours, and ease of getting to care (1).[11]

11. This finding appears to be contradictory to Aday and Andersen's other finding that rural people are somewhat more satisfied than urban people with the quality of medical care they receive. Although a contradiction may exist, it is also possible that while rural people find care more inaccessible, when they eventually receive care, either the quality is higher or their expectations regarding quality are lower.

5. *Physician and population mobility.* Physician-population ratios for a particular geographical area assume that the area is a closed system. While this is a reasonable assumption at the national level, it loses its validity among smaller geographical units.[12] For example, physicians based at one location may travel on a "circuit-rider" basis to other communities and counties (14; 24; 76, pp. 34–35). More importantly, rural residents can and do travel beyond their local communities to secure the services of physicians—especially nonprimary care specialists (3, 12, 58, 81, 83). Nor is the rural-to-urban travel pattern the only pattern in evidence. A recent study of 119 small-town Georgia physicians, most of whom were in primary care, shows the existence of an urban-to-rural travel pattern. Although these physicians were located 15–70 miles from the nearest urban areas, 10 percent of their patients—most of whom appear to be "regular patients"—were from urban areas (33).

Another type of migration involves those who are not regular or planned patients of the area in which they use services. The resort area of Sun Valley, Idaho, provides a good example of this. Sun Valley is located in Blaine County which had 9 active, nonfederal physicians in patient-care activities in 1972 for its tiny permanent population of 6,100 (63, pp. 182–83). This translates into 148 physicians per 100,000 population—a ratio well above the national average (Table 4.6) and most suggested ratios (Table 4.8).[13] However, the influx of large numbers of pleasure-seekers greatly deflates the physician-population ratio based on year-round or permanent residents.

The insensitivity of physician-population ratios to both physician and population mobility may be their greatest limitation. This limitation may acquire greater significance as more people have more leisure and mobility to further accelerate such a phenomenon as urbanites teeming into the hinterlands on weekends and holidays.

12. Selecting the proper unit of analysis poses a real dilemma between the analytical problems caused by mobility and those caused by aggregation. If the nation or even a state is selected, the analytical problems caused by physician and population mobility become rather unimportant. However, in using these large units we overlook problems of physician distribution within these geographical units; the problem of overlooking maldistribution within the unit of analysis can be severe even in small geographical areas. For example, in Washington, D.C., which has an overall physician-population ratio of almost 200 active nonfederal physicians per 100,000 population, a predominantly black neighborhood in the northeast section of the city has only 27 physicians per 100,000 population (62, p. 5).

13. This type of evidence is frequently used to support the argument that physicians are not "profit maximizers" but locate where noneconomic amenities, including leisure and recreation, are abundant. As the population of this type of area swells from 5 to 20 times normal size with affluent vacationers, a physician who locates in such an area could very easily be "profit motivated." After all, there is probably no community in the United States with a higher incidence of broken and sprained limbs than Sun Valley, Idaho.

6. *Geographical size, contiguous areas, and population density.* Variations in these three factors have important considerations for the optimum distribution of physicians that are not reflected in physician-population ratios. These considerations are directly related to the problems of accessibility and mobility but deserve separate attention. To illustrate the effect of geographical size, assume the unit of analysis is the county. In inventorying the physician-population ratio for all U.S. counties, we find that Owyhee County, Idaho, and Robertson County, Kentucky, have the same number of physicians per 100,000 population—namely zero. Owyhee County is 6,100 square miles and Robertson County is 101 square miles (63, p. 10). Although neither county may be a good place to become ill, most of us would probably prefer Robertson County without knowing anything else about the two counties.

With most types of retail and public services we think of nearness in terms of distance. In the case of physician services—especially the services they deliver in emergency situations—time is frequently a more meaningful factor than distance.[14] Although persons in sparsely populated areas are a greater distance from physician services than those in densely populated areas, they may not always be remote in terms of time. For example, a heart attack victim in downtown Manhattan at peak rush hour may be no better off than if he were in the middle of Owyhee County, Idaho.

It may be that a county without a physician has neither a normative nor an economic shortage of physician services if surrounding counties have services that are easily accessible. Hence the adequacy of physician services in a particular area must also consider the availability and accessibility of services in contiguous areas.

There is need for further research and work on alternative ways of measuring the adequacy of physician services. The indirect approaches discussed earlier for assessing the effects of normative and economic shortages are possibilities. Other promising possibilities have been or are being pursued. In 1971–73 the Health Services and Mental Health Administration, Department of Health, Education and Welfare, identified "health service scarcity areas"—defined as "geographic areas where health and related services in the area and contiguous area are not available to a substantial portion of the population" (77, p. 10). The term available as used in the definition was com-

14. Time is also important in nonemergency situations from the standpoint of wages foregone, especially for many nonprofessionals such as farm workers and domestics who usually have no sick-leave provisions with their employers. This represents an indirect cost of using health services. Another indirect cost is transportation, a factor that will increase in importance as energy costs rise.

prehensive and included (1) a quantitative lack of health and related resources and services, (2) inaccessibility of existing health and related services, and (3) ineffective utilization of existing health and related services. Under this definition a scarcity area could be a combination of census tracts, a minor civil division or census county division, or an entire county. The actual identification process had a grass-roots flavor. Areawide and statewide comprehensive health planning agencies, relying on their own knowledge of local situations and additional local inputs, were asked to identify and carefully document (on a form provided by HEW) scarcity areas. As of December 31, 1972, 1,333 areas had been identified; the raw data indicated that "a significant number . . . of them are rural" (64, p. 26). This program was terminated in 1973 after identifying approximately 1,500 scarcity areas. A thorough analysis of these areas is now under way.

Another approach in progress within HEW's Bureau of Community Health Services is the development of an "index of medical underservice." The index is an aggregation of factors considered descriptive of medical underservice. Initially four indicators are being used: physician-population ratio of primary care physicians, infant mortality rate, percent of population age 65 and over, and percent of population with family incomes below the poverty level. These four indicators were selected and weighted by individuals knowledgeable in the fields of health care administration, health service delivery, health status and health service measurement, and other relevant fields. As reported to Congress, the rationale for using an index approach rather than simply considering a number of separate indicators was:

> to allow for simultaneous consideration of all the criteria used. The indicators of underservice chosen are weighted according to their importance in identifying medical underservice. In that way, the measured value of a given indicator of underservice is considered along with its relative weight for measuring underservice. Because of this interdependence of the indicators or criteria, it is unlikely that any single indicator can be used to show that an area or population group is or is not underserved. As a result, the index should be a more predictive tool than separate criteria.[15]

Radtke, in a study of physician manpower in the Pacific Northwest, developed another alternative to the use of physician-population ratios. Using an econometric model he estimated the economic benefits of bringing an additional physician to each Comprehensive Health Planning (CHP) district in the Pacific Northwest. The economic bene-

---

15. Report to Congress on the Criteria to Be Used for Designation of Medically Underserved Areas and Population Groups as Required by the Health Maintenance Organization Act of 1973, June 6, 1974, p. 1.

fits were cast in terms of the gain in economic productivity by preventing early mortality. Current physician income was used as the cost of bringing an additional physician into a CHP district. If the benefits of an additional physician exceeded the cost, then an additional physician was said to be justified.[16] On this basis Radtke determined that 23 CHP districts could justify additional physicians and 12 CHP districts had an excess of physicians (i.e., costs were greater than benefits) (59, 60). The 23 districts in which an additional physician could be justified were much more rural in nature than were the 12 districts having an excess of physicians.[17]

LOCATIONAL DECISIONS OF PHYSICIANS. Increasing the quantity of physician services available to those in rural areas can occur by (1) better transportation and communication linkages with existing services in urban areas, (2) increasing the number of physicians in rural areas, or (3) increasing the efficiency and productivity of those presently practicing in rural areas.

These three basic approaches are not mutually exclusive, and each is of considerable importance in reducing shortages of physician services in rural areas.[18] The problems and policies germane to improved access to urban services and greater productivity and efficiency from rural physicians are considered in other chapters (5 and 8). Hence this section will briefly describe what is presently known and unknown about the locational decisions of physicians. Obviously our capabilities for increasing the number of physicians practicing in rural areas is based on understanding the factors that influence their locational decisions.

Two different types of research strategies have been employed in attempts to isolate those factors influencing where a physician chooses to locate. One is that of asking physicians why they are practicing where they are or asking students, interns, and residents what factors they will look for in a practice location. The other is correlation of the physician-population ratios of geographical areas with various characteristics (e.g., social, economic, and demographic factors) of these

16. This justification is based solely on economic grounds. Radtke is quick to point out, and correctly so, that decision makers are also concerned with other considerations (e.g., decreased suffering) in allocating physician manpower.

17. Hans Radtke, personal communication.

18. There are ways of reducing either a normative or an economic shortage of physician services other than increasing the quantity of services available. For example, in the case of an economic shortage, effective demand can be reduced by raising prices. In the case of a normative shortage, human need can conceivably be reduced by countless factors including safer highways and autos, environmental improvements, and changes in life-styles such as more exercise and less smoking.

areas. Although the first approach deals more directly with the question of physician motivation, it is limited by the accuracy of physician recall and other problems (including cost) associated with primary data collection. The second approach allows the researcher to amass a large body of data rather inexpensively (at least when secondary data is used) and to analyze it through the use of theoretical models and sophisticated statistical techniques. The obvious limitation of this approach is that the identification of *correlates* does not necessarily mean these correlates are *causal* factors. Despite the respective shortcomings of both approaches, we are not completely at sea. On the basis of existing research it can be hypothesized that three sets of factors are of considerable importance in influencing physicians' locational decisions: pecuniary motives, professional considerations, and personal and family considerations—some of which are related to physicians' backgrounds.

Pecuniary motives suggest that physicians embody at least some semblance of economic rationality and tend to practice where the effective demand for their services and their incomes will be high. Effective demand for physician services will generally increase with population growth and as per capita income, educational levels, and the number of elderly increase. A number of studies show one or more of these factors to be strongly correlated in a positive direction with the number of physicians (7, 8, 28, 30, 34, 35, 39, 43, 45, 50, 52, 56, 59, 70, 84).[19]

However, some anomalies have also surfaced. For example, Yett and Sloan's multivariate analysis of new medical school graduates found a negative relationship between "percent elderly" and the probability of physician location (84); Radtke found a negative relationship between education and the physician-population ratio in the Pacific Northwest (59). When physicians are asked for the factors influencing locational decisions, economic considerations are not mentioned as often as might be expected. In a study by Taylor et al., economic factors were not even mentioned (73); in studies by Bible, Peterson, Hassinger, and Cordes and Barkley, economic factors ranked well below nonpecuniary considerations (10, 20, 36, 57). On the other hand, the rural physicians (but not the urban physicians) in Parker

19. Most of the factors associated with a strong effective demand are also associated with urbanization. Although degree of urbanization undoubtedly explains much of the variation in the geographical distribution of physicians, it is not a very insightful or easily manipulated variable from the standpoint of policy decisions. Urbanization is a proxy for countless factors including greater cultural opportunities, more medical schools, more crime, and more pollution. What we really want to isolate are the specific factors associated with urbanization and rurality that physicians find attractive and unattractive.

and Tuxill's study gave high priority to "ease of getting started" in selecting their practice location (53). Similarly, economic considerations were the most frequently mentioned factor in an Illinois survey cited by McFarland (49).

Professional considerations include such factors as proximity to hospitals and training facilities, ease of consultations with and referrals to other physicians, and opportunities for professional growth. A number of studies have shown these types of factors to be important in physicians' locational decisions (8, 11, 13, 20, 28, 34, 39, 49, 53, 56, 57, 59, 66, 73). In addition, Bible found a greater tendency for physicians to express concern about the adequacy of factors related to professional satisfaction, growth, and development as degree of rurality increased (10). A similar inclination was reported by Champion and Olsen (17). However, Yett and Sloan found a negative relationship between the probability of physician location and number of beds in teaching hospitals (84). This led the researchers to conclude that new graduates view teaching hospitals as competitors. In most studies factors associated with professional considerations appear to be more important to specialists than to general practitioners (28, 43).

Personal and family considerations are sometimes interwoven with professional considerations. For example, the type of practice arrangement can influence the amount of leisure and privacy available to the physician—an important factor associated with physician satisfaction, according to some studies (10, 20, 22). Greater leisure and privacy are frequently cited as alleged benefits of group practice. At the same time group practice generally provides greater opportunities for consultation and other professional advantages. However, the list of personal and family considerations is much more extensive than just the amount of leisure and privacy available to the physician. If there are no leisure-time outlets in a community other than the rocking chair, the community may be very unattractive to physicians. Existing research indicates that the quantity and quality of recreational and cultural amenities and public services such as the educational system are important in selecting a practice location (8, 11, 49, 53, 71, 84). In addition, Elesh and Schollaert's study of Chicago's physicians suggest physicians—especially general practitioners—avoid nonwhite neighborhoods for both economic and personal reasons (28). Another personal consideration cited in some studies is the importance of practicing near friends, family, and relatives (10, 36). Peterson's findings suggest this is a more important factor for urban than rural physicians (57). The importance of friends, family, and relatives may be related to the tendency for physicians to practice in the same region, state, or community in which they have had prior exposure. Yett and Sloan have shown quite conclusively that the number of events (birth, medical education, internship, or residency) a physician experiences in a state greatly increases the probability he will ultimately practice in that state (84). Others have reached similar conclusions (13, 17, 20, 36, 49, 53, 65). Results by Taylor et al. indicate that urban doctors are more inclined to practice in the same community in which they were reared than are rural physicians (73). However, even if the physician does not locate in the same community in which he has had prior exposure, there is a strong tendency for him to locate in the same size community in which he spent his early years (10, 17, 20, 26, 36, 53, 73).

These correlates are extremely interesting but also create some vexing interpretative and policy-related problems. For example, what if the decision to select a particular place of practice is made before the internship or residency and the location of the internship or residency is selected on this basis rather than vice versa? In addition the tendency to practice in the same state in which the physician was born, went to medical school, and served his internship and residency does not mean that the physician will practice in the "right" place within the state. Although much progress is being made toward a better understanding of the factors affecting the geographic distribution of physicians, much additional research and clarification are needed.

FUTURE RESEARCH NEEDS. There can be little question that substantial normative and economic shortages of physician services exist in many rural areas. Much more precision is needed in measuring more accurately the extent of these shortages, changes in the magnitude of these shortages over time, and comparing the magnitude of rural shortages to those found in urban areas. One reason for the present lack of precision is the heavy reliance on physician-population ratios. Much imaginative and innovative thinking and research are essential if the measurement of shortages is to take on added precision.

Another research area of high priority is a better understanding of why physicians locate where they do. Future research efforts can improve on the past record in this area if (1) physicians are studied by type and (2) consideration is given *simultaneously* to pecuniary motives, professional considerations, and personal and family considerations. For example, there is certainly no a priori reason to believe the following typologies of physicians respond in the same way to the same stimuli: general practitioners and specialists,[20] pediatricians and neurosurgeons, physicians graduating in 1937 and those graduating in 1973, graduates of foreign medical schools and graduates of U.S. medical schools, women and men physicians, physicians from different racial and ethnic backgrounds. Another typology of particular importance and interest includes physicians who either migrate or are considering migrating from one area to another. Although most physicians do not change their geographic locations once established (10, 20, 36), a significant minority do. Studies also show a higher rate of discontent among rural than urban physicians (10, 17). More research is needed to isolate the reasons for this discontent and to determine what can be done to alleviate it so the existing stock of rural physicians is not depleted further.

With respect to the second point, many research efforts focus singularly on pecuniary, professional, or personal and family considerations. Although all three sets of factors are likely to be of importance, a more comprehensive or integrative research approach is needed to determine simultaneously their relative importance among different types of physicians. The recent work by Yett and Sloan is one of the few if not the only research effort to fall into this category.

Evaluative research regarding policies and programs designed to attract physicians into rural areas is in its infancy (46, 48); more of this type of research is needed. Related to this is an assessment of the unintended effects on physician distribution of existing and proposed policies and programs not specifically designed to alter the distribution of physicians. For example, DeVise argues that the impact of medicaid, medicare, and federal grants to medical schools has widened the disparity between "physician-poor" and "physician-rich" states and is fearful that federal subsidization of Health Maintenance Organizations will further accelerate the disparity (25). Butter and Schaffner argue that relaxation of immigration policies has contributed to the rural-urban disparity because of an apparent tendency for graduates of foreign medical schools to locate in urban areas (15). What will be the effect on physician manpower in rural areas if a national health insurance program is enacted and if medical schools continue to emphasize the recruitment of women and racial and ethnic minorities?

Research on the supply of physician services must not be viewed in isolation. The results of being preoccupied with the number of

20. Most of the studies that have separated general practitioners from specialists are less able to explain the variation in geographic distribution of general practitioners than of specialists (7, 39, 84). This relative inability to explain the location of general practitioners is particularly germane to rural health policy in that general practitioners constitute the bulk of physician manpower in rural areas.

physicians in rural areas can be disastrous. For example, if medical professionals and policymakers decide that X number of physicians are required to meet the human need for services in rural areas, their location in these areas would be an unbelievable waste if the population were not able or willing to purchase the quantity of services others felt they needed. Such a costly error can be avoided if we remember that our ultimate concern is not the number of physicians but the utilization of physician services in quantities sufficient to meet the human need for these services. In short, research on ways in which physicians can be attracted to rural areas must be balanced with an analysis of (1) the demand for physician services and (2) programs and mechanisms for translating existing human need into demand. Only when this balance is struck can researchers make their maximum contribution toward solving the problems of rural medical care delivery.

—

CHAPTER FIVE

TRANSPORTATION AND COMMUNICATION AS COMPONENTS OF RURAL HEALTH CARE DELIVERY

BRADFORD G. PERRY

THE FIELD of health care delivery may be thought of as a social system which exists along with other social systems—e.g., the economic system, the religious system, the family system. The health care delivery system, like the other social systems, attempts to meet certain needs of society. Included in the overall health care delivery system are several components or subsystems: private office practice, group health care, hospital and clinic, public health, and the support subsystem of which pharmacists are an example. Transportation may be considered another subsystem within the total health care delivery system.

Transportation may be further divided into two categories: transportation for emergencies and transportation for primary care. The former has recently received much interest with the passage of the Emergency Medical Services Sytems Act of 1973 (Public Law 93-154). The latter, while not receiving such fanfare, is still an integral component of the health care transportation system.

Under ideal conditions the medical care delivery system functions to (and in practice appears to) meet the needs of the population. The general system is usually effective and to some extent accomplishes its established goals. However, part of the system appears to either break down or be nonexistent in rural areas. It is not a "nonsystem" but functions at less than optimum effectiveness.

To alleviate this systemic dysfunction we must search for possible causes and provide suitable alternative measures. One such measure is to be found in the transportation network. As a subsystem, transportation is dependent on and vital to the existence of the general socio-

BRADFORD G. PERRY is assistant to the Associate Director, National Center for Health Services Research, Public Health Service, Rockville, Maryland.

medical system. Medical transportation cannot be conceptualized in and of itself but rather as a component of a larger integrated entity.

HISTORY OF MEDICAL TRANSPORTATION. The mode of medical transportation that first comes to mind is the ambulance. Originally bearing the connotation of mobile field hospital, the word ambulance has assumed the meaning of a specially equipped vehicle for transporting the sick or wounded. Precursors of ambulance teams existed in Italy at least 1000 years ago (22). Animal-drawn ambulances were used in the 1850s in the Crimean War (7) and by Napoleon's armies in 1795 (24). Standardized horse-drawn military ambulances were introduced in the United States during the Civil War by Dr. Johnathan Letterman (7). The first U.S. motorized ambulance unit operated in Mexico during the American expedition against the Mexican general, Pancho Villa (7). Since the signing of the Geneva Convention in 1864, ambulance units and the wounded in their care have been considered neutrals on battlefields.

Civilian ambulances generally are built for speed and smooth riding while carrying one or two patients and an attendant to a hospital. Because of rugged field conditions, military ambulances are designed for sturdiness rather than for speed. They are usually equipped for emergency treatment of the wounded on the way to collecting stations. The military ambulance, called a "cracker box," usually has a load capacity of six ambulatory or four stretcher patients (7).

Documentation of the degree of effectiveness of ambulances and their role in health service delivery has been rare, and an incomplete picture is provided by the relatively few published studies. Probably the first formal ambulance service in rural areas originated in 1912 at the Washington County Hospital of Washington, Iowa. As the first rural county hospital in the United States (12), this still-functioning unit paved the way for a new era in medical care.

Since its early development ambulance service has made increasing use of available technology, and today many vehicles utilize rather sophisticated medical equipment. The ambulance takes a variety of forms, ranging from the ordinary station wagon to the huge jet-powered U.S. Air Force C9A. It is not uncommon for accident victims and those in need of acute care to be flown to and transported between medical facilities via helicopter. Such developments, however, are more prevalent in urban than in rural areas.

Since the ambulance was designed to be used primarily for emergency services, it is only recently that vehicles have been developed for the medical transportation of nonemergency cases. Patient transportation for primary care has long been neglected, and most sophisticated efforts on this front have taken place in urban centers. However, transportation for nonemergency care has become more important as comprehensive health facilities and services for rural people have become more concentrated in few locations.

Several cities and some rural areas presently have programs for the transportation of the aged, the disabled, and the indigent to medical centers. For the most part this has been accomplished through joint utilization of existing mass transit facilities such as school buses and commercial vehicles and, more recently, through the use of the minibus.

Thus far we have discussed transportation as it relates to the physical delivery of the patient to the medical facility. Complementary to that is the delivery of medical personnel to the patient. John Flynn, a Presbyterian minister, was an early pioneer in this field. Impressed by the many medical tragedies he had seen during his rural Australian ministry, Flynn proposed in 1912 the use of an airplane to bring swift medical attention in time of trouble (23). What originally appeared as the idea of an impractical visionary became, through the development of suitable aircraft and communications technology, the Royal Flying Doctor Service. Making its first flight from a single base in 1928, the service now comprises fourteen bases, each staffed by qualified medical and technical personnel. In addition to handling emergency evacuation situations, the service makes routine monthly clinic flights to isolated areas, many of which have no medical service at all (23, p. 172). Applications of this technique have been studied and are now being used in some rural areas of the United States.

A more recent development in the delivery of medical services to rural people has taken place through the Kentucky Pioneer Visiting Nurse Program. The program uses all-terrain vehicles to convey medical teams to patients as well as to mobile medical care units. Equipped with relatively sophisticated medical equipment and staffed by trained personnel, these vehicles usually take the form of converted motor homes or step vans. Many conduct scheduled visits to isolated rural areas and act as points of referral for other than routine care.

Discussion of a medical transportation network and its relation to the larger social system dictates the adoption of a multidimensional perspective and necessitates further definition. For the purpose of this chapter, transportation will be viewed as any means through which patient and medical care are brought together, whether through physical movement of the patient, medical practitioner, or both.

THE PROBLEM OF RURAL HEALTH CARE DELIVERY. A
clear-cut definition of the present problem is rather difficult, since a multitude of factors have contributed to its existence. To say

it is caused by a dearth of physicians in rural areas is an oversimplification. To say it is caused by a lower population density is also blatantly obvious and can lead only to tautological reasoning. The problem comprises time, distance, and geographic and demographic factors and can be stated thus: How might we utilize our existing transportation system or develop innovative methods of transportation to deliver health care to rural areas in an efficient, equitable, and effective manner?

Since rural areas are sparsely populated, emergency services are often scarce and in many cases nonexistent. This is additionally compounded by a higher rate of emergencies in rural areas. Nationally it is estimated that automobile accidents result in 53,000 deaths and 4 million injuries per year (8). Although figures are generally not available by rural-urban differentiation, auto accidents pose special problems in rural areas whether they occur to rural or urban motorists. Due to the dearth of readily available medical services and time-distance factors, the survival rate among rural residents and for victims of auto accidents occurring in rural areas is believed generally lower. In a Louisiana study of rural-urban accident victims, significant differences were found in notification time and mode of transportation of rural and urban accident victims, with the urban victims generally having a greater chance of survival (14).

Likewise the need for emergency medical service to rural areas is emphasized when one considers the farm or farm-related accident. Fatal farm and farmhouse accidents rank high in occupation-related deaths. Certainly many fatalities might be prevented by adequate emergency medical care.

A discussion of emergency medical services must also consider the nonaccident-related patient. Many acutely ill rural residents die as a result of the nonavailability of medical service. It is estimated that heart and artery diseases result in 55 percent of the total U.S. death rate (3). Means must be found to deliver adequate care to the coronary patient and patients in various other categories to whom this type of care is an absolute necessity.

Although the immediacy of emergency care is apparent and often given greatest consideration, no medical system can function without adequate primary medical services. The delivery of primary medical care to rural areas because of its lower priority often receives inadequate attention.

THE PRESENT SITUATION. About half the country's ambulances and most rural ambulance services are operated by funeral directors; the remainder are operated mostly by police and fire departments (15). Few rural hospitals and fewer health departments provide

ambulance service, so rural communities suffer to a greater extent than
do their urban counterparts. Increasingly, funeral directors are unable to offer such services because expenses outstrip profit. Moreover,
most services operated by funeral homes are lacking in trained personnel and properly equipped vehicles. Although many rural police
and fire departments operate ambulance services, here again many
personnel are either untrained or lack adequate training. At the
same time, many rural towns simply cannot afford to purchase and
operate an ambulance. Since the passage of the Emergency Medical
Services Act, many additional ambulances have been placed in service, but so far the situation has not changed appreciably.

Nationally the use of ambulance services is rapidly increasing,
and at the same time a higher proportion of their services are for
transportation of nonemergency patients. A study of Boston's City
Hospital during 1965 and early 1966 revealed that, of a sampling of
432 emergency trips, only 120 were considered true emergencies (21).
It is reasonable to assume that this type of utilization may also be
taking place in the rural community.

Many medical transportation systems lack adequate manpower
and vehicle design. The American College of Emergency Physicians
recommends that an effective ambulance emergency service include:

1. Casualty-treating vehicles of a design that provides adequate
space for equipment, the patient or patients, and attendants
2. Proper equipment for all life-threatening emergencies
3. Properly trained emergency attendants
4. Properly staffed emergency departments to receive the patient
5. Central area dispatch and two-way radio communication between ambulance and emergency department
6. An adequate reporting system (25)

The ambulance, however well equipped, does not stand alone as
a life-support vehicle. To be effective it must be supported by the
entire sociomedical transport system. An example of one such type
of transportation system is presently in operation in Illinois serving
highway accident victims and acutely ill residents of rural areas. While
predominantly centered around main highway arteries, the program
utilizes the transportation media of surface ambulance and aircraft
linked to a central dispatch center via radio communication. The
system also links 37 Illinois hospitals and borrows from medical evacuation techniques practiced in Vietnam, using flying ambulances, well-
trained emergency crews, and on-the-spot field communications. During its first year of operation, the system cared for 15,000 patients and
boasted a 98 percent survival rate (19).

Several other states have similar plans for the management of

trauma. Maryland is presently operating an emergency medical evacuation service directed by its State Police Department and coordinated
through the University Hospital at Baltimore. This service also uses
ground ambulances and aircraft linked through the State Police radio
communications network. Personnel report a high rate of patient
survival; although accurate figures are not available, costs are said to
be "manageable." The operation deals primarily with the evacuation
and interhospital transfer of accident victims, but it has often delivered
care to the acutely ill and to rural residents.

This type of medical transport system, although costly, might
have implications for the delivery of emergency service to rural areas.
However, such an innovation will require time and a reordering of
societal priorities before its possible implementation in rural areas.

Primary Care Transportation. Although emergency care vehicles are
vital to the health service delivery system, they are only part of
the total picture. To adequately deliver service to rural areas requires the establishment of an effective system for the delivery of primary care. Here again transportation becomes an important component of the health delivery system.

To receive primary care many people in rural America must drive
long distances. Although most rural roads are adequate, a person in
need of medical attention may be unable to undergo the stress of a
long auto trip. In the absence of available medical care, the individual
often simply "waits till he is no longer sick." To deal with such
problems, some rural communities have purchased minibuses which
make scheduled trips to medical centers. Others have chosen to
utilize existing school buses. Many communities use similar vehicles
not only for patient transportation but also for transportation of the
elderly to recreation centers.

A system of transportation for primary and routine medical care
is presently being developed by the RRC Corporation of Troy, New
York, to serve health and social service needs of clients in the rural
lower Naugatuck valley region of Connecticut. At an estimated cost
of $568,000, the three-year program seeks to establish a minibus trans-
portation network in an area where no such system presently exists.

The most significant operational innovations include a fleet of
six minibuses designed to accommodate individuals in need of special
services (the wheelchair patient, the elderly, the paraplegic, the handi-
capped) and the "Fairtrain System"—an automated fare-collection procedure based on the use of credit cards, which allows charges to be
matched closely to transportation services provided.

Other rural areas are studying variations of this type of transportation system. However, because initial costs are high, many com-

munities are not capable of such an undertaking, and progress will probably be slow. Bringing individuals to medical services is only one aspect of medical transportation for primary care; to satisfy other requirements of the health care delivery system, we must find means to bring medical services to the rural inhabitant.

One such innovative delivery system is presently being studied in rural Dry Creek, West Virginia. Under a $2.1 million grant from the U.S. Department of Health, Education and Welfare, the Mountaineer Family Health Plan is attempting to deliver health care to sparsely populated Beckley County, a 610-square-mile "health wasteland." The transportation component of the Mountaineer Family Health Plan is a jeeplike all-terrain vehicle, driven by a trained nurse on her daily rounds. Although one individual cannot be expected to attend to all of the area's medical needs, this stopgap measure results in many referrals of individuals who otherwise would receive no medical care at all.

Mobile Medical Care Units. More sophisticated versions of the previous method, called Mobile Medical Care Units, are being tried in some rural areas. Often equipped with advanced medical equipment and specially trained personnel, these self-contained motorized vehicles bring medical care to isolated and semi-isolated rural areas.

Mobile health units were initially developed during the epidemic of trypanosomiasis (sleeping sickness) in Africa between 1915 and 1940 (4). Due to their high degree of success, they are now being used throughout the world, particularly in rural areas. In a 1969 article in *Medical Care,* Dr. Thomas Bodenheimer classified mobile units as follows:

> Mobile health units can be classified according to the presence or absence of mobile equipment. Traveling medical personnel carrying only small amounts of supplies are called mobile teams. Mobile services including equipment in addition to personnel are known as mobile facilities. When speaking in general of mobile personnel, facilities, or both, the term mobile unit is used.
>
> Simple mobile units can be jeeps or cars for the transport of personnel with basic equipment and drugs. Ambulances with oxygen, stretchers, splints and bandages are a form of mobile unit. A more complex mobile unit may contain a sink with running water, cabinets, a generator for electricity, refrigerator, examining table, simple laboratory facilities such as a microscope or centrifuge, x-ray equipment, dental equipment, and so forth. Of course, as the unit becomes larger, its mobility, especially on the muddy narrow roads of many underdeveloped countries, decreases. Units must be chosen, therefore, by balancing the need for facilities and the requirements for mobility. Different types of mobile units also have different purposes. Some are designed to provide primary com-

prehensive care to people who have no access to stationary facilities. Others are for more limited specialized care, such as immunization, x-ray diagnosis, dental checkups, or multiphasic screening (4).

Complementary to the roving self-contained mobile unit concept is an unusual venture initiated by residents of Buckingham, Cumberland, and Fluvanna counties in central Virginia. Funded by a U.S. Office of Economic Opportunity grant to the Central Virginia Community Health Center, the project will use four medically equipped house trailers brought into this rural area. Designed as a family care clinic, the center expects to serve 7,000 patients with a rotating full-time staff of four physicians living in the area and having university medical faculty status. A central figure in the clinic's delivery of care will be the nurse practitioner or nurse clinician trained to relieve the physician of routine duties (5). Long-range plans call for permanent buildings to house the clinic with several auxiliary posts in the outlying areas. If a permanent facility is constructed, the medically equipped trailers may be relocated to another rural area.

Efforts to provide mobile medical services are being made in several categorical ways, illustrated by the fact that mobile medical care is becoming increasingly more specialized. Among the variety of mobile units in existence are coronary care, intensive care, surgical, intensive nursery care, and a host of others, all of which could have significant impact on the delivery of health care to rural areas (20).

Air Transport. Linked closely with and acting as an adjunct to the previous modes of medical transportation is air transport of both patients and medical personnel. Development in this field has resulted mostly as an outgrowth of methods proven under military situations. Today many wartime evacuation methods are receiving civilian application. The previously mentioned trauma management program of Illinois exemplifies one such application.

Modes of air transport vary from the helicopter to fixed-wing jet-powered aircraft, depending on the nature of the service provided The helicopter is used largely for short-run immediate service and for the interhospital transfer of emergency and acutely ill patients. Many medical helicopters are equipped for the performance of in-flight treatment for several patients; others are equipped only to transport patients.

Light fixed-wing aircraft are used for medium-range patient transportation (about 100–300 miles) and generally are equipped to accommodate one or two medical personnel and one or two patients. These and helicopters are also used to transport physicians and medical personnel to rural areas.

Larger aircraft, such as fixed-wing jet-powered aircraft, are used almost exclusively by the military for mass patient transport to regional hospitals or medical staging areas. Most of these are equipped for in-flight casualty treatment and, in many cases, in-flight surgery. Some experts attribute the reduction in wartime mortality among hospitalized casualties (from 4.5 percent in World War II to 2.5 percent in the Korean conflict to less than 1 percent in Vietnam) in large part to the fact that the wounded reached medical facilities more rapidly through aeromedical evacuation (11). Air transportation of rural patients is still in the embryonic stage; factors such as lack of trained manpower, money, and societal interest are serving to retard its growth.

The rural northwest portion of South Dakota presently has an air ambulance network consisting of 18 air taxi services. Although it has met with some success, problems of trained manpower and financing appear to threaten its continuation. During 1968 a total of 203 patient flights were made. Most were to transport patients to or from hospitals outside the area, such as to the University of Minnesota Hospital (2). In order to continue, the air ambulance service must recruit an adequate supply of trained manpower. One air taxi service has no trained medical personnel at all. Moreover, most aircraft lack medical network radio communications and can have only limited contact with medical facilities. In many emergency situations this program has used the air transport facilities of nearby Ellsworth Air Force Base at Rapid City, but this is expensive since patients must reimburse the Air Force for total cost of the aircraft operation (2, p. 4).

In addition to the transport of patients to and from medical centers, we must consider also their transport between hospitals. In a study of medical transport needs in rural communities, Jacobs has hypothesized: "Certain classes of patients may have a more favorable health outcome if transferred to a facility with more resources . . . improved transport services may facilitate and be necessary for these transfers" (10). To offer such service in New Hampshire, Jacobs suggests the need for improved medical transport of patients between community hospitals and a regional medical center in the northeastern part of the state. His suggestions follow the general trend of many others and center around the use of helicopters and STOL aircraft.

Manpower. Thus far we have discussed transportation as a means of bringing patient and medical facilities and personnel together.

However, whatever type of system is available will be virtually ineffectual in the absence of capable personnel.

A spokesman for the American College of Surgeons reports that approximately 20,000 victims of automobile accidents alone could be

saved annually if they were to receive prompt, trained medical attention at the scene of the accident and adequate care in transit to hospitals (9). It is estimated that perhaps 5 percent of today's ambulance
attendants meet the minimum National Academy of Sciences recom-
mendation of 70 hours training for emergency paramedical technicians (9, pp. 14–15). In rural areas where funeral directors provide
emergency transportation as a sideline, turnover is so great that only
a small percentage receive even first-aid training.

Under shadow of the previous statistics, the implications for
medical manpower in rural areas appear grim. It is impossible to
imagine even the best transportation system being at all effective in
the absence of trained personnel. Few rural communities have provided paramedical training even for police and fire department personnel. Some hope may be offered in the form of the physician's assistant, but until such time as problems of task definition, accreditation,
and licensure are solved, major problems will exist. Research must be
performed to determine means of providing adequate training of
medical and paramedical personnel and adequate incentive to warrant their remaining in rural areas.

Communications and Technology. Medical transportation is one
function of the subsystem of communications and technology.

The presence of two-way audio communications may reduce the
need for some transportation and increase system effectiveness. Broad-
band communications (two-way audio, two-way video) may serve to
further reduce the need for patient transportation and increase the
quality of medical care delivered.

The value of two-way closed circuit "interactive" television to
health care has been demonstrated. Many remote rural areas are
using such technology and have met with success. The Vermont–New
Hampshire Medical Interactive Network presently interconnects 20
hospitals scattered over four states. The system uses existing micro-
wave sites of the area's educational television network (16). Under
ideal conditions this interactive system should allow:

1. Practicing physicians at the community hospitals to participate in education activities at the medical schools
2. Patients at community hospitals to be seen by specialists working elsewhere
3. Remote physician consultation and increased interaction
among medical and paramedical practitioners of the area
4. Exploration of new areas of cooperative agreements which
might result in better delivery of quality medical care to remote areas.

Other technologies presently available include patient self-operated notification systems. The Soviet Union has long utilized a telephone service whereby the patient need only dial the digits "03" to be placed in touch with medical aid. The United States has the "911" central dispatch service, although it is presently available in only 150 communities (9, p. 14). Recently an organization in New York City called Medical Alert, Inc. developed a device called the Sendar medallion. Worn around the neck, the device is placed in operation by slight pressure on the medallion, which in turn activates a radio-telephonic signal alerting the Sendar office via special telephone line. The alert is a recording of the patient's name, address, telephone number, and Sendar file number. The operator at Sendar consults the patient's file or personal and medical data and makes the necessary telephone calls to dispatch medical assistance (6).

FINANCIAL CONSIDERATIONS. A serious question about the ability and willingness of communities to support a comprehensive rural health transportation system involves priorities in the use of resources. Most medical delivery systems are costly; often they are more expensive in rural areas when adjusted for patient number and utilization. It is not the intent of this chapter to suggest methods for financing the delivery of care to rural areas but rather to allude to the sociological aspects of the problem and to suggest some areas for future research.

Today's medical transportation systems in rural communities are generally limited to ambulance services and are financed through various means. Some choose to subsidize funeral directors to operate ambulance services. This is the least expensive method but has the disadvantage of utilizing untrained personnel. Some communities prefer to let police and fire departments operate medical transportation systems. Some have established volunteer services, and still others have organized new departments of local government (1).

Several rural communities contract with city ambulance operators. Although personnel are more highly trained and vehicles well maintained, this method is expensive and available only to more affluent areas. Still others have established local franchise operations, which is perhaps one of the best plans if the community is small enough to be serviced by one or two ambulances. This method has the possible advantages of familiarity in the community and a higher level of training of emergency medical technicians.

Air ambulance services and medical minibus systems are not yet established in a sufficient number of rural communities to assess financial mechanisms. Most are funded by federal and state agencies.

Financing of transportation systems depends ultimately on social priorities. We must seriously ask ourselves: Do we want to pay for medical services to rural areas? Do we really want a comprehensive medical transportation system if we must pay for it? In short, does society perceive the rural health problem important enough to support a solution to it?

FUTURE DEVELOPMENT. The future of medical transportation in rural areas may well be presaged through presently existing yet little-applied innovation. Perhaps some insight may be gained by an examination of the highly developed military system of medical transportation and a program that is developing as an outgrowth of that system—the U.S. Air Force aeromedical evacuation program. "Air Evac" falls under the purview of the Air Force's Military Air Lift Command and is headquartered at Scott Air Force Base, Illinois. The highly integrated system uses a variety of military aircraft ranging from the helicopter to the C-141, a jet-powered converted cargo plane. Air Evac is responsible for the evacuation of battle casualties and for the transport of military patients within the United States. Integral to the system are the military hospitals, some of which serve as referral and specialty treatment centers. Coordination of air travel and patient movement takes place at a central dispatch station at Scott Air Force Base. Using trained medical personnel and advanced communications and technology, this patient transportation system has met with major success.

In light of Air Evac's success, it is natural to think in terms of its application to the civilian community. Rural communities have utilized this military system to transport patients needing emergency and specialty medical services. Although the service is costly, attempts should be made to determine the feasibility of its application to the civilian community.

A variation of Air Evac is presently in effect in Texas, Colorado, Washington, Arizona, and Idaho. Called MAST (Military Assistance to Safety and Traffic), the program uses military helicopters and medical corpsmen as adjuncts to the existing local emergency medical service system. The program is organized primarily for the purpose of providing assistance to civilian victims of traffic accidents or other medical emergencies (13).

Existing personnel and equipment from active-duty army aeromedical and Air Force Aerospace Rescue and Recovery units are part of the program. These military personnel work in cooperation with local health care providers and law enforcement officials according to locally developed plans between the civilian and military communities.

The program is sponsored by six government agencies forming the MAST Interagency Executive Group, with administration assigned to the MAST Intergency Coordinating Committee. This committee comprises representatives from the Departments of Defense; Health, Education and Welfare; and Transportation.

The program is attempting to provide better patient care in medical emergencies and reduce the more than 55,000 deaths occurring annually as a result of highway accidents by transporting patients from the scene of the emergency to the appropriate medical facility, by interhospital transfer of critical patients, and by transporting medical specialists and equipment to the emergency scene.

From its beginning until May 1972, the program had flown 1,049 missions and transported 1,297 patients, logging a total of 2,224 hours of flying time. Costs are being covered by funds already available for operations and training. No special funds have been allocated, nor have existing funds been reapportioned. No charge has been made for any assistance provided.

Serious consideration should be given to the possibility of even more widespread application of these military techniques. With the demise of the Vietnam engagement, the possibility of devoting some military flying time to such uses should be explored.

Future rural systems may well utilize all forms of vehicular transportation. Paramedical personnel may assume a greater degree of responsibility, and mobile facilities may be linked to central dispatch and consultative centers via telemetry and broad-band communications. Some authors have conceptualized regional life-support centers linked to elaborate transportation and telecommunications systems, but most such plans are intended for urban application. Patients may be able to self-summon medical attention through the use of personal transmitters and other devices, but we must consider the practicalities of the rural situation.

At this time little information is available relative to the impact of the energy crisis on transportation for health care delivery. However, as energy becomes less available for general transportation, both emergency and routine health-related transportation become a more critical consideration. As the difficulty of transportation increases, alternative innovations such as two-way visual and audio communications will increase.

To develop adequate health care transportation systems for rural areas, research is indicated in the following categories:

1. *Demographic analysis*—In terms of population and special distribution characteristics which type of transport modes are appropriate?

2. *Manpower*—Are the supply of and demand for trained man-

power sufficient to staff a transportation service and other facilities linked to that service?

3. *Vehicle design*—With the concept of ambulance service rapidly changing from merely a means of transportation to a means of patient treatment, what types of vehicles (ground, air, STOL, VTOL) are most appropriate to rural areas?

4. *Mobile medical care units*—Considering types of services required and vehicle design, what is the possibility of using this type of vehicle in rural areas?

5. *Regionalization of rural medical care*—Is it feasible to establish regional medical care facilities in rural areas and link them with medical transportation systems?

6. *Communications and technology*—What technologies presently exist and which may be applied to medical transportation systems in rural areas?

7. *Application of military transport systems*—Which military transport systems are appropriate for rural areas and how can they be applied?

8. *Financing*—What existing and future innovative financing mechanisms might be applied to rural medical transport systems?

9. *Consumer health education*—How can consumer health education affect transportation system design and usage?

CHAPTER SIX

FINANCING RURAL HEALTH SERVICES

SYLVIA LANE

UTILIZATION of health services depends to a notable extent on their financial accessibility. Hardy states, "It appears many potential patients delay visits to a doctor's office until they become seriously ill because of the high cost" (5). The negative effects of coinsurance on utilization are documented in Scitovsky and Snyder (12) and Phelps and Newhouse (10).

Of the $71.9 billion spent in fiscal 1972 for personal health care, direct payments by consumers constituted 34.9 percent. Sources of the remaining 65.1 percent, provided indirectly, were: 26.4 percent from group and individual insurance plans, 24.7 percent from federal general revenues, 12.5 percent from state and local taxes, and about 1.4 percent from philanthropy and industry (3).[1] Consumers bore all of the indirect costs through payments for insurance premiums, taxes, contributions to philanthropic agencies, foregone compensation for employment, or higher prices.

METHODS OF FINANCING. Currently payment for personal health care is made directly by consumers, using their income or savings under fee-for-service arrangements or prepayment plans;

SYLVIA LANE is a professor of agricultural economics, an agricultural economist in the experiment station, and a member of the Giannini Foundation, University of California, Davis.

The author is indebted to Wesley Musser, doctoral degree candidate in the Department of Agricultural Economics, University of California, Berkeley, for valuable insights on occupational distribution of and trends in rural development affecting income of rural residents; and to Professors Milton I. Roemer, Ivan Hansen, James Copp, and Helen L. Johnston for their valuable comments on the draft of this chapter.

1. The difference between expenditures for personal health care and the total amount of public health expenditures to achieve or promote "health" in the United States represents mainly administrative and research costs.

by private insurers for those consumers covered by health insurance, with premiums paid directly by the insured or on their behalf by employers; by private nonprofit groups or agencies or by industry, on behalf of recipients of services; and by government agencies. The proportion of consumer expenditures met by private health insurance varies by type of care (28, p. 96), but there has been a marked upward trend in this proportion over the years.

The post-World War II development of fringe benefits through collective bargaining and the growth of union-management health and welfare funds have been major forces behind the tremendous growth of voluntary health insurance in the United States (9, 13). It is estimated that over 75 percent of health insurance is purchased on a group basis under employee-benefit plans (7). At year-end 1970 more than 80 percent of the population under age 65 had some form of private health insurance, but the amount and types of coverage are often limited. Eighty-three percent had hospital coverage; 81 percent had some protection against surgical costs; and 75 percent were at least partly covered for in-hospital physician visits. The percentages were lower for nonhospital-associated health care: 74 percent were covered for x-ray and laboratory examinations; 48 percent for office and home visits; 53 percent for out-of-hospital prescription drugs (both subject to deductibles and other limitations); 15 percent for nursing home care; and 10 percent for dental care (28, p. 96).

About 17 percent of the civilian population under age 65 (representing some 31 million persons) were still wholly unprotected by private health insurance in 1970. However, medicaid protection applied to about 9.5 million poor families with children at the end of 1970 and an additional 1.25 million poor, disabled, or blind. The percentage of persons aged 65 and over with private health insurance was generally much lower than that of other age groups, largely because of their coverage under the medicare program (28, p. 96).

Among persons in the labor force (age 17–64), white-collar workers had higher health insurance coverage rates than blue-collar workers. Persons who were "usually working" were more often covered by health insurance than the retired or those keeping house or engaged in some other nonemployment activity, such as attending school. Persons with a disability that prevented them from doing productive work in or out of the home often lacked coverage. In 1968 only 48 percent of the 2.6 million persons with such a disability had hospital insurance coverage. Only 64 percent of the unemployed members of the labor force had hospital insurance, compared with 84 percent of those who were currently employed (14).

Those most likely to be without hospital insurance were children, the poor, men 17–24 years of age, those with less than 8 years of education, nonwhites, the farm population, private household work-

Table 6.1.   Annual Costs of Medical Care in Nonmetropolitan Areas, Autumn 1971

Budget Category	Total Consumption Expenditures	Costs of Medical Care	
		dollars	percent
Lower budget	$ 5,464	517	9.5
Intermediate budget	7,746	521	6.7
Higher budget	10,385	543	5.2

Source: U.S. Department of Labor, Bureau of Labor Statistics, *Handbook of Labor Statistics, 1973*, GPO, Washington, D.C., 1973, pp. 328–31; *Three Budgets for an Urban Family of Four Persons, 1969–70*, Suppl. Bull. 1570–5, GPO, Washington, D.C., 1972, pp. 10–12; *Three Standards of Living for an Urban Family of Four Persons, Spring 1967*, Bull. 1570–5, GPO, Washington, D.C., 1969, pp. 44, 45.

ers, and hired farmworkers. As with hospital insurance, income is probably the most important factor in determining whether a family has surgical insurance. Only about 33 percent of the poor compared with 90 percent of those in the $10,000-plus income bracket had surgical insurance in 1968 (28, p. 97).

Only 37 percent of farm laborers and foremen were covered by any form of health insurance, compared with about 75 percent of the persons in all occupations. Moreover, relatively few rural people had sick pay or other income maintenance benefits. In fact, as rurality increased the proportion wholly uncovered by health insurance increased; for those covered, the size of the gap between what was covered and full comprehensive coverage also increased.[2]

In industry those least likely to have health insurance coverage were plant workers in selected service areas (e.g., janitorial, dry cleaning, laundries); the least prevalent form of health insurance provided by industrial establishments is "castastrophe" or major medical insurance (30, p. 242). Similar data could not be located for nonmetropolitan areas.

CONSUMER COSTS. To answer the questions of who and how many will have an adequate quantity of health services financially accessible in rural areas, it is first necessary to determine what constitutes an "adequate package" of health services for a person or a family for a given period of time. The Bureau of Labor Statistics has defined an adequate package of health care services for a family of four (employed husband age 33, a wife not employed outside the home, an 8-year-old girl, and a 13-year-old boy, living in places with populations of 2,500–50,000) for three budget standards (Table 6.1). In all three budget standards, the medical care allowance in-

2. Helen L. Johnston, Chief, Rural Health Section, Office of Rural and Migrant Health, HEW, letter, Jan. 3, 1973. Also see (17).

cludes the same basic hospital and surgical insurance for all family members, obtained by the husband through a group contract at his place of employment. The Health Insurance Association of America estimated the costs of a standardized contract for commercial carriers in the areas priced for the budget. The contract provides full care for 70 days in a room of two beds or more for each hospital confinement, all supplies and ancillary services normally provided, and surgical benefits. Costs also were obtained for the Blue Cross–Blue Shield contracts most nearly comparable to the commercial insurance provisions.

Budget costs were based on the lower of the two premiums (for either the commercial or Blue Plan contracts) in each area. A majority of families of the budget type do not bear the full cost of their health insurance, since the employer pays part or all of the premium. The cost of the contract selected for each area, therefore, was weighted by the following proportions of families: 30 percent paying the full cost of their insurance, 26 percent paying half the cost, and 44 percent making no payment since the employer pays the entire cost.

The higher standard budget also includes a supplementary major medical insurance contract, which covers all family members and was obtained by the husband through a group contract where he worked. Costs of a standardized contract in all budget areas were estimated for the commercial carriers by the Health Insurance Association of America (Blue Cross–Blue Shield contracts were not included). The contract can supplement either the Blue Plan or commercial insurance basic hospital-surgical contracts. The terms include:

1. An initial deductible of $100 per person per contract year.
2. Coinsurance, the contract covers 80 percent of the charges beyond the basic policy plus the $100 deductible.
3. Benefit maximums of $5,000 in any illness or during the benefit year and $10,000 lifetime for each person. The maximums are restorable on proof of insurability.

The charges covered include hospital, surgical, nonsurgical prescribed drugs and medicines, x-ray services, laboratory tests, oxygen, physiotherapy, radium, radiation isotopes, equipment and applicances, and local ambulance services.

As with the basic hospital-surgical contracts, the cost of the supplementary major medical contract was weighted to reflect those costs borne by the employer (using the same weights described above).

Quantities for medical care not covered by insurance were derived from two sources. Physician's visits and dental care were estimated from 1963–64 utilization data from the National Health Survey and are the same for all three standards. (Due to the $100 per person deductible in the major medical insurance for the higher standard budget, the cost of physician's visits cannot be deleted from that budget.) Allowances for eye care, prescription and nonprescription drugs, and other miscellaneous medical care were developed from the 1960–61 Consumer Expenditure Survey data. The costs in the latter group are the same in all three budgets except for eyeglasses, where the cost of eyeglass frames varies from budget to budget.

None of the budgets considered "hidden costs" such as transportation (which may be especially high for rural individuals or families) or time away from the usual occupation (for which there is seldom compensation in the case of many rural workers).[3]

If an adequate package of health care services is that as defined above and the percentages of their total budget allocated by families for medical care are those assigned by the bureau, about half the families in nonmetropolitan areas had annual incomes below those specified for the intermediate budget and thus could not afford the cost of the package in that budget. About two thirds were below the income level of the higher-cost budget and thus could not afford the amount allocated in that budget. Changing the income level or the percentage allocated for medical care would move the budget or financial constraint point.

Since incomes in nonmetropolitan areas have been increasing at the rate of 7.4 percent a year for the last four decades and medical care costs have been increasing at the rate of about 7 percent a year since 1966 (2, 30, p. 268), a greater percentage of nonmetropolitan residents should have been able to afford the higher-cost package for the next decade—assuming no change in methods of financing and no acceleration in the price of health care. Health care costs did accelerate, however. Consequently, unless methods of financing change, the majority of nonmetropolitan residents may not be able to afford the intermediate or higher-cost medical care packages in the future. Also health care expenditures are not spread evenly among the population nor from one year to the next (but being predictable on the average for large enough groups, they are an insurable risk). In any one year the chances are one in five that medical bills will exceed 10 percent of the family income; chances are one in fifty that they will exceed half of the income (8). Thus some insured families with relatively high incomes who budgeted recommended percentages for health care services but did not carry major medical insurance—which is included only in the higher budget by the Bureau of Labor Statistics and is carried by the smallest percentage of those insured (7)—may find themselves medically indigent.

3. Johnston.

HEALTH MAINTENANCE ORGANIZATION. The President's
National Advisory Commission on Rural Poverty recommended
in 1967 "that the Federal Government encourage and promote
the development of group practices, especially prepaid group practices
in rural areas, and assist in establishing facilities to be used for this
purpose" (33). This raised the question of the feasibility of establishing Health Maintenance Organizations as a means of improving
financial accessibility and consequent utilization of health services in
rural areas.

A Health Maintenance Organization (HMO) has been defined by
HEW as "an organized system of health care which accepts the responsibility to provide or otherwise assure the delivery of an agreed-
upon set of comprehensive health maintenance and treatment services
for a voluntarily enrolled group of persons in a geographic area and is
reimbursed through a prenegotiated and fixed periodic payment made
by or on behalf of each person or family unit enrolled in the plan"
(34, pp. 9–10). Apparently there are many variations that fit this definition. Examples of existing HMO type organizations range from the
Kaiser Foundation Medical Program with a prepaid membership of
2,247,000 to the Family Health Plan of Southern California which
serves a few thousand families in the Long Beach area (11; 34, p. 45).
In general, according to HEW, an HMO should have the capacity to
provide or arrange for any health services a population might need
to reasonably maintain its health. In some instances this may constitute simply a referral of the patient to needed care from some other
source. As a minimum there must be formal arrangements either to
provide directly or to secure from some other source: ambulatory
physician services, preventive services, inpatient hospital care, and
emergency care. For medicare populations HMOs are required to go
further and provide or arrange for "Part A and B benefits," including
extended care, facility care, home care, and psychiatric care (34, p. 49).

Whether the HMO must serve a minimum of 10,000 or 25,000
persons to be economically viable, it will be necessary that it serve
multicounty areas in many of the rural areas of the United States (24);
thus geographic availability and the related matter of transportation
for low-income rural people will become problems. The likelihood of
persons becoming members of HMOs will depend partly on their acceptance of the concept.

The HMO is not necessarily a less-expensive solution or even a
financially accessible solution for many consumers.[4] Typical membership charges for a subscriber family with two or more dependents in

4. When full costs are considered, it may be the lowest cost alternative for
providing health services under our present arrangements in the United States.
See Somers (13, pp. 140–42).

the Kaiser Foundation Medical Program in northern California in 1972 were $50.57 a month, and usually an employer paid $12 of that amount (although many employers paid more). There were additional charges for pregnancies ($60), visits to the doctor's office ($1.00), house calls ($3.50 or $5.00 depending on the time), interrupted pregnancies ($40), and drugs and prescriptions. There was no provision for dental care and limited provision for several other types of health care.[5] This is a far more inclusive package of services than that provided under the Bureau of Labor Statistics' higher budget, but it would still cost the consumer $462.84 a year before the additional charges in the typical case.

Currently HEW is attempting to encourage the establishment of and create demand for HMOs in rural areas

> through the HMO provisions of proposed legislation and through encouragement of prepaid Medicare contracts. In the long run, the Department plans, where possible, to convert categorical grant dollars to premium dollars for similar services to pay the premium of that population not covered by Medicare, Medicaid or employer's sponsored health plans and who are unable to pay for HMO premiums out of personal resources (34, p. 106).

Obviously not everyone could be enrolled in an HMO under present methods of financing health care. The Harvard Community Health Plan's spokesman (in responding to a questionnaire from the Subcommittee on Health of the Committee on Labor and Public Welfare of the United States) stated:

> It is difficult to see how individuals *not* now covered by health insurance would be able to participate in HMOs under arrangements currently available or those proposed in the Administration program. . . . In fact, it is difficult enough to provide access to individuals who do have health insurance coverage because of the categorical nature of health insurance financing in this country. In most cases reaching a reasonable cross-section of the population requires multiple and complex arrangements with Blue Cross and commercial insurance carrier plans . . . and various public agencies to provide enrollment of Medicare beneficiaries and the poor. Millions of people who are poor, marginally employed, or even self-employed are still excluded (33, Ch. 1).

Short of a universal compulsory national health insurance program, under which payments would be made to HMOs, it is difficult to see how everyone would be able to participate in an HMO (34, p. 82).

"If there is no national health insurance program, then the only way persons not now covered by some insurance program could be

---

5. Information from Kaiser Foundation Medical Program.

enrolled is either on a geographic or individual basis. Such an approach is not only costly but may also be actuarially risky" (34, p. 83).

FACTORS AFFECTING ABILITY TO PAY. The general economic problems of providing health services in nonmetropolitan areas can be focused by examining specific problem areas. In 1969 the median nonmetropolitan area family's income was approximately $8,000 for the year compared to the metropolitan family's median income of $10,261 (25). Generally lower average incomes in rural areas were associated with being over 65, being a woman, being a nonwhite, having a relatively low level of educational attainment, holding a lower rung in the occupational structure, or having fewer and lower-wage employment opportunities in particular locations (18). These categories of rural deprivation were for the most part the same as those found in urban areas, but the rural or nonmetropolitan component in each category tended to be more disadvantaged than the urban or metropolitan component. Furthermore, some of these high-poverty categories (notably elderly, low-education, and low-occupation status) represented a larger proportion of the rural population than of the urban population (20, 22, 26).

Sources of income are changing in rural areas. Most rural people are employed in nonfarm work; farm residents acquired 48 percent of their total per capita personal income from nonfarm sources in 1970. This proportion has been steadily increasing since 1960 (16). Farm residents rely increasingly on wages and salaries from employment in manufacturing plants, from government employment, or from employment in wholesale and retail trade or other nonagricultural industries (27).

Although there is increasing employment in commerce and industry in nonmetropolitan areas, the metropolitan-nonmetropolitan income gap remains. Manufacturing plays a significant role in both areas, but "fast-growing industries" (exceeding the overall national growth rate of 23.8 percent) grew faster in metropolitan than in nonmetropolitan areas in the 1960s. The only fast-growing industry with a notably higher growth rate in nonmetropolitan areas was construction. According to the Economic Development Administration, the nonmetropolitan lag in employment and income is accounted for by the industrial mix which favors metropolitan areas and is abetted by the continued decline in agricultural employment in nonmetropolitan areas (19, Part 1, p. 52). Although overall per capita personal income in nonmetropolitan areas has been rising at an average rate of 7.4 percent per year during the past four decades, rates of growth in income have not been the same in the various regions in the United States. The improvement in nonmetropolitan per capita income has been largest in the Southeast, which accounts for more than one fourth of all nonmetropolitan income in the United States (19, pp. 30, 33).

There are recognizable concentrations of rural counties with declining populations and declining personal income (19, p. 28). According to Edwards and Beale, "they extend from the central Appalachian counties westward through the Ozarks and then fan out to include large portions of the plains and mountainous states and to part of the lower south and the cut-over west of the Great Lakes" (4). These are mainly counties where the population is predominantly engaged (often unprofitably) in farming or in mineral extraction, forestry, or fisheries. Edwards and Beale also indicate that from 1962 to 1967 only about half the rural counties added at least enough private nonfarm jobs covered by Social Security to offset losses of farm jobs.

IMPLICATIONS OF ECONOMIC SITUATION. As growth of income in nonmetropolitan areas continues, the percentage of the nonmetropolitan population that will be able to afford health insurance (and consequently the health services covered in policies) will increase. However, the greatest percentages of increases in income categories in nonmetropolitan areas over the last decade have been in the $12,000–12,999 and the over $20,000 per year income brackets (23). Health insurance coverage for persons in these income brackets is already relatively high (28, p. 97).

In 1973–74 prices for medical care rose 12 percent (2, p. 455). Reiterating, the average long-run rate of growth in per capita income in nonmetropolitan areas in recent decades has been 7.4 percent (18, p. 30). Under these cost-income conditions, lower percentages of nonmetropolitan families will be able to afford the levels of health care described in the Bureau of Labor Statistics' budgets as time goes on. To maintain the level of services (again assuming the same cost-income conditions) an increasing proportion of the budget would need to be allocated for medical care.

As manufacturing and construction activities expand in nonmetropolitan areas, group contracts will cover an increasingly higher percentage of persons. The rate of increase in coverage, however, depends largely on the type of manufacturing or construction firm moving into these areas. Firms in heavy industry with union contracts are more likely to have employee-benefit plans that include health insurance and more comprehensive coverage than others.[6] As yet these are a minority among the firms offering new jobs in nonmetropolitan areas, but their proportion is increasing (13). And the farm population, which is least likely of any industrial group to have any type of employee-benefit plan, is decreasing (15).

Occupational categories increasing most rapidly in rural areas (25) for males are largely the ones with higher earnings and fringe benefits (professional and managerial, service workers, and operatives). Occupational categories increasing most rapidly for females (clerical and sales, craftsmen, operatives and laborers, and other service workers) are generally lower-wage, lower-benefit categories (25). Of all occupational categories in nonmetropolitan areas, the service category for females is increasing most rapidly, and this is a relatively low-wage, low-benefit category.

Other categories of the population in rural areas may not benefit equally from changes in the nonmetropolitan employment situation. These are the classic poor with excessive numbers among the elderly, black, and poorly educated. These groups may be separated even more from the rest of the population by changes in the employment structure.

CONCLUSIONS. Those in rural areas of the United States who cannot afford the quantity and level of health services specified in the lower budget of the Bureau of Labor Statistics without increasing the percentage spent on this category are and will be (and the following are not mutually exclusive categories) those whose incomes are relatively low (below about $6,000 for a family of four in 1971 and commensurately higher as prices for health services increase); those not likely to be covered under group health insurance contracts because they are unemployed or employed in lower-wage paying, lower-employee-benefit industries; nonwhites; those with relatively low levels of educational attainment; female heads of households; those living in farm households in counties that are not experiencing economic growth; or children of persons in the listed groups. For those over 65 and on medicare, the amount budgeted for medical care by

6. See (29). Table 70 shows medical care benefits in 353 of 620 agreements: 213 of 306 in manufacturing, 140 of 314 in non-manufacturing industries. Employee-benefit plans with over 100,000 workers covered for medical benefits in manufacturing (listed in order of number of workers covered) were in transportation equipment, primary metals, electrical machinery, and apparel; in nonmanufacturing they were in communications, construction, retail trade, transportation (excluding railroads and airlines which would swell the number), and services. All these industries are expanding in some rural areas (6) but are still far from predominant.

the Bureau of Labor Statistics in autumn 1971 is financially accessible only to those close to the median income for this age group if they budget 10 percent for this expenditure category (21; 31; 32). The above-mentioned groups are the ones that profit least from economic growth in the United States. If present trends continue, they will be fewer, but they will tend to be the "people left behind" in the rural areas not experiencing economic growth (1).

The HMO will be, as it is now, financially accessible to those in the higher-budget income categories (i.e., those well above median income levels in the United States) and to those covered under group contracts where the employer pays a sufficient portion of the premium. Industries with such contracts are apparently increasingly moving into rural areas. The HMO will not be financially accessible to many members of lower-income groups, whether they are in urban or rural areas (how many should be the subject of further study), unless they are directly subsidized by the government or unless there is a system of national health insurance covering everyone in the United States.

CHAPTER SEVEN

COMMUNITY-STRUCTURE CONSTRAINTS ON DISTRIBUTION OF PHYSICIANS

WILLIAM A. RUSHING and GEORGE T. WADE

MOST WOULD agree that one aspect of the so-called medical crisis in the United States is the uneven distribution of physicians in various segments of the population. Discussions frequently focus on the wide discrepancies between communities. In 1971, 143 counties in the United States had no active nonfederal physician, and many others had ratios of less than 25 per 100,000 compared with 143 per 100,000 for the nation as a whole (1).

Several systematic studies of the problem have been conducted, with regions, states, metropolitan areas, and counties as the units of analysis. Findings consistently show that population size and urbanization, wealth of the population, and hospital facilities (as indexed by the ratio of general hospital beds to the population) are significantly associated with the distribution of physicians (2–13). Most approaches view the distribution in individualistic terms, i.e., in terms of the values and attitudes of physicians. A prevailing assessment focuses on the economic motivation (13) and business orientation (14) of physicians; physicians are seen as concentrating in high-income areas in order to maximize their income. Others contend that physicians concentrate in areas with hospital facilities and medical schools so they can have access to needed facilities and association with professional colleagues (3).

WILLIAM A. RUSHING is Professor of Sociology, Vanderbilt University. GEORGE T. WADE is a graduate assistant, Vanderbilt University.

Reprinted (with permission from Hospital Research and Educational Trust, Chicago, Ill.) from *Health Services Research*, 8:283 (Winter 1973). Research reported in the chapter was supported in part by PHS Grant HS-0007 from the National Center for Health Services Research and Development. The material is based on a paper presented at the 1973 Annual Meeting of the American Sociological Association, New York.

This article also investigates some of these factors, but the focus differs from other studies in three respects. First, the interpretative framework is different. The relationship between the distribution of physicians and various population characteristics is interpreted not in terms of the motives, values, and interests of physicians but with emphasis on a general social and economic process (which, however, may involve physicians' motives, values, and interests). Second, the factors associated with the distribution of physicians are viewed as not unique to physicians but as part of a macrosocioeconomic process that imposes significant constraints on efforts to modify the distribution of physicians in the United States. Third, the unit of analysis is the county, which is considerably smaller than that used in other nation-wide studies of the distribution of physicians. This is a limitation on the study, since counties do not always constitute meaningful communities as defined by cultural, social, and economic criteria; they do, however, constitute significant political units.

DATA. The major sources of data are the 1967 AMA publication by Theodore, Sutter, and Jokiel on the distribution of physicians by county in 1966 (15) and census publications on socioeconomic characteristics of counties for 1960 (16, 17). County physician ratios are for nonfederal physicians providing patient care, thus excluding medical faculty, medical administrators, research scientists, and inactive physicians but including interns and residents. Unless otherwise indicated, figures for county population are based on the estimates of Sales Management, Inc. for 1966 as given in the AMA publication (15).

All counties from the 48 contiguous states are included in the analysis with the exception of counties in Virginia; these are excluded because of the presence of "independent cities" within counties, which are included in the census data but not in the AMA data. (The District of Columbia is also excluded.) The total number of counties is 2,971. In addition, more intensive data are available for the 95 counties in Tennessee and the 87 counties of the Tennessee Mid-South region (74 counties in central and eastern Tennessee and 13 counties in southwestern Kentucky).

FINDINGS. Two of the most frequent findings in research on the distribution of physicians are the associations between physician ratio and levels of wealth and of urbanization in a population. With the exception of a study for the 1923–38 period (10), all studies have been based on regions, states, selected metropolitan areas, or counties from selected states.

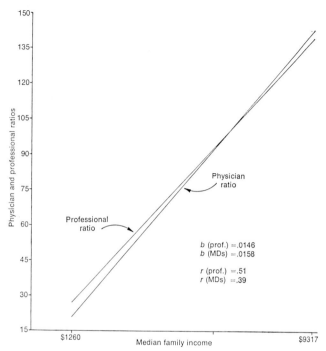

FIG. 7.1. Regression of physician ratios (per 100,000 population) and professional ratios (per 1,000 employed males) on median family income of county, 1960.

Figure 7.1 gives the regression line, regression coefficient, and correlation coefficient for the relation between median family income per county and the county physician/population ratio for 2,958 U.S. counties, with the range of income values indicated on the abscissa. (Median family income is not reported by the census in 13 instances.) As can be seen, the physician ratio increases as community wealth increases, and the correlation coefficient is moderately high for these types of data.[1] Results are thus consistent with studies that have used larger units of analysis. Figure 7.1 also shows the regression line for the ratio of all employed males in the county who are classified in "professional and technical" occupations to all employed males in the county, as reported by the 1960 census (16). The two regression lines are strikingly similar.

1. Since findings are for the entire population (all U.S. counties rather than a sample of counties), tests of significance have questionable meaning. Moreover, given the large number of cases, a very small correlation is statistically significant; with $N = 2958$, an r of .05 is statistically significant at the .01 level.

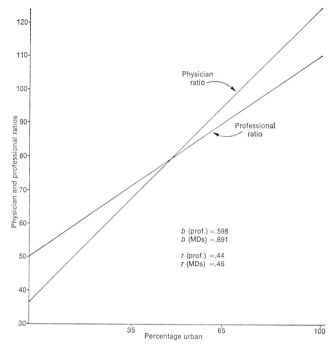

FIG. 7.2. Regression of physician ratios (per 100,000 population) and professional ratios (per 1,000 employed males) on population size-density index (proportion of residents living in areas defined as urban), 1960.

The physician and professional ratios are also regressed on the proportion of county residents classified by the census as living in urban areas (17), as shown in Figure 7.2. Again the resemblance between the two regression lines is clear. The maldistribution of physicians thus appears to be part of a more general process that influences the distribution of professionally and technically trained persons in general and not just physicians.

This is not to say that the process is exactly the same for physicians as for male members and most other professional and technical occupations. Many professional and technical groups (e.g., university professors and research scientists) are limited in their location by the location of industrial firms and other bureaucratic organizations that employ them. Since most physicians are independent (solo) practitioners, they are subject to fewer such constraints—although many other males classified in the professional and technical census category (lawyers, architects, veterinarians, dentists) are also independent practitioners engaged in solo practice or some form of partnership arrangement.

But the differences between the independent professionals and those who are rigidly tied to bureaucratic organizations can easily be overstated. The tendency for organizations that employ many professions to be located in affluent and urban-type communities is determined largely by the external economies (e.g., large populations) such communities provide. The locational decisions of the independent professionals are probably influenced by the same kinds of considerations. In the case of physicians, high-income urban-type communities provide the types of external supports (e.g., a critical mass of population) that the practice of most forms of medicine requires, especially practices associated with narrow specialization. Moreover, an emphasis on differences in processes between the independent professions and bureaucratically based professions may cause us to lose sight of the fact that the different processes are themselves part of a more general process that involves them both. In both cases the consequence is the same: wealthier, more densely populated communities have more than their proportionate share.

The data for Tennessee and Tennessee Mid-South make it possible to compare the distribution of physicians with that of other health-care personnel. First, physicians are compared with registered nurses for the 95 Tennessee counties. Numbers of physicians (excluding military physicians) and active nurses by county for the year 1962 are obtained from Pennell and Baker (18). The population figures used to compute rates are for 1960 (17). Rates per 100,000 population were computed and the relationship of each to median county income (1960) investigated. Results are shown in Figure 7.3. Both the regression coefficient and the correlation coefficient are higher for nurses. (With 95 cases an r of .25 is statistically significant at the .01 level.)

A second source of data is equally informative. In a 1969 survey of all 105 general short-stay hospitals in the Tennessee Mid-South region with membership in the American Hospital Association, information was obtained on the number of personnel in each of several occupational categories for 91 hospitals (19). Occupational categories include registered nurses, practical nurses and nurse technicians, and aides-orderlies, expressed as the number per 100 beds. Regression slopes and coefficients of correlation between each category and the median family income (1960) for the county in which the hospital is located are compared in Figure 7.4. (With 91 cases an r of .26 is statistically significant at the .01 level; hence all coefficients in the figure are significant.) It is clear that the effect of community income on health manpower varies directly with the professional development and technical expertise of the occupation. Even the semiskilled

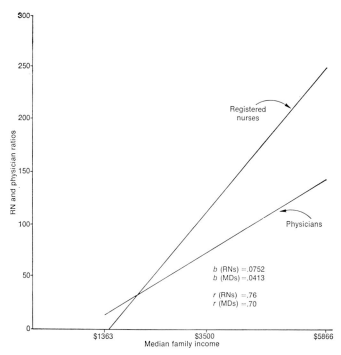

FIG. 7.3. *Regression of active registered nurses and physicians (1962) per 100,000 county residents (1960) on median family income for Tennessee counties.*

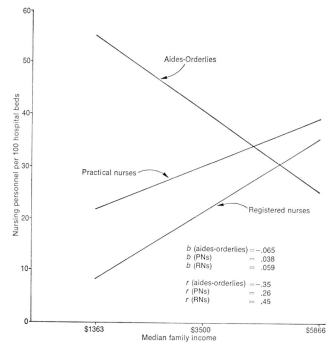

FIG. 7.4. *Regression of three nursing ratios on median family income of county for hospitals in the Tennessee Mid-South Region.*

practical nurses and nurse technicians tend to be concentrated in the more affluent communities, though slightly less so than registered nurses. To the extent that the quality of care depends on the professional qualifications of nursing personnel, it is clear that quality of care is directly related to the socioeconomic structure of the community.

To this point the following conclusions may be drawn: (1) physicians are unequally distributed in communities in the United States depending on the socioeconomic characteristics of the communities; (2) the distribution of physicians as patterned on these characteristics resembles the distribution of other technically trained personnel, both within and outside the medical field. This raises serious questions concerning the strategy of using professional and semiprofessional personnel—paramedics—to supplement and substitute for physician services in rural and economically deprived areas.

Such data do not tell us anything about the physicians' motives in concentrating in more affluent communities. But motivation aside, the distribution of physicians appears to be patterned on aspects of community structure, implying that efforts to redistribute physician manpower will be *constrained* by community structure. This can be seen from county differences in the relation between county hospital facilities (indexed by the ratio of general hospital beds to county population and the physician ratio).

Hospital Facilities, Physicians, and Community Constraints. In studies of the correlates of the physician ratio, the relations between several independent variables (including the hospital-bed ratio) and the dependent variable (the physician ratio) are usually examined as to what extent two or more of the independent variables are able to predict physician manpower better than one variable alone or to determine which among the several independent variables is the best predictor of physician manpower. In such studies the following kind of question is asked (6, p. 431): "Given the units of analysis under consideration [metropolitan areas], what single predictor variable will give us a maximum improvement in our ability to predict values of the dependent variable [number of physicians per 100,000 population]?" Different authors have arrived at different answers to this question. Some contend that community income is the most significant factor (10), others that population size and urbanization are (2); still others emphasize the possible significance of hospital facilities (20). In all cases, however, the predictor variables are viewed as independent of one another and their effects as additive.

This perspective is misleading, because the effects of one independent variable do not operate in isolation from the effects of other independent variables. Stated differently, the values of one variable provide a *context* within which the effects of other variables operate. This is especially true with reference to hospital facilities. Community hospital facilities are important in attracting and retaining physicians, and some communities with low physician ratios appear to have established such facilities in an effort to attract or keep physicians. At the same time, however, the same set of facilities may have a different effect depending on the type of community in which they are located. When a relationship between hospital-bed and physician ratios is reported, investigators are usually careful to indicate that several factors besides hospital beds are involved, such as population size, urbanization, and socioeconomic factors. Nevertheless, there is a tendency to assume that because hospital beds explain a portion of the variance in physician ratios not explained by other factors, hospital beds have an effect independent of other factors (6, 7). The point is explicit in the early work of Mountin, Pennell, and Nicolay (10, p. 1952; emphasis added):

> *Regardless* of income class of the county, the presence of a large number of hospital beds reflects more attractive locations for physicians. . . . Such facilities *alone* afford attraction for establishing medical practice apart from other factors such as wealth, population expansion, and urban characteristics of counties.

The hypothesis here is different. The effect of hospital facilities in attracting physicians to (or at least retaining them in) a community is believed to vary with the economic and urban character of the community. Stated differently, the effect of community hospital facilities in attracting and retaining physicians is constrained by the community context in which those facilities are located.

The hypothesis is tested for all 2,971 counties. The numbers of general hospital beds per 100,000 population are computed from AMA data (15). The correlation between the physician and hospital-bed ratios for all counties is .52, which provides at least some modest support for those who contend that hospital facilities can be a means by which communities are able to attract and keep physicians. Further analysis indicates, however, that the relationship is variable, depending on the community context.

Counties were classified in the census classifications of Greater Metropolitan (GM), Lesser Metropolitan (LM), Adjacent to Metropolitan (AM), Rural (R), and Isolated Rural (IR)—a classification used largely because it was readily available but reflecting to a large extent the socioeconomic and urban development of the county. The county types were arbitrarily scored from 1 to 5, with IR = 1 and GM = 5; correlations were computed between these values and the proportion of county residents classified as urban and the median family income of the county. Product-moment correlations were .62 and .51 respectively.

The regression coefficients of physician ratios on hospital-bed ratios systematically increased from IR to GM counties, except for a reversal between R and AM counties:

County Type	Regression Coeff.
GM $(N = 104)$	31.95
LM $(N = 289)$	18.50
AM $(N = 866)$	8.32
R $(N = 991)$	13.22
IR $(N = 721)$	4.74

(For ease of interpretation, regression coefficients are multiplied by 100; thus the coefficient of 31.95 means that an increase of 100 hospital beds per 100,000 results in an average increase of 31.95 physicians per 100,000.)

The significance of community structure is especially clear from Figure 7.5. County types are scaled on the abscissa according to the average median family income for counties in each county type, and the regression coefficients are placed on the ordinate. Although small numbers of cases always raise questions about the magnitude of a correlation coefficient, inspection of the plots leaves little doubt about the contextual effect of community socioeconomic structure on the relation between hospital-bed and physician ratios. Essentially the same results are obtained when the regression coefficients are plotted against the average proportion of urban residents in each county type $(r = .95)$. The extent to which hospital-bed ratios exert an actual effect on the physician ratio—that is, the difference in the slope of the regression line—is clearly constrained by the socioeconomic structure of the community.

In drawing this conclusion it is recognized that the relationship between physicians and hospital facilities is more complex than pictured here, since physicians are frequently instrumental in getting hospital facilities established in a community and the relationship is to some degree reciprocal. The assumption in the regression analysis that the direction of the relationship is from hospital facilities to physicians is an oversimplification. It is also recognized that the hospital-bed to population ratio is an imperfect measure of hospital *facilities*. A community of one million population may have the same number of beds per 100,000 as a community of ten thousand. It is probable, however, that the former will have a much wider range of facilities (e.g., coronary care units, intensive care wards, radiology

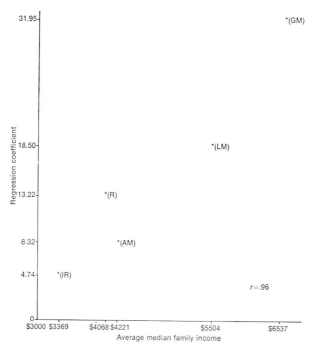

FIG. 7.5. Coefficients of regression of county physician ratios on hospital-bed ratios plotted against average median family income (1960) for county type.

facilities, pathology laboratories, and cobalt treatment facilities). Despite this limitation (which this study shares with a number of others) the results would seem to support the hypothesis that community structure is an important constraint on the relationship between community hospital facilities and community physician manpower. The weaker the social and economic resource base of the community, the greater the constraints.

Change over Time. The findings imply a longitudinal hypothesis: over time, physicians will increasingly concentrate in more affluent urban-type communities. Mountin, Pennell, and Brockett conclude that this was true between 1923 and 1938 (11). Examination of data for Tennessee indicates the same thing. Data available by county for 1950 from Pennell and Altenderfer (21), based on 1950 census figures, include physicians in faculty, administrative, and research positions as well as physicians in patient care; all nonmilitary federal physicians are also included. Data for county population are

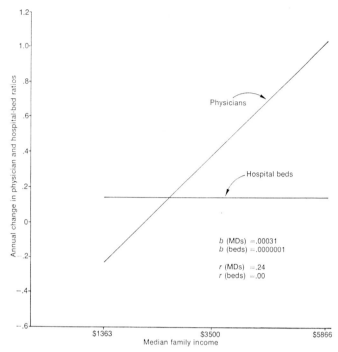

FIG. 7.6. Regression of average annual changes in physician ratios (1950–62/66) per 1,000 population on median family income for Tennessee counties (1960).

from 1960 census tabulations (22). The latest figures available that include the same categories of physicians are for 1966, based on a survey conducted by the Tennessee Mid-South Regional Medical Program in that year, which unfortunately included only 75 of the 95 Tennessee counties. Data for the other 21 counties—from Pennell and Baker (18), based on the 1962 AMA questionnaire—include essentially the same categories as the 1950 figures. Since the time period is 12 years for 21 counties and 16 years for 74 counties, the change in county physician ratios for the period is expressed as the average change per year. Figure 7.6 gives the results for change in the ratio regressed on county median family income for 1960, roughly the midpoint for the 1950–1962/66 period. As can be seen, increases in the physician ratio are directly related to county wealth.

A similar analysis was conducted for hospital beds, with the number of general hospital beds per county for 1950 and 1966 obtained from American Hospital Association publications (23, 24). The regression line and correlation coefficient for the relationship of hospital-bed ratios and community wealth are presented in Figure 7.6. The almost horizontal regression line and the correlation coefficient of zero indicate that community wealth was not related to change in the distribution of hospital facilities between 1950 and 1966. The contrast with changes in the physician ratio is clear. The lack of such a relationship for hospital beds is due no doubt to the influence of the Hill-Burton construction program, one aim of which was to bring about greater equity in the distribution of hospital facilities among communities across the country. This program provided funding for most of the new general hospital beds that were established in Tennessee during the 16-year period (25).

Two conclusions are indicated. One is that while the Hill-Burton program has been reasonably successful in resisting the constraints of community structure in the distribution of hospital facilities (at least it did not assist wealthier communities to improve their position over poorer communities from 1950 to 1966), it has not brought about a more equitable distribution of physician manpower. The other conclusion is that since hospital facilities do help to attract physicians to communities, even though the effect is not so strong in deprived communities as in affluent ones, the distribution of physicians would probably be still more uneven today if the Hill-Burton program had not existed. The program did not neutralize the social and economic forces originating in community structures and hence did not reverse the trend toward greater concentration of physician manpower in the richer, more populous communities, but it probably did slow the trend somewhat.

DISCUSSION. The findings are consistent with frameworks emphasizing the urbanization process, in which differences between communities in physician manpower are viewed as another reflection of urban-rural differences (15, p. 16). This interpretation is quite general and fails to indicate what the specific factors are that contribute to such differences. However, both theory and empirical results from economic and sociological analyses of community (25–27) are sufficiently developed to provide the basis for a framework in which causal factors are identified with somewhat greater specificity. The framework postulates that strong local service sectors (of which physician manpower is a part) are part of a broader complex of social and economic forces such as industry mix, overall community wealth, and external economies associated with large populations. For example, large populations provide important external economies to industry in the form of access to buyers, suppliers, and labor market; in the case of industries that require high-level technical skills, they provide access to a labor market that can supply those skills. (Universities, research parks, technical institutes, and the like are apt to be located in areas of high population concentrations.) This in turn attracts more population, more technically and professionally trained persons, greater community income in the form of higher salaries, and consequently an increase in the number of persons to provide services —including medical services—to the population.

The distribution of physicians, therefore, is intertwined with a complex of demographic, social, and economic factors. These factors work in the direction of keeping rich communities rich and poor communities poor. Community social and economic advantages (or disadvantages) are cumulative, and physician manpower is just one part of this cumulative pattern. This pattern imposes important constraints on any program designed to redistribute medical manpower in the United States. If this conclusion is accepted, the findings presented here have important policy implications for programs designed to reduce community inequities in medical manpower. The implications for two such programs, of the many proposed, may be considered illustratively.

One proposal emphasizes an increase in the overall supply of physicians. The assumption seems to be that with an increase in the number of physicians, physicians will gradually be "pushed out" into rural and economically deprived areas. This assumption appears to be erroneous on several grounds. First, if the larger supply of physicians continues to be patterned on the same factors as outlined above, the *relative* difference between advantaged and disadvantaged communities will continue and perhaps increase. Moreover, the *absolute* supply of physicians in rural, economically depressed areas may actually decrease. With increased specialization, physicians need access to larger populations in order to find a sufficient number of patients, and populations must have enough financial resources to afford the increasingly expensive treatment that increased specialization leads to. Also, an increase in third-party payers (either major medical private insurance plans or national health insurance) may actually make community inequities larger. In the first place, insurance plans do nothing to change community structure, and this is crucial in the distribution of physicians. In addition, universal insurance coverage will increase the demand for health services in wealthy urban areas as well as in poor rural areas. There are, after all, many underprivileged persons in affluent communities who, because of limited economic resources, are not now receiving medical care. These financial barriers will be eliminated as third-party payment becomes universal or nearly so. Consequently a larger cohort of physicians will be able to find an effective demand for medical services in areas where the physician-population ratio is already high and where, for whatever reasons, physicians are attracted to live.

The belief that an increase in the supply of physicians in itself will lead to a more even distribution of physicians is inconsistent with trends of the past twenty years. According to the 1950 census there were 64 counties without even one civilian physician (21). In 1959, according to Stewart and Pennell's analysis of data from the AMA (28), 74 counties were without an active nonfederal physician; the figure grew to 98 in 1963 and 126 in 1968 (29), and in 1971 the number of counties without an active federal *or* nonfederal physician in patient care was 133 (30). Although the types of physician included in the tabulations vary (in the 1950 census *all* employed physicians except those in the armed forces are included; the 1971 AMA figure includes federal and nonfederal physicians in patient care only), it is clear that the number of counties with zero physician manpower consistently increased over that 21-year period. And this has occurred during a period in which the overall national active civilian physician/population ratio appears to have increased: from 124 per 100,000 population in 1950 (21, p. 34; 31) to 143 per 100,000 in 1971 (31, population estimated). Thus the number of communities with zero physician manpower was increasing over this 21-year period while the overall supply of physicians was apparently increasing. An increase in the supply of physicians cannot in itself be expected to result in a more even distribution.

Another type of program is the development of so-called physician assistants (including the Medex and Primex programs). Some persons view personnel trained in such programs as supplementing or substituting for physician services, often in areas where the physician supply is low. The first problem with this view is that as long as such persons are the physicians' *assistants,* they will be close to the physician in a *spatial* sense and hence will be distributed much as physicians are. But the basic question is: What are physician assistants going to find attractive about communities with low physician supply that physicians, nurses, and technically trained persons in general have been unable to find? Rather it is to be expected that physician assistants will become part of the general social and economic process that encourages the concentration of technically trained persons in richer, more populous environments.

In general any program designed to redistribute physician manpower based on increasing the supply of manpower alone probably will not be very successful, because professional manpower is one aspect of a macrosocioeconomic process that tends to favor these communities which have most in the way of social and economic advantages. If this is so, efforts directed to modifying the distribution of physicians must focus on the causes of the distribution rather than on the distribution itself. One might argue that in the long run a community can probably best increase its physician manpower by attracting more and higher-paying industry, which in turn will increase the population and the overall standard of living and hence the physician/population ratio. This, however, is not realistic, since most private industry realizes important economies by locating in communities with large populations in which the skill mix is already high.

We would suggest instead that programs should focus on *organizational* changes in medicine in which *service* rather than physician manpower is the central focus. Mechanisms need to be developed through which the reach of medical personnel and organizations in high-manpower communities can be extended to communities where manpower is scarce. Such efforts might be patterned on area health education centers and would involve the development of intercommunity medical networks through which citizens of low-manpower communities could be referred to appropriate physicians in high-manpower communities on a systematic basis. The approaches used in different settings would differ depending on the needs and requirements of those settings. In all such programs, however, two elements would be central: (1) the location of centers in communities where the social and economic resources are sufficient to sustain a medical community and (2) the development of medical organizations that would assume responsibility for the medical welfare of citizens in a specified number of communities.

The difficulties involved in such programs are many and obvious, and the ideas are certainly not new. But in the light of the results reported here and the interpretation of those results, such programs would appear to be more realistic than the alternatives of trying to bring about a redistribution of physician manpower or attempting to develop the social and economic resource base of communities. The latter approaches might work for specific communities, but as generalized approaches their failure is almost guaranteed by the socioeconomic forces of society.

It is not our purpose to propose a solution to the problem of community differences in physician manpower. Rather our purpose is to show that the distribution of physicians is part of a macrosocioeconomic process, that other professionally and technically trained personnel are part of this process, and that any attempt to modify existing inequities in the distributional pattern of physicians will be constrained by this process. Programs designed to create a more equitable distribution of physicians that ignore this are not likely to have the consequences their designers intend.

CHAPTER EIGHT

ORGANIZATION OF HEALTH SERVICES FOR RURAL AREAS

CHARLES O. CRAWFORD

SERVICES DELIVERY MODEL. In analyzing the organization of any community service, it is useful to employ a services delivery model. For any human service there is a provider or group of providers and a consumer or group of consumers. The provider focuses on and engages in the process of provision; the consumer's interest is primarily in utilization. (Consumers are, however, becoming increasingly involved in the provision process through consumer participation.

From a social organization standpoint it is important while analyzing community services to give adequate consideration to the relationship between structure (consumer-provider) and process (or function) and the intended-unintended and functional-dysfunctional aspects of social action (37). These aspects or dimensions apply to many health services: the *provider* may be the physician, dentist, hospital, nurse, or other personnel, facility, or service; the *consumer* is the individual. (However, labor unions and other third parties sometimes mediate between provider and consumer.) The two structures of provider and consumer interact through the processes of provision and utilization within some geographic area or within some other meaningful context of community. In diagrammatic form this model can be portrayed as a triangle (Fig. 8.1).

CHARLES O. CRAWFORD is Associate Professor of Rural Sociology, Pennsylvania State University.

This chapter is a revised version of an earlier publication, "Organization of Health Services for Rural Areas." University Park, Pa.: Department of Agricultural Economics and Rural Sociology, A.E. & R.S. No. 106, 1973. The author gratefully acknowledges the comments and suggestions made by Sam Cordes and Samuel Leadley on an earlier draft of this paper.

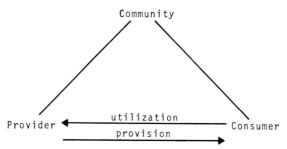

FIG. 8.1. Interaction of provider and consumer within a community context.

Significance of Community. Community dynamics is an important but often overlooked part of service delivery. Blum asserts that "the bulk of community health activities occurs at the local level even when provided by state agencies" (11). The National Commission on Community Health Services (NCCHS) stresses the need to focus on the community and points out that operational definitions of communities can vary when discussing health services (44). As a consequence, the concept of "community of solution" (the local area in which a problem is solvable) is advocated. Illustrations of such communities include mental health "catchment" areas, environmental health "shed" areas, and health service marketing areas.

It is important to realize that any definition of community is conditioned by the level of service being discussed. Primary care is provided on a local basis; secondary care usually encompasses a larger geographical area; and tertiary care, the most sophisticated level, is provided on an even larger geographical basis.

Location of services represents consideration of frequency of use, cost, and distance. Primary care is more frequently needed and involves less cost per unit than tertiary care. Thus proximity to primary care tends to be a more important consideration in its utilization. It is important, however, that services at all levels taken together provide a regional network with sufficient linkages to insure that individual patients not miss any care needed at any of the levels. These linkages depend on an intricate professional referral system. Unfortunately such linkages are not always present.

Questions of where to locate services can be perplexing to planners and policymakers. Some recommendations are in terms of location at "growth" nodes (38). Other research seems to indicate that there are scalable patterns of services appropriate for different sizes of communities and that attempts to develop services in a small community that are found only in larger and/or more differentiated communities will likely fail.[1] Both these approaches tend to overlook what Cordes and Crawford have labeled "normative need" (17)—the fact that in spite of homogenization in society, communities differ in terms of beliefs and values, and these in turn affect accepted ways of defining and handling community problems. A process and/or structure found suitable for solving a problem in one community may not be appropriate in another. Thus normative variations in community settings call for flexibility in organizing community health services.

Provision Process. The two major processes in the services delivery model are utilization or consumption (dealt with elsewhere in this volume) and provision of services. A community-based service needs four broad types of resources: (1) organization, (2) manpower, (3) finances, and (4) facilities. These categories are somewhat analogous to the economist's notions of management, labor, capital, and land.

Although organization is treated with manpower, finances, and facilities, it is on a somewhat different level. It is the process of putting resources together in such a way as to produce a desired output in the most efficient manner. In a specific example of cultural lag, Blum asserts that "effective delivery of health services and information is often decades behind the actual knowledge or techniques of rendering specific service . . . the creakiest part of the health delivery service has been the administrative vehicle which is neither able to carry the necessary load nor proceed at an adequate pace" (11). Numerous organizations are involved in the delivery of health services, although these health-related organizations are less numerous in rural than in urban areas. Interorganizational relationships in health contexts are worthy of research attention.[2]

There are many types of manpower providing health services. In terms of income and training, physicians could be taken to represent one end of the spectrum and custodial workers and health aides the other, with numerous other health professionals and paraprofessionals between.

Financing health services is proving to be a major national issue. Most experts predict some form of national health insurance in the near future. Somers points out that "intelligent analysis and effective

1. Paul Eberts, Frank Young, and some of their colleagues at Cornell University are conducting research on community differentiation and service array in which this point seems to emerge.
2. See Baker and O'Brien (9), Milio (39), and White and Vlasak (62). Also see Gerald Klonglan and Steven Paulson, "Interorganizational Coordination as a Policy for the Delivery of Health Services in Nonmetropolitan Areas," a paper presented at the 1971 Annual Meeting of the Rural Sociological Society in Denver, Colo.

control of costs must take account of the entirety of how we finance, organize, and deliver health services as well as the external economy" (55). Currently financing is a particularly relevant component of organization for health service in rural areas; rural families are less likely than urban families to have health insurance, with farm families having the lowest rate of coverage (32, p. 23).

Facilities needed for provision of health services include buildings, transportation, communication, and care technology. The quantity of these resources needed varies considerably by primary, secondary, and tertiary levels of care. Although communication equipment is an important facility in health care, especially in emergency health care, the *process* of communication is just as important. Communication among providers and between providers and consumers is a major problem in providing and utilizing services.

Levels of Health Care. In reviewing the organization of health services in rural areas it is important to consider levels of services.

Elinoff has outlined three levels of care (21). The service delivery model outlined earlier can be applied to primary, secondary, and tertiary care. Further, it seems appropriate to apply the model to one level at a time rather than to the total health care system. Such an approach is even more justified in rural areas where primary care is most common. Secondary and tertiary services are likely to be found outside the rural community and frequently at considerable distance.

Primary care has been defined in a number of ways:
—"first contact care" (60)
—"that kind of care that most of the people need most of the time" (5)
—"range of services adequate for meeting the great majority of daily personal health needs" (15)
—"basic and preventive level of health care" (21)

Writers like White (60), Appel (8), Garfield (23), and NCCHS (44), who view primary care as the first point of entry for a patient, overlook a significant fact—that many persons go directly to specialists after having diagnosed a problem themselves (10, 27).

Secondary care includes most surgical procedures and more complicated medical diagnoses and procedures usually rendered by specialists and requiring more complex technology. Care of this order is usually found in general hospitals and at points fewer in number than primary care sources.

Tertiary care is at a more sophisticated level. Because of the complex and expensive care involved at this level, tertiary care centers cover a much wider geographic area than primary or secondary health care services. Extensive cardiac care and cancer therapy are examples

Table 8.1. Number of Physician Visits per Person per Year by Area of Residence and Age, United States, 1969

	Age				
	All Ages	Under 17	17–44	45–64	65+
SMSA	4.4	3.8	4.3	4.9	6.2
Outside SMSA					
Nonfarm	4.0	3.2	4.0	4.5	6.2
Farm	3.1	2.3	2.6	3.7	5.6

Source: National Center for Health Statistics, *Age Patterns in Medical Care, Illness and Disability,* Ser. 10, No. 70, 1972, p. 10.

of tertiary care. It is not uncommon for some secondary care centers to attempt to provide complex cardiac and cancer therapy without the complete array of needed resources; as a consequence they may provide incomplete and underutilized services. Tertiary care of adequate quality is usually found at medical schools and medical centers.

PRIMARY CARE NEEDS. We can get some idea of the need for and use of health services of rural and urban residents by examining data from the National Health Survey. The data in Table 8.1 indicate that nonmetropolitan persons visit physicians less often than persons from metropolitan areas. The average number of physician visits per person in 1969 was 4.4 for metropolitan persons, 4.0 for nonmetropolitan nonfarm, and 3.1 for farm persons. This trend held for all age groups except those 65 and over where the metropolitan and nonmetropolitan nonfarm ratios were the same.

The data in Table 8.2 reveal further patterns of lower utilization. Although the differences between people in SMSAs and nonfarm people outside SMSAs are small, it is clear that farm people were more likely to have longer intervals since the last physician visit.

The data in Table 8.3 indicate, however, that the lower rate of physician visits among nonmetropolitan persons portrayed in Tables 8.1 and 8.2 was not the result of fewer health problems. Table 8.3 demonstrates that as one moves out from metropolitan areas, the percentage of persons with some limitation of activity due to chronic illness increases. This pattern did not hold true for all ages; children on farms had a lower rate of limitations than did children from metropolitan areas or children from nonmetropolitan nonfarm areas. It may be that rural people are not aware of their health problems until these problems interfere with their normal patterns of living. This, coupled with lower incomes and geographic isolation, undoubtedly influences utilization patterns. The data in Table 8.1 indicate that there was a greater possibility of undiagnosed illness among rural

Table 8.2. Percentage Distribution of Persons by Time Interval since Last Physician Visit, by Residence, United States, 1969

| | Population | Length of Interval | | | | | | |
		Less than 6 mo.	6–11 mo.	1 yr.	2–4 yr.	5+ yr.	Never	Unknown
SMSA	100.0	55.9	14.9	11.7	10.9	3.9	0.5	2.1
Outside SMSA								
Nonfarm	100.0	52.6	15.1	13.0	12.1	4.5	0.9	1.8
Farm	100.0	44.5	16.0	14.6	14.6	7.0	1.3	2.1

Source: National Center for Health Statistics, *Physician Visits: Volume and Interval since Last Visit*, Ser. 10, No. 75, 1972, p. 15.

Table 8.3. Percent of Persons with Some Limitations of Activity Due to Chronic Conditions by Age and Area of Residence, United States, 1968–69

	All Ages	Age			
		Under 17	17–44	45–64	65+
SMSA	10.4	2.4	7.0	17.1	38.9
Outside SMSA					
Nonfarm	12.7	2.4	7.7	21.8	47.4
Farm	13.8	1.6	8.4	21.0	50.2

Source: National Center for Health Statistics, *Age Patterns in Medical Care, Illness and Disability,* Ser. 10, No. 70, 1972, p. 15.

persons since they had fewer visits to physicians. As rural persons get older, previously undiagnosed illness begins to have its impact on various types of role performances. Then, at later ages, dealing with health is perceived as necessary. The effects of available financial assistance (medicare) may also create the smaller differences at older ages by reducing the income problem.

Supply of General Practitioners. One common argument as to why rural areas have lower physician utilization rates than urban areas is that there are fewer physicians in rural areas. Rural areas do have a considerably lower total supply of medical physicians than urban areas, due primarily to a relatively smaller number of medical specialists in rural areas. When types of areas are compared with regard to relative ratios of general practitioners, rural and urban areas do not differ appreciably.

In comparing physician supply for primary care in rural and urban areas, it is important to keep in mind that some specialists provide primary care. This is especially true for internists, pediatricians, and obstetricians. When we consider that these three categories comprised 35 percent of all specialists in 1971 (43, p. 194), it can readily be seen that urban areas are likely to have a greater number of functioning primary care practitioners than rural areas.

An analysis of primary health care practitioners needs to consider osteopathic physicians as well as medical doctors. Osteopathic physicians are increasingly being recognized as qualified practitioners as their training approaches that of medical doctors. In 1967 there were 10,067 osteopaths in private practice in the United States (43, p. 192), and 85 percent of these were in general practice. Thus the number of primary care physicians is increased almost by the number of osteopaths in practice. The distribution of osteopaths is also important when considering primary care in rural areas. In 15 states with MD/ population ratios lower than the national ratio, the ratio of osteopaths to population was equal to or greater than the national ratio (45, p. 54). These tended to be more rural states where osteopaths helped meet a need for general practitioners.

In terms of organization for primary care, osteopathic and medical physicians tend to be in solo practice in rural areas. As the preference for colleague affiliation and regular hours of employment among younger physicians increases, we may see more physicians practicing together in partnerships or groups or employed in hospital outpatient departments. Federal support for establishment of Health Maintenance Organizations may also lead to changes in the organization of primary care. At present, though, solo practice is the modal form of practice of rural medical and osteopathic physicians offering primary care.

As forms of group practice develop in rural areas, we will see a trend for primary care being provided at greater distances from rural residents than has been true in the past. Thus the health services community for primary care may increase in geographic size.

Supply of Other Manpower. There are other significant categories of manpower and various organizational forms through which primary care is provided to residents in rural areas.

CHIROPRACTORS. Chiropractors represent a primary care resource in many rural communities. Although they are viewed as marginal practitioners by a number of health care professionals (58), they may be viewed by some of the public as quite appropriate for some tasks (27). One report of use of chiropractors revealed that the percentage of persons making visits was higher for rural families, especially farm families (4.3), than it was for urban families (1.9) (42). In a study of use of chiropractors in rural Iowa, McCorkle found that chiropractic practice fits well with beliefs and behavior of rural residents (33).

In terms of their distribution, 44 percent of all chiropractors in the United States in 1971 were located in five states: California (20 percent), New York (7 percent), Texas (6 percent), Missouri (6 percent), and Pennsylvania (5 percent) (43, p. 73). Roemer has cited a tendency for chiropractors to settle in rural areas (48). Chiropractors are generally found in solo practice and operate as independent practitioners.

The role of chiropractors in primary care should not be overlooked, since support and attention given to illness by someone with perceived authority can be an important factor in overcoming an illness. Treatment involves a good deal of "psycho" as well as "somatic" care (36). White and Skipper note that chiropractors may provide a more personal relationship than medical physicians (61).

DENTISTS. Roemer points out that "the urban-rural distribution of dentists is even more skewed than that of physicians" (48). Cordes presents 1962 data showing that the ratio of dentists per 100,000 persons in greater metropolitan areas was more than 2.5 times the ratio for isolated rural areas (16).

Organizationally, dentists are largely in solo practice. Investment in office equipment is usually larger for dental practice than for medical and osteopathic office practice.

NURSES. Nurses are playing an increasingly important role in primary care. New titles which reflect this broader role include pediatric nurse practitioner, nurse practitioner, and primary care nurse (13). With additional training and authority to practice, some nurses can work very effectively as supplementary primary care practitioners.

Cordes presents data indicating that metropolitan areas had nurse/population ratios more than twice those for isolated rural areas in 1962 (16). With unmet needs for primary care personnel in rural areas, greater experimentation is taking place with other types of providers. This recognizes that some tasks performed by physicians can be performed by persons with less but special training in primary care.

PHYSICIAN'S ASSISTANTS. Another new type of medical practitioner is the physician's assistant. Both the expanded nurse role and that of the physician's assistant offer many opportunities for providing a type of primary care in rural areas where there are no general practice physicians. This is particularly true if mobile or "outreach" units are used to deliver services where the cost of transporting support personnel is less than that of transporting physicians. Paramedical personnel can also assist physicians in their offices. Jacobs and his colleagues in a recent study of Medex personnel found certain tasks were successfully allocated to physician's assistants (29). Their research indicated that a greater division of labor in primary care is possible.

The integration of paramedical personnel into the organization of primary care creates a number of problems yet to be resolved (1). Role relationships between them, the physician, and other health personnel are not always clearly defined. Patients may view assistants' care as inferior and expect to see a physician (31). On the other hand, where no care is available, acceptance may be higher (6).

In view of the declining availability of general practice physicians, the use of paramedical personnel in rural areas should continue to be seriously considered and evaluated. Such evaluation should attempt to analyze role relationships, satisfaction, acceptance, alternative modes of care, and other questions from an organizational standpoint.

Other Organizational Forms. Selected alternatives to solo office practice of medical and osteopathic doctors for providing primary care to rural residents have been explored. Some of these, like the use of paramedical personnel, have been provider-initiated. Another provider-initiated alternative is formation of partnerships of group practices. Group practices have possibilities of attracting and keeping physicians since they provide more opportunities for regular hours, vacations, colleague interaction, sharing equipment, and participation in continuing education programs.

However, group practice in rural areas poses problems for patients. Common facilities at fewer locations means more patients will have to travel greater distances; thus transportation problems may inhibit seeking care. Perhaps development of group practice with paramedics at outposts could be a viable alternative.

Another alternative in primary or ambulatory care—one that has been patient-initiated—is the use of hospital emergency rooms as a substitute for primary physicians in private office practices (8, p. 150; 49; 51; 55, p. 29). Finding that a physician is unavailable at certain times, especially evenings and weekends, patients are increasingly seeking care at emergency rooms. The use of the emergency room sometimes places a burden on the hospital and the patient, especially if there are no house doctors. Use of the hospital emergency room does, however, present an opportunity to organize primary care along lines advocated by some experts, i.e., hospital-based primary care (3; 8, p. 150). By having primary care outpatient services or ambulatory care centers or departments attached to a hospital, physicians have greater access to facilities needed to provide higher-quality care. Again, though, the adaptation of this organizational mode to rural areas is limited, because transportation problems emerge as a potential barrier or at least a factor limiting its use. The problem of sorting emergencies from nonemergencies and dealing with each in an effective, efficient, and appropriate manner is also unresolved.

Two other solutions to provision of primary care reflect governmental initiative. The National Health Service Corps (NHSC) is a program designed to place physicians and other health professionals in certain communities having critical manpower shortages (4). The goal of the program is to minimize continued NHSC involvement in any given community with the hope that once a physician establishes a practice in the community and is accepted he will remain there.

A second government-initiated mode of care consists of limited care provided through local public health departments. Public health departments have traditionally provided preventive and educational health programs—well-baby clinics and immunization and educational programs. However, when public health agencies move into the treatment stages on their own initiative, private practitioners usually exert their power to force the agency to withdraw, since this encroaches on their domain (64, p. 235). As a result, public health agencies do not play a major role in primary treatment.[3] In areas where there are no physicians in private practice, however, the movement of public health agencies into treatment phases of primary care is not altogether lacking.[4] More thought needs to be given to the responsibility and role of public health agencies (local, state, or federal) in providing care when factors that usually attract private physicians (i.e., proximity of colleagues and diagnostic laboratories) are nonexistent.

The involvement of public health agencies in primary care, however, is dependent on strong local public health organizations. Such well-organized local health activity does not exist in many parts of the country. In Pennsylvania, for example, in 1970 only five of the 67 counties had local health departments (18), and all of these were located within three SMSAs. In rural areas public health activity was left to the state health department, operating its limited resources in four administrative regions.

Other parts of the country vary in terms of strength of local public health departments and activities performed. In general the Southeast has strong county health departments; other parts of the country are less well organized (25). Establishment of local health departments is often accomplished by local referendum, and rural areas are less inclined than urban areas to vote for such organizations (18).

Bodenheimer (12) has pointed to yet another alternative for rural primary health care. He maintains that in areas where population density is low, mobile units staffed by physicians or auxiliary personnel can be used to make periodic scheduled visits and/or serve on a telephone or radio response basis. Making the mobile unit a part of a well-organized comprehensive care program and staffing it with paramedical personnel would seem to hold considerable merit in providing health care to rural areas.

Another type of organization for primary care involves the placement of primary care in a fairly tight network of comprehensive primary, secondary, and tertiary care provided through group practice. This is the increasingly popular form of organization known as Health Maintenance Organization (HMO)—typically a prepaid, group practice, comprehensive care program.[5] The suitability of HMOs to

3. A directory has been prepared listing and describing the many programs in which physician support personnel are being trained (46).
4. A discussion of these concepts as they relate to development of a team approach can be found in Rubin and Beckhard (53).
5. For an extended discussion of the relationship between the private and public realms of health care see Allan (2) and Rogers (50).

rural areas seems questionable in view of the points that have been made so far—low density population and low incomes. However, it should not be ruled out as an alternative organizational form, especially if transportation and financial problems can be overcome.

Primary care provided by university medical centers represents a variation of centralized organization for primary care. Much of the primary care delivered in this manner is found in urban areas where neighborhood health centers are established as part of an outreach mission of a medical center (41). With increasing frequency, however, medical centers are establishing community-based outreach care centers in rural areas.[6]

Medical care foundations, an organizational form originally developed in California in 1954, are being established as another way of providing patient care. As of November 1973 there were nearly 80 such foundations in the United States, and passage of P.L. 92-603, containing a provision for Professional Standards Review Organization (PSRO), has stimulated further development of medical foundations (14). Donabedian cites a number of studies evaluating this form of organization (20).

PRIMARY CARE CONSIDERATIONS. Three additional considerations, which cut across all organizational forms of primary care previously discussed, are: (1) importance of personal touch, (2) emerging emphasis on the activated patient, and (3) need for systemic linkages.

Importance of Personal Touch. Provision of health care is both a technical and a sustaining process (35). On the technical side treatment is given to specific illnesses and conditions ranging from cuts and sore throats to the most serious illnesses. At the same time, however, health care by its nature is designed to deal with personal, emotional, psychological, and other aspects of the individual.

In organizing health services, attention needs to be given to preserving the sustaining part of health care. This does not mean that this is the exclusive responsibility of the primary care physician. However, allowance must be made for it to be performed by someone—a nurse, a social worker, a family health specialist, or other professionals. "Those items of medical practice that can be organized in the manner of the assembly of an automobile constitute only a small fraction of contemporary medical care" (35, p. 4). The sustaining and psycho-

6. Kohn (30), in his review of Canadian health programs, mentions this point in relation to the sparsely populated northern provinces of Canada. Donabedian also stresses the potential of governmental health departments (20, p. 168).

social or emotional component of health care has been cited as one that might be more effectively provided to rural residents if primary care services are developed in rural areas rather than have the residents seek this care outside their familiar communities (6).

These considerations become increasingly serious as attempts to apply rational systems theory to health service delivery becomes popular (3). Care must be taken not to rationalize the health system to the point where it can no longer carry out one of its basic functions. However, "systemization and personalization are not necessarily antithetical" (55, p. 87). In a sense, what we need is an efficient system of health care delivery that preserves the personal, all-encompassing concern of the "old country doctor." I would stress again, however, that this does not necessarily have to be carried out by a physician.

Role of Activated Patient. A second general consideration to which increasing attention is being given is the need to utilize the patient's capacity to deal with some of his own day-to-day health problems. Wilson has labeled this the need for the "activated patient" (63). Others point to the need for increased "individual responsibility" for one's health (24) and to deal with emergencies (26). An article in an AMA publication for laymen suggests that patients can and should make some decisions regarding the seriousness of their symptoms before automatically calling a physician (54). Many recognize the need for health education (47; 55, Ch. 5), but its integration into primary care programs in rural areas needs considerable strengthening.

This need for a more informed patient has two significant dimensions. On the one hand it requires the individual to adopt recommended practices that would reduce his risk to certain diseases. Control of diet, maintenance of exercise, elimination of smoking, and weight control are a few examples (56).

Secondly there is need for greater understanding of the health care process. What can the person do for himself and what should he not do? What and where are the components of the complete primary health care program? How does the person get access to health care? What should be done in an emergency? In terms of the services delivery model outlined earlier, this emphasis on making the consumer more active is in essence an attempt to bring the consumer into the provision process.

In adult education an agency that comes to mind is the Cooperative Extension Service of land-grant colleges. Through the extension service an educational team has been established in virtually every county in the United States, traditionally consisting of a county agricultural agent, a home economist, and a youth worker.

In recent years some state extension services have added county staff in new subject matter areas, among which is health education. Questions have been raised regarding the qualifications of the extension service to carry out health education programs. Critics maintain that the extension service does not have the trained manpower or the research base to support a health education program. Supporters maintain that cooperative extension has an educational delivery mechanism at the local level and that by developing appropriate linkages it can carry out an effective health education program (57). Some state extension services have actively begun specialized health education programs; evaluation seems to indicate that if linkages with health agencies are developed, an effective job can be done.[7]

Systemic Linkages. A third important consideration in primary care is concerned with the provider side of the service delivery model.

This is the necessity for systemic linkages, both among various organizations providing different services and among communities in provision of a common health service. This is a classic sociological problem of interorganizational relations to which Loomis's social systems model might be applied.

Often overlooked are linkages of health service organizations with organizations from other institutional spheres of community life. School health services can play important roles in providing child health care, although benefits of these programs have been questioned (28). Clergymen, with some additional training, can be important agents in providing services for persons with emotional problems. These nonhealth manpower and facility resources take on special significance in rural areas where highly trained health manpower is scarce.

Warren raises the question of whether the element of competition (and therefore domain overlap) among agencies should not be encouraged so that the consumer, through his selection process, will be assured of a higher quality of service (59). Will a monopoly lead to poorer or better service? Anderson has also expressed the view that competition among health agencies, particularly the bargaining process, should be encouraged (7). Much of the discussion of this issue does not seem relevant to rural areas, since clientele to support such competitive services is nonexistent. Direct health services in rural areas have been (and in the future may have to be) of a monopolistic nature, with the important interorganizational questions being in terms of interinstitutional linkages.

7. A nationwide study was completed by the federal government in which it was found that the American public lacks considerable knowledge about proper health practices along the lines of those cited. The implications of some of these findings for the public are discussed by Furlong (22).

SECONDARY AND TERTIARY CARE FOR RURAL AREAS.

One definition of primary care—"that kind of care that most people need most of the time" (5)—helps put secondary and tertiary care in perspective. Secondary and tertiary care represent less frequently used services but generally those for which more specialized skills are needed. Secondary care can be found in community-type hospitals and often involves specialists; tertiary care is usually provided in medical centers and involves the superspecialties.

Since community hospitals and most specialists render secondary level services (although specialists also provide tertiary service and some primary care service), one way to consider secondary care service is in terms of these resources.

It has been noted that the number of hospital beds in rural areas has substantially increased in the past 20–30 years as a result of the Hill-Burton hospital construction program (25, 48). However, the number of hospital beds alone is not an indicator of quality of service. "Sparsely populated, low-income rural and semi-rural counties have relatively more hospitals than do urban, high-income counties, but the rural hospitals tend to be smaller and less adequately staffed" (19).

Also in terms of surgery performed, rural hospitals may be inferior. Bylaws of rural hospitals permit the rural general practitioner to perform surgery that would not be permitted in urban areas (48). Another indication of the poorer quality of rural hospitals is that in 1966 only 45 percent of nonmetropolitan hospitals, compared to 78 percent of metropolitan hospitals, were accredited by the Joint Commission on Accreditation of Hospitals (16, p. 40).

Although it is desirable in many cases, merger or coordination of small rural hospitals with other hospitals remains a difficult problem. Several approaches have been tried, but the general result seems to be failure. The route of voluntarily merging community hospitals appears to have severe limitations because of community pride and reluctance to give up autonomy (52).

At the conclusion of a study of one rather well known and well planned five-year program of regionalization of rural hospitals, the investigators stated: "In essence, regionalization, with its signed agreements, remained on the whole a paper achievement" (34, p. 156).

The idea of coordination, however, remains attractive. Government action has been taken to strengthen coordination among hospitals and other health facilities through Comprehensive Health Planning. Through the establishment of areawide planning bodies and statewide agencies, it is intended that some degree of order, rationality, and effectiveness will emerge in health care delivery.

It was pointed out earlier that many specialists are providers of secondary health services and that they are heavily concentrated in metropolitan areas. A major part of the explanation is that since the conditions they treat are relatively uncommon, a larger population is needed. The requirement of more supportive services and more elaborate facilities in secondary care is also related to specialists' location in metropolitan areas The same reasoning on a magnified level applies to specialists providing tertiary care. It appears that it is not feasible to get specialists into rural areas as providers of secondary or tertiary care. What is needed is access to these services through the primary care resources that are available in rural areas or could be developed there.

CONCLUSIONS. Twenty-five years ago Mott and Roemer, in discussing rural health care, asserted that "the economic and geographic features of rural life . . . are the basis of the problem" (40, p. 149). More recently Wilson expressed the same view: "Rural health is a problem of two basic dimensions. These are financial status and geographic location" (63, p. 1623). A third factor that needs to be explicitly recognized is consumer health education.

The solution of the geographic, economic, and educational problems requires focusing on the community, provider, and consumer and the processes of provision and utilization—on the *organization* of delivery of health service. If problems of transportation, financial support, and consumer education can be solved, the problem of manpower may prove to be less serious than it is often perceived to be. Additional manpower resources may be needed, but sufficient improvement of the three other inputs will minimize the need.

CHAPTER NINE

PUBLIC POLICY OF RURAL HEALTH

BERT E. SWANSON AND EDITH SWANSON

IT IS difficult to single out the unique health care problems of rural Americans from those of other Americans. There is no clearly discernible separate rural health delivery system, nor is there a systematic accounting of health conditions or care, nor are there any general organizations or programs centered about rural health policy. It may be that the concern for rural health cannot and should not be separated from the health problems facing Americans in general. In any event it seems fruitless to discuss rural health without placing it within the general framework of the crises facing the national health system.

Leading policymakers, key administrators, analysts, and commentators have generally proclaimed a health crisis. Former President Nixon stated there is "a massive crisis" in our medical care system requiring both administrative and legislative action (49). Senator Edward Kennedy has referred to the health system as the fastest growing failing business and points to the double disaster of family sickness and bankruptcy (24). Similarly former secretary of HEW, John Gardner, chastised the present system of medical care as "outworn, expensive and outrageously inefficient" (20). For emphasis, another former secretary, Abraham Ribicoff, pinpoints a critical factor when he states:

> The country does not now have, and never has had, a national policy on health and medical care, or at least not a policy that represented any clear, specific, and positive statement about the medical care that the citizens of this country were entitled to receive, and the financial and social conditions in which they were entitled to receive it (35).

BERT E. SWANSON is Professor of Political Science and Urban Studies, University of Florida. EDITH SWANSON is Research Associate, Community Health and Family Medicine, University of Florida.

The sense of crisis, however, is not shared by all. Harry Schwartz, a *New York Times* journalist, declares that American medicine is not so grievously ill as it is made out to be and that the radical social surgery proposed as a corrective measure constitutes a cure that may be worse than the disease (38).

American health policy has witnessed three major shifts toward the medical care system, with several incremental changes adopted from time to time. The first was the adoption of public health measures through the use of police powers to control and eradicate major threats to health from unsanitary and epidemic outbreaks in the late 19th century. The second shift focused on reform of medical schools with the purpose of upgrading the quality of trained physicians early in this century. The third shift, following World War II, placed most of its attention on the development of medical research and training. Incrementally the federal government has chosen specific target populations to be included under a government care or insurance program. More recently the focus is on how to determine need and deliver adequate health care to individual patients. The first reform was adopted in response to the health knowledge of the time, i.e. sanitary engineering. The second was initiated and conducted by forces within the medical profession to develop medical skills and apply medical knowledge. The third reflects the quarrel between the dominant medical profession and the many voices of diverse consumer interests that demanded expansion of the scope of government to include better medical care for individuals in need, whether through voluntary or government-sponsored insurance.

These demands or preferences for government intervention—sporadic at times and more insistent lately—have placed the authorities, especially federal, into a partnership with the growing medical industry. However, government's role has been carefully circumscribed to that of providing financial support for basic research, training health care personnel, subsidizing medical facilities, and providing medical services for special populations. The last has extended to such groups as those on public assistance (welfare), veterans, members of the armed forces and their dependents, coast guardsmen, merchant seamen, federal employees, the aged and disabled covered by the Social Security program, crippled children, prison inmates, Indians, Eskimos, those essentially under federal guardianship, and persons quarantined by the immigration service.

CONTEMPORARY NATIONAL HEALTH POLICY ISSUES. The major contemporary health issues have shifted to place a greater emphasis on extending medical care to individuals believed to be in need and on the organizational, financial, and logistical problems of improving the health care delivery system. These not only carry the vestiges of earlier issues and policies but also involve the constellation of status roles and the relative degrees of power and influence over public policy. The key decisions relate to whether the scope of government should be further expanded in providing health care and what specific role government—national, state, and local—should play. The advocates of an increased governmental role have articulated their demands since the turn of the century. A government-sponsored health insurance was proposed during the New Deal in conjunction with the Social Security Act in 1935. Failure to adopt the proposal at that time has kept it an issue ever since, and other means have been devised for government to support the essentially private health care system.

Many proposals are pending before the U.S. Congress at any one time, all of which contain two essential elements—who is covered and who finances the insurance. For example, the American Medical Association has put forth the Medicredit plan which would allow federal income tax deductions of insurance premiums for those financially able, while the poorest one third of the population would receive government vouchers entitling them to purchase health insurance.

In the 1970s there have been three essentially different approaches to a national health insurance program. One is a system of incentives to encourage individuals to *voluntarily* purchase private (commercial) or government-regulated (Blue Cross–Blue Shield) health insurance. The second approach, the Rockefeller plan, requires the *mandatory* purchase of private health insurance. It would have both employer and employees share the cost of premiums; the government would pay the premiums of the unemployed and the poor out of general revenues. The third approach, the Reuther plan, calls for *compulsory health insurance* as part of the Social Security system which supplants most of the coverage now offered by private insurers. Two thirds of the cost would be paid by employers and employees and one third would come from general tax revenues. The Reuther plan, while recognizing the need to reorganize the entire health delivery system, is not specific about what kind of new organization should be established to administer to the poor.

While the issue of determining the financial role of government remains essentially unresolved except in providing high levels of support for research and training and for direct medical care to the selected population groups, there are several other policy issues that require attention. These are the matters of who governs or controls the health care system and how it is to be organized. Although the

Private ——————→		(a continuum)	——————————→	Public
	Self-Regulation	Regulatory	Distributive	Redistributive
How organized?	cottage industry (physician's office)	public regulatory/ planning agencies	Public Health Service	community-based clinics
		Health Maintenance Organizations (HMO)		
Who governs?	provider associations	health planning administrators	public authorities	resident community control boards
		consumer protection advocates		
Who pays?	fee-for-service (individual patients)			government (general revenues)
	commercial insurance	Blue Cross/ Blue Shield	medicare	medicaid

FIG. 9.1. Policy map on alternatives for the American health care system.

latter appears to gain most attention, the former is implicit in most policy discussions. The question of organization may be easier to specify and less threatening to the vested interests to resolve. Or the focus on organization may be used to discuss indirectly the more controversial issue of who should govern the health care system. Or it may be that the pragmatic American approach encourages incremental changes in selected areas serving target populations without much consistency or comprehensiveness on the essential variables of the health care system itself.

A policy map (Fig. 9.1) attempts to provide an overall view of the variety of operational and proposed policies and programs to expand the scope of government in the American health care system. The key questions are: (1) How is the health care program organized? (2) Who governs it? (3) Who pays for it? In addition the health care policies and programs have been placed on a private-public continuum with self-regulation activities the most private, regulatory policies less private, and distributive policies involving the most extensive use of government with redistributive programs the least private.[1] The most complete private health care system would be self-regulatory by the providers—physicians, hospitals, etc.; the most public health care system would involve efforts by government to redistribute elements of health care from those more able to pay to those in need.

1. For a useful discussion on types of policies, see Lowie (27).

The provisions for health care system organization range from self-regulation of the private "cottage industry" of individual physicians serving individual patients in their offices to the redistributive development of community-based clinics providing direct patient care by a community-chosen professional staff, with some important variations in between. One such approach is to have the distributive public health service deliver medical care to selected target groups. Another is a partnership of providers and consumers in such organizations as Health Maintenance Organizations (HMOs). Still another is regulative through planning-agency activities over a given community or geographic jurisdiction.

The provisions that determine who shall govern range all the way from exclusive provider control to community control boards, with a number of combinations of health planning approaches which involve public and provider representatives as well as consumer protection advocates. The United States has gradually been modifying the exclusive control by providers through planning but has not moved the full distance to government control of the health care system. Nor has recent advocacy of community control of certain hospitals and clinics been widely accepted. Moreover, a sizable public health service to provide direct health care has not been established, even though a more prominent role has been given to government to provide payments for specific groups (such as those on public assistance programs). Furthermore, state and federal commissions have the authority to regulate the quality of health care through licensing personnel and setting safety standards for the production of food and pharmaceuticals. It should be pointed out that quality control through certification and licensing is only quasi-governmental; it is essentially self-regulation in that the nongovernmental professional interests are strongly asserted and protected, using the government's legal means for self-regulatory aspirations. In an attempt to bridge the gap between the production and the distribution of medical technology, priorities were briefly given to the Regional Medical Program (RMP), which focused on an effort to provide a more rational, coordinated, and equitable distribution of health care generated by both the private and public sectors. Aside from providers and government, we have introduced third-party and consumer interests to participate in the deliberative processes. These include primarily the insurers (both commercial and nonprofit Blue Cross/Blue Shield) as well as the Social Security agency of the federal government and consumer advocates. While these interests have been primarily concerned with the costs and distribution of health care that rely heavily on payments from the beneficiaries, they differ in their objectives: third-party insurance interests have been closely associated with, if not influenced by, the providers; consumer advocates are strenuously attempting to represent a wide range of consumer needs.

The provisions for the form of financial support of the health care system range from the traditional "fee-for-service" of the private practitioner to the government assumption of financial responsibility for providing direct medical care to all Americans through general revenues. Primary attention is being given to formulating some alternative health insurance with broader, more comprehensive coverage. At least the debate of the 1970s is to find some means acceptable to most of the influential or politically relevant forces which include not only providers; consumers; and insurers but also management and organized labor; hospitals; pharmaceutical and other suppliers; and representatives of federal, state, and local governments. The major form of medical payments today is through voluntarily subscribed-to third-party insurance programs. In addition both medicare and medicaid have recently become important programs. The former, a distribution approach, is part of the Social Security system and covers those over 65 who have participated in Social Security while gainfully employed. The latter, a redistribution approach, covers the indigent receiving public assistance who need medical care.[2]

While some analysts or interests prefer to concentrate on one dimension or another of this policy map, one cannot help but see the interrelationship between organization, control, and finance. Yet it appears most difficult to formulate policy in all three areas simultaneously so that a well-integrated, coherent, comprehensive, workable, feasible, and acceptable health care system can be created. Any penetrating assessment of the monumental efforts of post-World War II is disheartening to some:

> The empires, the medical-industrial complex, and the money which spawned them (federal government) are still big. But the "Health New Deal"—the mid-sixties gesture towards a more rational and egalitarian health system—lies in wreckage across the land. Medicare is a disappointment; Medicaid is a scandal. Regional Medical Programs and Comprehensive Health Planning are two new overlays of irrationality on top of the system they were to restructure (22).

A more generous view is offered by Ann Somers, who describes the paradoxical situation facing the health system—the major domestic issue of the 1970s—by contrasting the astonishing progress against constant allegations of inadequate medical care. The progress is

2. Somers refers to the two programs as, "medicare—popular and expensive; medicaid—expensive and unpopular" (41).

distinguished by miracles in the discovery and application of drugs, cures, and diagnostic and surgical techniques; imaginative health care systems—public and private; medical protection for 20 million elderly —at least against the most expensive medical care; several million additional indigent and medically indigent now receiving charity medical care; more rigorous quality controls and drug testing; and additional medical educational programs. The inadequacies are marked by unfilled health needs, exorbitant rises in costs, galloping inflation, and widespread discontent with most medical institutions. The present paradox as Somers sees it is the product of continuing progress with serious dislocations and need for adjustment created by a more rapid advance of knowledge in the fields of science and technology than in social and economic organizations.

IDENTIFICATION OF RURALITY. The central question that comes to mind is whether the paradoxical situation described above significantly affects rural America differently from other parts of the country to warrant special policy and program attention. For those who analyze the health system the answer is not clear. Some proceed with a very general analysis of the nation's health system wherein rural conditions are largely ignored. For example, a recent national commission made some 150 recommendations; not one focused on rural health directly, and in fact the commission chose to focus on "urban design and health" (31). Other commissions have had at least a separate panel or task force to explore the special health problems of rural inhabitants, but even these have emphasized that "a national program for rural health is not a thing apart, it is interwoven into every program to raise the health standards of the nation" (32, 33). On the other hand, some have concentrated with a sense of urgency exclusively on rural health, comparing its condition to those found in underdeveloped countries. In making such a comparison, however, Doherty introduces the poverty factor and the circularity of rurality, poverty, and health: "In rural areas, income is generally lower and medical services are generally poorer and less accessible than in urban areas and at the same time, the incidence of chronic illness, which limits work activity and thus reduces income, increases with both rurality and low family incomes" (14).

This linkage has received further corroboration by Roemer, who posits the reciprocal relationship between health and social well-being —poverty causes disease and disease causes poverty. He states that this relationship operates in all types of geographic and social settings, but "it probably applies to rural areas more than urban ones, because in such areas . . . the resources for preventing and treating sickness are less developed" (36). The Dohrenwends, in pursuing their study of social selection versus the social causation of psychological disorder, found little to suggest that rural versus urban settings account for the variations in rates of disorder (15, pp. 10–13).

No one has found (nor presumably expects) astonishing medical progress to have been created from rural medical sources. The development of medical science and technology has emanated from essentially a few select urban centers where our most advanced medical research and training take place. Similarly the decisions to evolve improved health care systems (especially for the elderly and the medically indigent) as well as the support of additional research and training programs and quality controls come primarily from the national and state policymaking centers. However, the other half of the paradox—constant allegations of inadequate medical care—consistently stems from the concern with *both* rural and urban health, especially for the poor and even more so for blacks. It is not clear, however, whether rural residents have greater unfilled health needs, are more adversely affected by rising medical costs and general inflation, or are more discontent with their medical care than other human services when compared to other Americans.

One of the major analytic problems facing any study of rural America, and more specifically rural health, is the lack of a data bank with common "rural" units of analysis. On population characteristics the Census Bureau reports variously in terms of rural (farm and non-farm) and urban; places of specific population sizes; and nonmetro-politan-metropolitan for other purposes. On governmental revenues, expenditures, and manpower it reports on selected sizes of counties, cities, and towns with no aggregate data on rural places. On a number of economic indicators, rural and urban America is all but lost in national aggregate reports. Reports on rural health indicators are also inconsistently applied when attempting to relate health status to available health resources and utilization patterns. Similarly the many special studies conducted by scholars and analysts range widely in the amount of useful knowledge generated about rural areas—small communities—as well as the outputs of a number of policymaking centers at the county, state, and regional levels.

Yet we expect policymakers—legislative and administrative—at the national, state, and local levels to focus special attention and formulate specific policy prescriptions concerning rural health. If we want these policy expectations fulfilled, we should attempt to specify contrasts in rural-urban health conditions and demonstrate the unusual health problems facing rural residents, dramatizing their unique adverse effects as well as indicating the selective difficulties involved in securing satisfactory resolutions. We should also prepare for the policymakers' perusal an inventory of the knowledge available and draw upon the insights gained from the many studies and operational experience in the organizational control and financial aspects of the health system and its changing form and procedures. This is not to say that this rather rational, more comprehensive approach of marshaling data and knowledge is the only or even the best way to persuade and influence policymakers. The open display of protest and electoral strength can and has alerted elected policymakers to the need for policies and programs and has stimulated them into action. The occurrence of an epidemic or a sense of crisis is, unfortunately, probably a more persuasive factor in gaining public or community action. In addition, the informal exercise of power and influence in decision-making centers is often the most reliable and effective means by which to gain action. But as policymaking becomes more complex and sophisticated, less monopolized by those in the private sector and more subject to public and consumer scrutiny, a rational knowledge base with carefully integrated strategies will be more likely to enhance its users.

A POLICY SCIENCE APPROACH. This chapter adopts the approach of the policy sciences in providing knowledge *of* and *in* the decision processes of the public and civic order.[3] The former implies systematic, empirical studies of how policies are formulated and put into effect; the latter anticipates the needs of policymakers and the mobilization of knowledge when and where it is useful. The three major attributes of the policy sciences are: (1) a problem orientation comprising the intellectual activities involved in clarifying goals, trends, conditions, projections, and alternatives in the specific policy area; (2) a contextual mapping of decisions as part of larger social processes; and (3) a synthesis of the diversity of research methods to combine dependable techniques of investigation with a degree of participatory activity in the policy processes. This perspective is concerned with the selection of data—variables and indicators—and generalized knowledge for use in policy that calls upon anticipating the future. What data and knowledge are recognized as pertinent to formulating a specific policy? What kind of reliable data and knowledge are available or missing; what can be collected, assembled, and presented when needed? What important sources of data and knowledge are overlooked due to the narrow cognitive maps of policymakers? How can these maps be modified? Can policymakers be supplied with critical estimates on what will likely happen if they make no

3. For a cogent, detailed discussion on policy sciences, see Lasswell (25).

changes in policy or what may happen as they modify or proceed with a particular policy option? Can policy analysts supply creative suggestions about policy alternatives that might further or achieve agreed-upon goals and objectives?

A cursory review of health policies suggests there is little or no rural health system or subsystem, public or private, at least as distinct from being part of the larger health system. On the other hand, there is a vital and recognizable rural influence over a host of policies that affect the farm as an economic unit of production. The failure of farm and rural leaders to formulate more comprehensive social policies as they pertain to health should be investigated as an important research focus. Here significant comparison might be made with other economic dominants who have appeared reluctant if not highly resistant to consider the social consequences of their economic activity. They have also been slow to choose or rely on an expanded scope of government to resolve problems that are created or left unattended by private activity except for selective economic issues such as farm subsidies. For health there simply may not be significant public support within rural settings to stimulate demands for social concerns nor the organizational capacity with few professionals; little information; and limited facilities, services, and resources—public and private—to generate sufficient effort to mobilize support for improving the rural health delivery system.

In applying a policy approach to rural health, the intent is not to be definitive but exploratory—discovering deficiencies and gaps in our data and knowledge base, concepts, measures and measurements and assessing policy outputs and impacts.

HEALTH CONDITIONS: STATUS, UTILIZATION, AND RE-SOURCES (SUR). Health conditions contain three interrelated dimensions. The first, health *status,* is a variety of epidemiological measures of ill health in its many forms and occurrences. The second is patient *utilization* rates of physician visits and hospitals' patient-days. The third, health *resources,* includes manpower, facilities, and services. All three are essential variables of a health care delivery system as they reflect the need, ability, and willingness to use available health resources.

Several recent studies provide information about the health indicators of the nation, which occasionally distinguish and contrast urban-rural health status, resources, and utilization. Lerner and Anderson maintain that the "differences in the general level of health and well-being between city and country have narrowed almost to the vanishing point" (26, p. 109). This contrasts sharply with conditions at the turn of the century when mortality was much higher in the cities than on farms. The following statements should guide policymakers in selecting priorities for programs and action.

Status.

1. Social and economic conditions exert maximum influence on variations in mortality during the post-neonatal period of infancy (second through twelfth months) (26, pp. 109–10).

a. Mortality from all causes in the eastern south central states was 94 percent higher than in the Atlantic urban and northern rural states.

b. For causes of death most readily amenable to control—the infective parasitic and digestive diseases—mortality in southern rural states was about twice as high as in the other two regions.

2. Variations in infant and maternal mortality are inversely associated with the variations in the use of modern medical facilities for births (26, p. 110).

a. Ninety-nine percent of all live births in the Atlantic urban and northern rural states were attended by a physician in a hospital, compared to 85.0 percent in southern rural states.

b. The least use of modern medical facilities occurred among nonwhite births in Mississippi where over half of all live births were attended by a midwife.

3. The major communicable diseases—influenza, pneumonia, and tuberculosis—take their largest toll not (as formerly) in the heavily congested Atlantic urban states but in the economically least well off southern rural states (26, p. 110).

4. Mortality from accidents (motor and nonmotor vehicles) was lowest in the most urbanized areas (26, p. 110).

5. Mortality during the middle and later years of life is higher in the Atlantic urban states (26, p. 110).

6. Mortality from the degenerative diseases—major cardiovascular-renal diseases and malignant neoplasms—is higher in the northern Atlantic urban states (26, p. 110).

7. The burden of chronic disorder is clearly higher in rural than in urban populations (26, p. 113).

Utilization.

1. People at each end of the urban-rural continuum (urban residents in the SMSA and rural farm residents) are generally less likely to have used a hospital day than other residents (3, p. 15).

2. Yet rural nonfarm residents have a higher rate of hospital admissions (3, p. 17).

3. The number of visits to physicians and dentists is appreciably lower for central city and rural residents (3, pp. 8, 24).

4. The rural poor, both white and black, have fewer physician contacts per 100 disability days than all others (3, p. 31).

Resources.

1. The health facilities (hospital beds) of the southern rural states lagged far behind the Atlantic urban states. (However, the hospital beds per $100 million personal income after taxes are approximately equal and lower for the most metropolitan and isolated rural counties.) (26, p. 244)

2. A similar disparity prevails for physicians and nurses, especially full-time specialists (26, p. 228).

Perhaps the best way to summarize the mosaic of findings on health conditions, including those not reported here, is to quote Anderson et al. in their recent study of trends and variations:

> In conclusion we suggest that while great improvements in health care for disadvantaged groups have occurred over the last ten to twenty years, these groups are still not equal to the remainder of the population in the utilization of health care personnel and facilities. In fact, in order to be "equal" they may well have to *exceed* higher income groups in their use of services to compensate for a greater rate of illness and disability (3).

POLICY CONTEXT OF HEALTH: SOCIAL, ECONOMIC, AND POLITICAL (SEP). Of the large number of possible contextual variables concerning the health of a given population, we have selected some social, economic, and political characteristics (SEP) that are most likely associated with the health status, utilization, and resources (SUR) available to meet the medical needs of the nation or a community. By social we mean the demography of counting heads and classifying the characteristics of people. By economic we mean the distribution of wealth and income and the allocations of public financial resources. The political aspect will review some of the decision-making arrangements, leadership, and citizen-participation patterns that shape the allocation of resources for the health care system. In order to determine whether there are any unusual features of rural America, we present some selective generalized statements contrasting urban-rural differences and pointing out some noticeable differences between farm and nonfarm characteristics. Further distinctions are noted about socioeconomic class or status and racial differences where data are available.

Social. Census reports reveal a number of important demographic characteristics about rural residents—farm and nonfarm. Each of the following statements pertains to ruralites in contrast to urbanites (46).

1. Median age is approximately similar except lower for blacks, especially farm blacks.

2. Greater dependent populations (those under 18 and those over 65), especially farm blacks.

3. Mean family size is approximately similar except higher for blacks, especially farm blacks.

4. Much higher fertility, especially blacks and more especially farm blacks.

5. Much higher "replacement index" (women 35–44), especially blacks and more especially farm blacks.

6. More stable families (as measured by the proportion of children 18 living with both parents and the proportion of male heads of households) except lower for blacks, especially farm blacks.

7. Less well educated, especially blacks.

8. More functional illiteracy, especially farm blacks.

9. Fewer college educated, especially farm blacks.

10. Slightly fewer males in the labor force, especially nonfarm blacks.

11. Fewer females in the labor force, especially farm whites.

12. Less unemployment, especially farm whites.

13. Lower median family and per capita income, especially farm blacks.

14. Much greater poverty (proportion of families with incomes below $3,000 per year), especially farm blacks.

15. Families receiving Social Security benefits are approximately similar except lower for blacks.

16. Families receiving public assistance are approximately similar except higher for blacks.

17. More disability, especially blacks.

18. Longer tenure (in same house all their lives), especially for rural blacks.

19. Much greater substandard housing conditions (lacking some or all plumbing), especially farm blacks.

20. Greater index of income concentration, especially farm blacks being at the lowest level.

These statements suggest that ruralites, declining in number, have lower incomes and greater poverty among them and a greater propen-

sity to reproduce their own population with much higher fertility
rates. While having more stable families, ruralites have a larger population dependent on fewer persons in the labor force who have somewhat more disability. They are also less well educated, and more live
in substandard housing. Blacks have the most adverse set of conditions, compounding their greater potential need for health care while
having less ability to secure medical attention.

Economic. Most of the above statements reveal greater disparities
when contrasting families having poverty-level incomes with those
in the general population. The following sets of statements focus
on the conditions of the rural poor in contrast to urban poor (46).

1. Larger families, especially among blacks.
2. More family stability except lower for blacks.
3. Fewer female heads of households in the labor force.
4. Much more substandard housing, especially among blacks.
5. Much greater reliance on public assistance, especially among
blacks.
6. More families on Social Security but fewer farm blacks.
7. Greater income deficit, especially among blacks (the largest
deficit is among rural nonfarm blacks who have incomes less than 125
percent of the poverty level).

Since medical care involves both private and public components,
it is useful to measure the assets earned and held by individuals as well
as the revenues made available through governmental policy. The
following statements attempt to contrast farm incomes and assets with
the general populations (47, p. 337).

1. Farmers own a higher proportion of the national wealth as
measured by tangible (physical and land) assets.
2. Farmers own and hold an insignificant proportion of the
intangible assets as measured by income and cash flow.
3. The personal income of farmers is significantly lower than
that of urbanites but not much below the rural nonfarm population,
even when taking into account the nonmonetary form of farm income.
4. The lowest income population segment is the rural black—
farm and nonfarm.
5. The farmer has disproportionately less disposable personal
income.
6. Farm production is disproportionately lower as measured by
its share of the gross national product (GNP).
7. The assessed valuation of farm acreage for local property tax
purposes is disproportionately lower.

Another aspect of the economic picture is public finance. Governmental revenue and expenditures data, meaningful reflections of public policy, are not available for rural areas as such. However, some rough approximations can be made by the population size of the county for which the data are available. That is, the small counties most likely are rural and may be essentially farm. Table 9.1 illustrates the revenues, expenditures (especially those for hospitals and health), and long-term indebtedness (45).

1. The smaller the county by population size, the lower the total revenues made available for public purposes except for the smallest (those less than 10,000).

2. The smaller the county by population size, the lower the local share of public revenues except for the smallest.

3. The reliance on intergovernmental transfers primarily from the states is relatively constant, except that it is much higher for the smallest and much lower for the second smallest.

4. Public expenditures for public education—a state and local responsibility—are relatively constant except for the smallest and largest counties which are equal and more than those of intermediate-size counties. (This may result from the prevalence of special districts to provide public education.)

5. Public expenditures for public welfare—a federal, state, and local responsibility—are relatively constant except in the largest counties (urban).

6. Public expenditures for hospitals are relatively constant except for the largest counties.

7. The smaller the county by population size, the lower the public expenditures except for the smallest county.

8. The smaller the county by population size, the smaller the long-term indebtedness.

Thus the average farmer, while not affluent in terms of earnings or in terms of holding his proportionate share of financial assets and cash flow, does own a disproportionately larger share of the tangible land assets. While the former places a limit on the ability of the farm population to purchase medical care in the private market, especially for the small marginal farmer, the latter places at the disposal of local government (if it chooses) a potentially larger base on which to tax for preferred public purposes. The fact that in practice this base has not provided greater public revenues except for the smallest counties (due to substantial intergovernmental transfers primarily from the states) suggests there may be considerable resistance to expanding the scope of government to include health-related functions as well as to increase the level of financial support to governmental programs al-

Table 9.1. Selected Items of Local Government Finances for County Areas by Population Size Groups, 1972

Size of County	National Percent Population	National Percent Revenue	Revenues per Capita (dollars)			Expenditures per Capita (dollars)				Debt per Capita (dollars)
			Total	Local	Inter-govern-mental	Education	Welfare	Hospital	Health	
Less than 10,000	2.5	2.0	414	252	162	221.07	13.80	24.09	3.08	242.32
10,000–24,999	8.2	5.9	373	209	164	207.53	15.44	25.31	2.69	278.36
25,000–49,999	9.8	7.1	377	215	163	207.97	16.41	24.11	2.97	317.27
50,000–99,999	11.4	8.8	401	236	165	221.34	19.22	24.01	4.13	330.44
100,000–249,999	15.4	13.4	453	280	172	242.98	28.56	18.21	5.63	428.18
250,000 or more	52.8	62.7	615	394	221	253.84	64.10	31.66	10.05	608.64
All counties			518	322	195	239.38	43.63	27.27	7.23	484.60

Source: U.S. Bureau of the Census (45).

ready approved—certainly something requiring further research and explanation.

Political. Since public policy is formulated, decided upon, and implemented through complex public-private collective decision-making structures and processes, it is necessary to examine a number of political considerations at various levels or extensions of the federal policymaking system. These include the formal-legal aspects of governmental processes relating to the delegations and exercise of authority as well as more informal processes relating to distribution and use of power and influence by nongovernmental leaders and other relevant segments of the population. It is critical to examine the working relationship between sets of participants in policymaking processes at local (community and county), state, regional, and national levels. Following are statements on citizen participation and representation in policymaking:

1. The major form of participating in the political arena for most Americans is voting and exposing oneself as a spectator to political stimuli.

    a. There appears to be little difference between metropolitan and nonmetropolitan rates of voter turnout.

    b. The major variation is accounted for by socioeconomic class status and racial background—fewer lower-income persons and blacks vote (47, p. 374).

2. The characteristics of farmer voting behavior are highly variable in presidential elections (7).

    a. The farm vote has an irregular turnout based on economic sensitivity issues.

    b. The farm vote shifts in partisan preferences depending on what position each party takes on the sensitive economic issues.

3. Voters in less populated areas (counties under 25,000) have significantly greater relative weight in the selection of representatives in state legislatures (12).

4. The nonmetropolitan voters are overrepresented in the U.S. Congress both in the Senate and House of Representatives (11).

COMMUNITY LEVEL. There are many community studies; unfortunately they have been undertaken with such widely varying concepts, measures, and methods that their findings provide little in common on which to base public policy. However, two recent developments have assisted in providing more generalized insights about American communities, their leadership patterns, and policy outputs.

One is the effort to conduct secondary analysis retrospectively on the many case studies carried on by sociologists and political scientists (19). The other is the growing number of comparative studies (1) and quantitative analyses on aggregate data (9) that have attempted to seek out warrantable assertions about community policymaking.

1. Population size and growth rates correlate with political attributes.

a. Very large cities are more frequently pluralistic in their leadership patterns. These same pluralistic systems have moderate, low, or negative growth rates; leadership is associated with high growth rates (1, pp. 38–39).

b. The less the city resembles a metropolitan center, the more it tends to have a concentrated power structure (19, p. 50).

2. The smaller the population of the community, the lower the participation of elected authorities in carrying out political functions; informal leaders (nongovernmental) are relatively more important in rural areas (19, pp. 39–40).

3. The smaller the population of the community, the less overt the conflict. Levels of conflict tend to be higher for industrial communities rather than residential suburbs and for rural farm rather than rural trade areas (19, p. 40).

4. The more centralized the decision-making structure (consensual elite), the more predictable the outputs and the more the outputs reflect the values and interests of the dominant sector of the system (9).

5. The more centralized the decision-making:

a. the higher the level of policy outputs over fragile decisions (newness of issues such as fluoridation)

b. the lower the level of outputs over less fragile decisions (expansion of existing programs such as reflected in general budget expenditures and established programs).

COUNTY LEVEL. The county and township are the most frequently used governmental units in rural America; yet they are among the least studied. There has been little contextual analysis of policymaking in county government. In an effort to formulate a more meaningful research agenda, Bollen has formulated an index of political vitality as a framework for the comparative study of county government (6). He discusses five components of data, knowledge, and research needs.

Resource utilization is the measure of how a county uses its capacity to generate revenue for public purposes. This capacity is measured by the taxes raised *(willingness)* from its economic base *(ability)*; the ratio between the two is the fiscal *effort*. Most counties rely on the property tax which has not kept pace with increasing populations, price levels, and costs of running more and more sophisticated governments. In addition, underassessment is a major problem and is subject to extensive exemptions from other governmental units and charitable and nonprofit institutions.

Volume of intergovernmental linkage involves the relationship with other governments vertically (state and national) and horizontally (other counties, towns, cities, and special districts). The county has become in many instances—especially in health—a major administrative mechanism for state programs. There is a growing number of national assistance programs involving county government. "The great increase in county governmental activity in the last generation has resulted directly from the expansion of state and state-federal programs that must be administered locally" (6, p. 50). Interlocal cooperation has been operationalized by (1) parallel action, (2) a joint agency performance, (3) a single agency performance for other agencies, (4) the service contract, and (5) the conference for discussions.

Changes in organization and processes have sought simultaneously greater unified activity, stronger means of productivity, and more autonomy of organization and management. These include the establishment of an executive officer, reduction in the number of elected officials, expansion of the scope of government, a merit system, and the development of a planning capability. Some analysts have begun to advocate that the county become the basic building block of regional development.

Adequacy of public accountability involves an equitable apportionment of the representative seats on the county governing body. Many counties have been undergoing reapportionment to correct maldistributions of representativeness. Bollen complains that counties have generated very little information about their operations, thereby making it difficult for citizens to develop a major interest in activities that are "tucked away in the form of legal notices in an obscure section of the newspapers—when they do appear at all" (6, p. 62).

Extent of voting and competition in elections includes ascertaining both the proportion of potential voters actually voting and the degree of competition among candidates for elective office. Martin challanges our idealized notions of rural democracy by describing the conditions of government in rural America as less hospitable to the development of a favorable climate of democracy than those of other environments. "Rural government has little magic to stir people's minds. It is too picayune, narrow in outlook, limited in horizon, and self-centered in interest to enlist the support of the voters" (29).

STATE LEVEL. There have been several important systematic studies
attempting to account for state legislature policy outcomes as
measured by the budget allocations between functional categories
of public finance. These studies have generally used a systems approach to formulate a model for the analysis of policy outcomes based
on aggregate data. Inputs include such socioeconomic development
variables as urbanization, industrialization, income, and education and
certain selected characteristics of political systems such as previous
budget expenditures, division of the two-party vote, level of interparty
competition, level of voter participation, degree of malapportionment
of the legislature, legislative professionalism, and innovations. They
have generally found:

1. Socioeconomic variables—levels of urbanization, industrialization, income, and education—appear to be more influential in shap-
ing policy outcomes on the level of public expenditures than political
system characteristics (16).
2. States with loose multifactional systems tend to pursue more
conservative policies. In states with competition between two cohesive
and enduring factions more liberal policies are adopted (13).
3. Increasing competitiveness will produce increased social welfare expenditures (10).
4. Interparty competition promotes the distribution of benefits
to lower income groups (18).
5. Economic development is important in determining measures
of private health care (physicians per population and hospital insurance) but is not related to variations among states in public hospital
facilities or death rates (16).
6. In the allocation of the burdens and benefits of state revenue
and expenditures across income classes, the political system variables
were considerably more powerful than socioeconomic variables (18).
The political variables were measured by mass political behavior (participation, Democratic party vote, interparty competition, and legislative inducement to participate); governmental institutions (legislative
apportionment, legislative party cohesion, gubernatorial powers, and
tenure); and elite behavior (interest group strength, percentage of
state employees under civil service coverage, Grumm's index of legislative professionalism, and Walker's innovation index (21, 48).

REGIONAL LEVEL. Regionalism in America is a relatively recent development. A growing interest has recently been generated on the
regionalization of smaller units within metropolitan areas and
the combination of county units within state and regional administrative units between a number of states. Some suggestive relevant findings are:

1. There are distinct regional variations in the expenditures of American states. In general, western states are high spenders and northern and eastern states are low spenders. Southern states are not distinctive in expenditures per capita but score high in expenditures per $1,000 of personal income (39, pp. 158–60).

2. Regional spending peculiarities are consistent in reflecting the influence of political-economic constraints (previous expenditures, tax effort, and federal aid) and of state-local centralization on expenditures (39, p. 160).

NATIONAL LEVEL. Surprisingly few comprehensive systematic studies have been undertaken on the policy context of health from a national perspective. There have been innumerable commission reports and White House conferences on the state of American health, studies on local community decision-making in regard to health, and studies on specific policies or programs and how they were decided upon. Perhaps this paucity of systematic studies on the public policy of health is because "to most experts, few people are less qualified than politicians in technical fields, and few considerations are more irrelevant (if not downright hostile) to technical decisions than are political considerations" (23). To modify this situation, Swanson has proposed a paradigm on the politics of health with seven factors: (1) system output, (2) levels of stress, (3) system inputs, (4) power structures, (5) political ideologies, (6) political focus, and (7) system change processes (44). Further, Marmor has used his case study of medicare to suggest the need for: (1) an underlying framework of analysis—rational acts, organization process, and bureaucratic politics models; (2) delineating the characteristics of various social policies and their beneficiaries, financing, administrative structure, source of entitlement, and the extent of departure with past practice; and (3) establishing the differences between legislative and administrative politics (28).

Studies of the U.S. Congress have shown the following relationships between political party and farm and rural interests:

1. Postwar Democratic and Republican congressmen differed in precisely the same manner in their approaches to all sets of domestic issues (farm, city, labor, and western). However, Democrats from "interested" districts (i.e., congressmen from farm districts have interests in farm issues) maintained higher cohesion than Democrats from "indifferent" districts, and the reverse was true for Republicans. "Interested Democrats" held higher party loyalty than "interested Republicans." Democratic leaders persistently championed their "interested" members (30, p. 149).

2. The Democrats were a party of "inclusive compromise" (separate programs do not conflict); the Republicans were a party of

"exclusive compromise" (separate programs do conflict) (30, pp. 150, 155).

3. The key to the success of the farm bloc lay in its ability to achieve a degree of bipartisan harmony among Republican and Democratic farm congressmen and then to enlist the aid of the Democratic party and its leadership in supplying the margin of victory for its programs (30, p. 29).

STRATEGY FOR EXPLORING LINKAGE OF SUR AND SEP.

The above discussion is a preliminary and incomplete survey of data and knowledge, but it is sufficient to guide efforts to synthesize knowledge and action concerning rural health. The socioeconomic and political (SEP) dimensions seem to provide significant effects on health status, utilization, and resources (SUR) and seem to play a critical part in the care of the poor and those with catastrophic illnesses. The relationship for research on linkages betwen health conditions and policy context might be expressed:

$$PO_H = f[(SUR)\ (SEP)] + e$$

where: PO_H = *policy output of health* concerning facilities, services, manpower, public finance, etc.

  SUR = *the health status, utilization, and resources* factors defined above with specific variables

  SEP = *the social, economic, and political* factors defined above with specific variables

  e = residual factors

To explore briefly this guiding relationship, we should locate the decision-making structures in their respective socioeconomic status systems. Thus a simple egalitarian social structure encourages participation of a consensual mass, which is historically associated with the small community where a large proportion of the population takes part in community decision-making (most often found in parts of New England). The well-defined hierarchical social system seems to experience monolithic or consensual elite decision-making with a few leaders at the top, such as we now find in small towns where inner cliques control or dominate community affairs. A complex hierarchical social system is generally believed to have a polylithic or competitive elite political system (big cities) where no single "power elite" can completely dominate all issue areas but where each set of leaders wields influence within a certain well-defined, firmly established institutional structure (such as health, education, or housing). Finally, the more complex egalitarian system is believed to generate a pluralistic or competitive mass political system where many leaders participate and bargain with each other in one or more separate influence hierarchies over distinct issue areas.

If we attempt to locate target populations in need of health care, the health (SUR) must be dealt with within the policy context (SEP). In some settings to meet the health needs of specific population segments leads to disagreements and the struggle for power over who should formulate health policy. For example, we should expect lower health status, utilization, and available medical resources among the lower portions of the social structure, which are in a position of least influence over public policy in the hierarchical system. This is particularly true among blacks, especially rural blacks. We should expect little improvement in health care for the lower-income families, unless those at the top decide to favor some kind of redistribution policies. In the simple hierarchical system (most probable in rural America), especially with provider control of health care, we should expect a great resistance to changing the pattern of services. This resistance would be even more intense if the policies were to improve the health conditions for blacks at the expense of whites in a racially polarized setting. Top leaders' concern for the low-income families is somewhat more likely or easier to induce in the competitive power structure, where access to influence in a specialized sector such as health is somewhat more open and responsive to meeting human needs. Thus the probability is greater for urban blacks to have some of their welfare—if not status—demands met, especially if external aid from the federal government is decisive. The well-organized interest groups appear to be most successful in competitive systems; the small egalitarian communities seemingly prefer caretaker minimal public and private service systems. Critically important throughout these considerations are the prevailing ideologies of leaders and citizens and their roles in different political systems.[4]

A speculative ordering of priority target populations in need of improved health care might flow from poor blacks in the greatest need to upper-class whites in the least need. Yet empirical investigations might reveal that, in a very discriminatory community, blacks throughout every stratum of their subcommunity will have greater unmet medical care needs than whites or that blacks in a racially mixed community have somewhat fewer needs than those in overwhelmingly black or white communities.

Further speculation is offered here in the paradigm linking health

4. For an exploration of the differing perspectives and roles on citizen participation, see Swanson (43).

Table 9.2.   Paradigm Linking SUR and SEP

Health Conditions	Policy Context		
	Social	Economic	Political
Status	Social disparities affecting social and economic status position in stratified systems affecting access to health care.	Wealth and income differentials with reciprocal effect: income affects health; health affects income.	Individualized sense of efficacy in sets of power struggles.
Utilization	Differential beliefs and attitudes toward self and health care providers.	Cost/benefit for financing health care as to efficiency and effectiveness.	Who controls or influences how much, and who is to be served by health care delivery system?
Resources	Cultural norms to convert private resources toward communal health needs.	Marketplace orientation (supply and demand) without measure of socio-medical well-being.	Ideological predisposition of leaders and citizens to use government to distribute and redistribute health care.

conditions (SUR) and policy contextual factors (SEP) (Table 9.2). Aside from the normal physiological or medical explanations of health status, the data suggest the social disparities affecting the socioeconomic status of a person are important factors in explaining access to medical care. Highly correlated are the wealth and income differentials with their reciprocal effects: low income affects health, and poor health affects the income potential of persons found in most communities. Both are involved in the theory of social selection versus social causation offered by Dunham and pursued by the Dohrenwends (15, pp. 125–26).

Less researched and perhaps more difficult to explore is the individual's sense of efficacy as he engages in the many power struggles within the family, at school, on the job, and in the community (37). Certainly there are associations of higher socioeconomic status with higher political status and sense of efficacy. Socially determined beliefs and attitudes toward oneself and the use of health care are highly variable and need much more research attention. Poor urban blacks, for example, hold physicians in high esteem, attributing to them great healing powers.

While such data necessarily generated through attitudinal surveys may be somewhat costly, it is a relatively simple research item. More difficult, because of the mobile nature of the consumers, is investigation of costs/benefits as to both efficiency and effectiveness of financing health care.[5] Although there have been some studies on the leader-

5. For an effort to measure differentials in use of health care, see Bashshur, Shannon, and Metzner (4; 5).

Table 9.3. Paradigm on Ruralities and Probable Preferences to Improve the Care System

| Ruralities | Policy Map Considerations | | |
	How organized?	Who should govern?	Who should pay?
Farm			
Corporate	cottage industry	provider	fee-for-service
Family	extends cottage industry	provider	third-party payments
Tenant	Public Health Service or externally imposed criteria	government control	general tax revenues
Nonfarm			
Small Town	extended hospitals/ clinics	provider	AMA medi-credit
Country Dwellers	HMO	consumer protection	AMA medi-credit
Marginal Income	Public Health Service	government control	general tax revenues

ship patterns in community health (34), little has been done to investigate under what conditions influentials decide to provide extensive and intensive health care to meet human need regardless of social status. Similarly, little research has been conducted on cultural and social norms that attempt to convert private resources toward communal health programs. Some attention has been given to the marketplace of health as the provider supplies and the consumer demands; some attention should also be given to the consequences of the economic marketplace and industrial activity on sociomedical well-being. The most ignored aspect of this paradigm is the ideological predisposition of leaders and citizens alike to use government to distribute and redistribute health care. As a pragmatic nation we have drifted into a mixed public-private health care system without fully understanding where we are going, why, and with what short- and/or long-range consequences.[6]

The complexity of the paradigm (Table 9.2) grows as one applies it to the policy alternatives of improving the health care for rural Americans. Here the SEP context suggests that there are subsets of ruralites with varying positions in the socioeconomic and political structure with different needs and differential ability to fulfill them. If we join these contextual considerations to the policy map on how the health delivery system should be organized, who should govern it, and who should pay, we develop the suggested paradigm in Table 9.3. Note the six major types of ruralites: farm—corporate, family, and

6. For some thoughts on intuitive and a counterintuitive processes in public policy, see Forrester (17).

tenant farmers—and nonfarm—small-town residents, country dwellers, and those living on marginal incomes.

Speculatively, both corporate and family farmers would seem to prefer the cottage industry organized health delivery system, provider controlled. However, the family farmer may wish to have the extended facilities and services to provide improved care. The corporate farmer, without an organized labor force, supports fee-for-service payments; the family farmer seeks some form of third-party insurance payments—preferably some private, nonprofit, or cooperative instrument. The tenant farmer, on the other hand, may prefer some form of direct government service. He more than likely needs the Public Health Service essentially as an external authority that can impose a set of criteria that specify under what circumstances patients are eligible for medical care. Tenant farmers, however, require considerable financial support from general tax revenues. The nonfarm ruralites who reside in small towns usually seek extended hospital and clinic facilities and services and accept a provider-controlled health system. They might favor the Medicredit tax system suggested by the AMA. The country dweller who does not work the land is somewhat more interested in consumer protection over rising costs and the need for quality control over health care. If given an opportunity he might join a Health Maintenance Organization (HMO) with Medicredit as a form of payment. Those ruralites with a marginal income might best seek an extended Public Health Service with government control and financed through general tax revenues.

Speculation is useful only up to a point; what is required is substantial policy-oriented research which explicates the priority health conditions (SUR) and the policy contextual factors (SEP): not only evaluative research (50) to assess the effectiveness of policy outputs but also carefully selected interventions of planned change (40) to learn how the policymaking system operates and thus gain the insights necessary to improve the health care system for those most in need.[7]

CONCLUSIONS. This cursory diagnosis has perhaps raised more questions than it has answered. Is there a rural health system? If there is, it is not highly visible except either for the health-related activities of agencies with other primary missions or as represented by the small-town rural doctor. Most evidence suggests there is no rural health system—public or private—distinct from the larger comprehen-

7. The confrontation over community control to share in power by urban blacks is examined in Swanson (42).

sive health care system of our society. This differs considerably from the visible, recognizable rural influence in legislative-administrative policymaking at all levels of government. Perhaps the so-called farm bloc has a narrowly defined interest in the farm as an economic unit of production.

Why is there a viable rural influence in policymaking regarding the farm as an economic unit which at the same time lacks the focus on health policy when rural health needs are as great as, if not greater than, these of the general population? One answer lies in the reluctance of producer-oriented interests to see themselves as consumers or to share the aspirations of other consumers. Instead they concentrate on those policy alternatives that will most directly enhance their production, resist considering the broader social cost of economic activity, and certainly wish to limit the expansion of the scope of government. Secondly, the farm bloc influence may be on the wane with legislative reapportionment. Thirdly, the relatively homogenous or farmer-dominated rural social setting does not nurture ideological diversity, which is often the mainspring of rising expectations and stimulates new demands for improved health care; nor does it tolerate dissent or strident efforts to expand the scope of government. Finally, in rural America there are few health professionals and little in the way of an organized health constituency that can provide information on health needs and mobilize demands for expanded health care.

If there should be a rural health subsystem separate from a general health care system, five intellectual tasks are essential for its design: (1) What should be its goals? (2) What sets of health conditions (SUR) is it trying to improve and what policy contextual associative factors (SEP) need to be considered? (3) What are the *trends* in both the sets of health problems and contextual factors? (4) What *projections* seem most likely to occur, given certain policy contingencies? (5) What *alternative* courses of policy and action are most acceptable and feasible? If there should be no rural health subsystem, is it reasonable to attach the concerns for rural health to the ongoing general health care system? Can the general health care system be persuaded or mandated, to turn its attention and divert some of its talent and resources to the needs of rural Americans? If this cannot be done, or if it is unreasonable to attach rural health needs to the general health system, then we should become concerned with the short- and long-range social costs emanating from the present drifting policies and programs directed toward rural health care.

CHAPTER TEN

PATHWAYS OF RURAL PEOPLE TO HEALTH SERVICES

EDWARD W. HASSINGER

THE PROBLEM of access to health services involves more than convenient location of facilities. It represents a complex interplay among beliefs, social organization, and patterns of behavior of health consumers as they relate to a complex health care system. To understand rural health consumer behavior, we need to consider the characteristics of rural society, the health care system, and the patterned behavior of people in seeking health care.

AMERICAN RURAL SOCIETY

Characteristics. About a century ago American society began to emerge as an industrial urbanized society. Today industrialization and its associated developments are the hallmark of the society, and they have wrought profound changes not only for the cities but also for the countryside. A consequence for rural society is to bring it closer to the institutions of mass industrial society. Often decisions are made and resources controlled outside of rural people and communities (14, 70).

But as we examine its characteristics, we see that rural society does not approach homogeneity. The rural segment of this vast nation is differentiated by geographical section, religious and ethnic composition of its population, economic base, and other socioeconomic divisions.

EDWARD W. HASSINGER is Professor of Rural Sociology and Community Health and Medical Practice, University of Missouri.

The author acknowledges John C. Belcher, Robert L. McNamara, Charles Carlton, Richard Hessler, and Daryl Hobbs for helpful ideas that have been incorporated into this chapter.

OCCUPATION. Agriculture is no longer the leading industry in rural
    areas. However, it remains central to rural social organization,
    and changes in agriculture in many ways exemplify the develop-
ments in the entire rural sector of American society. Agriculture has
changed from a way of life to a commercial enterprise; farms have
changed from relatively self-sufficient units to units of high capitaliza-
tion, specialization, and technological sophistication. In the process
the egalitarian ideology of frontier society has been seriously eroded.
A principal distinction can be made between those who have successfully made a transition to commercial agriculture and those who have
been unwilling or unable to do so and have been left in the economic
backwater (73). While the "culture heroes" of agriculture are large-
scale operators, the economic and managerial requirements of large-
scale farming has literally driven many from the land, encouraged the
accommodation of part-time farming, retarded the entrance of young
men into farming through traditional channels, and widened the socioeconomic differences among agricultural producers. Among the
most vulnerable to displacement have been small-scale operators, especially among tenants. Some of these poorer groups such as black
sharecroppers have become farm laborers, and many are currently in
the migrant labor streams.

The nonfarm component is by far the largest part of the rural
population. If the farm population appears diverse, the rural nonfarm population is even more so. It is a residual residential category
that includes open-country residents not living on farms, village populations of varying size up to 2,500, and urban fringe residents who
do not meet the density criteria that would otherwise place them in
the urban population. The great majority of rural nonfarm residents
find employment in commerce and industry and relatively few in agriculture either as farm operators or farm laborers (32).

AGE DISTRIBUTION. No factor is more consistently related to indices of
    health and use of health services than age of the population. It
    is also a major consideration in health policy. The median age
of the urban, rural nonfarm, and rural farm segments of the population are quite similar. However, within the rural population are differences of substantial proportion.

In the first place, the median age of the rural nonfarm population does not fairly represent the age characteristics of one of its components—the rural villages. Many of these villages are notable for
their high proportion of elderly people and have been characterized
as being "old folks' homes" (23).

In addition, when one looks at the counties of unusually high
median age on the one hand and unusually low median age on the

other, it turns out that both situations are found almost exclusively among nonmetropolitan counties (8, p. 417). The counties of high median age are concentrated in the Midwest. The age pattern results from migration of young people from the area together with a relatively low fertility level. The death rate in many of these counties now exceeds the birth rate.

Counties of low median age are characterized by high fertility and tend to be the location of sizable cultural, ethnic, or racial groups. In the South, aside from the Appalachian area, the young age of the population is largely explained by the high fertility of the black population. In the West three different cultural groups are apparent in the low median age counties—the Spanish-Americans along the Rio Grande, the Indians in the Four Corners area, and the Mormons of Utah and Idaho. With the exception of the Mormon area, the counties with low average age tend to represent some of the most severely deprived economic areas in the country (8, pp. 417–19).

INCOME. Income is an index of level of living, components of which are housing, nutrition, and water supply. These factors in turn are related to health and illness. Income is also associated with ability to obtain medical services. These concomitants of income are reflected in findings of the National Health Survey that people with lower incomes have more illness and obtain fewer health services (53).

There are differentials in rural and urban income levels to the disadvantage of the rural population, especially the rural farm population. In 1970 the median family income in metropolitan areas was $11,203; for nonfarm families in nonmetropolitan areas, $8,881; and for farm families in nonmetropolitan areas, $6,819 (72).

It is common to discount rural poverty to some extent because of supposed lower costs of living and the greater possibility of "in kind" or noncommercial exchange in rural settings. However, there is some question as to whether any adjustment is called for. Rural people are for the most part dependent on monetary exchange in obtaining the goods and services they use, and the costs of some services are increased—not decreased by distance from them. The President's Commission on Rural Poverty found that poverty in rural areas was indeed real and in many cases cruel (52).

The poor in rural areas are similar categorically in many ways to the poor in urban areas. The rural-to-urban migration has been in part a transference of the rural poor to the status of urban poor. Thus the rural black or Spanish-American or Indian, the elderly, the poorly educated, and those in families headed by females are more likely than average to be below the poverty level (71). The effect of rurality is in general to accentuate the problem.

Although poverty is found in all rural areas of the country, the incidence in some is exceptionally high. The South—including the Appalachians, the Ozarks, the eastern coastal plains, the Black Belt of the Old South, and the Mexican-American concentrations in the Southwest—comprises an area of high economic deprivation among rural people. Other areas notable for high poverty concentration are the Four Corners of Arizona, Colorado, New Mexico, and Utah; the cutover of northern Minnesota, Wisconsin, and Michigan; and portions of the New England states (52, pp. 3–4). The economic problems of these areas are long standing and contribute to "poverty as a way of life."

SPATIAL ISOLATION. The degree of spatial isolation of the population classified as rural by the census varies greatly. Much of the rural population lives in or near Standard Metropolitan Statistical Areas (SMSAs) (3). East of a line through eastern North and South Dakota and western Oklahoma and Texas practically no one is more than 100 miles from an SMSA. Between there and the West Coast states are vast areas outside the 100-mile range of a metropolitan area. Proximity to a metropolitan area in itself, however, does not eliminate isolation. Some metropolitan counties have areas quite remote from the principal center of the SMSA. An example is the Duluth, Minnesota, metropolitan area in which the city is located at one edge of a large county that extends to the Canadian border and contains populations quite isolated spatially and socially from the center. Almost the entire Appalachian area is within 100 miles of a metropolitan area but contains some of the more socially isolated sections of the country.

An example of temporal isolation within relatively close distance of a metropolitan center is the problem encountered in transporting youth from the hinterland of Charleston, West Virginia, to that city for a work training program. All the youth in the program were within a 45-mile radius of Charleston. Many of them lived in small communities of 20–50 families located up the "hollows." A typical trip to one of these communities 45 miles from Charleston was 35 miles by highway, then on to a gravel road for another 5 miles, followed by 3 miles along a dirt road. The last family in the community was reached by walking 2 miles up the side of a hill. On the other side of that hill about 3 miles away is another settlement, but to reach it by auto one has to retrace the route back to the main highway and travel over gravel and dirt roads—a distance of 23 miles (49).

SUBCULTURES. The diversity of rural society extends to identifiable cultural groups. These may be relatively small groups such as the Amish, whose survival techniques in a secular society are of interest; or they may represent substantial numbers of people of rural society such as blacks in the South, Indians concentrated in the arid West, Mexican-Americans of the Southwest, and Anglos of Appalachia. Each of these groups has subculture status within rural society. Characteristic of all of them are the impingements of the larger society to which they have responded in different ways. The migration of southern rural blacks urbanward and northward has transformed the residential-occupational base of that population; similar movement has altered the social base of the Mexican-American population. On the other hand, the institution of the reservation has retarded the urbanization of the American Indian (9, 48, 57).

VALUES AND NORMS. Values and norms of behavior cannot be separated from group organization and behavior. We have already observed that rural society is characteristically diverse in occupation, age structure, income, degree of physical isolation, and ethnic identity. Therefore, we would expect to find normative diversity.

However, a common feature of rural social organization that might produce common normative positions is the small size of rural groups and organizations. Small size contributes to more primary or gemeinschaftlike relationships as interpreted by Loomis and Beegle (44). Thus Weller found that rural mountaineers manifested a high degree of *person-orientation* in contrast to the more characteristically urban *object-orientation* (74). Stephenson, however, on the basis of a community study in the same general area, found that both orientations were apparent. "What I have found in Shiloh, and suspect holds for similar areas elsewhere, is that certain parts of the community participate in this (traditional) subculture more than do others and that in fact the traditional way is at many points engaged in a competitive struggle with a newer and quite different life style" (66). Stephenson interprets this as evidence of changes in the values of rural people.

Bennett found particularism (along with individualism and egalitarianism) to be a characteristic value of North American agrarian society in a study of the Northern Plains that extend from the Dakotas and Montana into Canada (11). Particularism, a concept similar to person-orientation, refers to the tendency of individuals to conduct private arrangements with each other and to act on the basis of unique situations rather than universal rules.

There is some evidence of overall rural and urban value differences. Glenn and Alston examined beliefs and values of people on the basis of national polls taken from 1953 to 1965 (24). They examined the stereotype that rural people (relative to urban people) are more conservative, religious, puritanical, work-oriented, ascetic, ethno-

centric, isolationist, intolerant of heterodox ideas and values, preju-
dicial, uninformed, authoritarian, and family centered. With some
qualifications they found the stereotype to be "surprisingly accurate,"
with major exceptions in conservatism and authoritarianism (24, pp.
394–95). However, the differences were quite low between rural and
urban respondents on many of the items; they probably represent variation rather than disjunctures of beliefs and values. Furthermore,
the responses showed a lack of value consensus among rural respondents.

The general distinctiveness of rural and urban beliefs and values
are likely to be overstated rather than understated. A danger is that
the rather weak rural-urban value positions will be maximized as
stereotypes and that health care policy will be developed on the basis
of such creations. While it is often useful or even necessary to let
stereotypes represent reality, these particular ones may serve to mask
intrarural differences and to suggest that rural and urban values and
beliefs are worlds apart. Another effect of the judgment of strong
rural-urban value differences is to divert attention from problems of
organization in the delivery of health services.

Structure of Communities. Institutional organization in nonmetropolitan areas tends to be based on trade center communities. In
much of the country, trade centers are located at close and fairly
regular intervals from each other. In the more sparsely settled western
plains and mountain states, the distance between centers becomes
greater. Traditionally trade centers have functioned as places of professional and commercial services for hinterland populations which
were quite well defined. Rural communities tended to be small in
area and population because of the transportation technology and
the general scale of organization when they were established. At the
same time they aspired to maintain a full range of services which were
relatively unspecialized. In this sense trade centers were to a large
degree alike; the characteristic institutions usually were the small
school of unspecialized curriculum, the general store, the general
medical practitioner, citizen government, and farmer-preachers.

On the basis of this mode or organization, interaction among
people in town-country communities tended to be face-to-face and informal. Incumbents of public offices and boards were generally selected on the basis of personal characteristics and family background
rather than on the basis of issues or political ideologies. Occupants
of leadership positions represented the "backbone" consensus of community norms of behavior. Professionals—including county agents,
school teachers, and doctors—were expected to conform to the norms
of the community.

COMMUNITY POVERTY. The rural heritage with its limited scale and
    mode of organization and its norms of behavior has contributed
    to what Ford calls "community poverty," which is manifest
among other ways "in the inadequate functioning of local systems of
social institutions such as government, school systems, health and
medical services, and so on" (18, p. 155).

> More firmly than the rest of the society [rural Americans] clung to the
> fundamental belief that public institutions could and should be run by
> ordinary citizens with a minimum of special technical qualifications and
> often as a part-time adjunct to their main occupation. Together with
> this went the belief that public institutions should perform only those
> functions that individuals and families could not perform by them-
> selves (18, p. 168).

The consequences of institutional poverty on program development is suggested by Levitan's assessment of the problems of implementing OEO programs in rural areas. "A major problem in funding
rural projects has been the lack of delegate agencies that are capable
of administering OEO's programs" (42). In testimony before the
President's Commission on Rural Poverty, a witness cited the difficulty of developing organizations to help the poor in rural areas,
which he attributes in part to opposition by local power holders (51).
Zeller and Miller come to a similar conclusion in their analysis of
problems facing community action in the Appalachian area (76).

CHANGES. Stability features are built into existing community organi-
    zation. The trade centers in nonmetropolitan regions represent
    the life work as well as the life ways of generations of families.
Centers were not built overnight, nor do they die quickly. Business-
men who have invested capital and years in a small-town enterprise
may have few, if any, alternatives except to remain because of losses
that would be incurred in selling the business in a declining community and the absence of other employment opportunities for middle-
aged proprietors. More than one local businessman has responded to
economic reversals by cutting overhead (symbolically turning out the
lights in the front of the store) and sticking it out. Similarly a physician who established a practice in a small town may find it difficult
to move after a few years because of community obligations and potential financial losses incurred in transferring the practice. The
middle-aged and older doctor, like the businessman, is not likely to
find mobility an easy matter.
    Important changes have taken and are taking place with regard
to the relationship of people to service centers and with service centers to each other. This is partly a result of changes in transportation,

technology, scale of organization, and rising aspirations of rural residents. The most obvious changes have involved adjustments to time-distance dimensions. A. H. Anderson points out that one-half hour's travel time was about 3 miles in 1915, but in 1961 he conservatively estimated it to be 15 miles. A 3-mile radius represents 36 square miles, a 15-mile radius 700 square miles (3, p. 6). Both areas represent approximately the same time-distance of their respective eras. With the greater mobility of people and their desire for more specialized goods and services, a commercial center no longer maintains an exclusive trade territory. Farmers and other rural residents in an area may use several service centers and use them selectively for different purposes. A study of Sherman County, Nebraska, showed that open-country residents used numerous service centers (3, pp. 29–31). A similar pattern of multiple use of centers was found to exist in a Montana study where "the majority of farmers and ranchers patronized three or more towns, visiting them with some degree of regularity," each town fulfilling different functions (59).

As a consequence the trade centers become differentiated in service functions, and some decline and others gain in importance. After such adjustments some trade centers provide only limited services for those in their immediate vicinity (i.e., bread and gasoline), whereas other places may develop specialized services for an expanded area (i.e., hospital and air service). This interrelationship among towns, although not planned and often resisted, is nonetheless real. These centers in combination provide the services used by people in multicentered communities.

One attempt to understand the relationship of centers to one another and to rationalize the pattern as a basis for planning services was done by Kraenzel in the Great Plains (41). The sparse population of the region imposes on it what has been called the social cost of space (4). This thinly settled area, however, is characterized by differences in concentration of population, with more than half the population counted as urban. Kraenzel has divided the population of the Great Plains according to its concentration. Much of the population is found along major avenues of transportation in stringlike fashion. Here are located the principal business, industrial, educational, health, governmental, and social resources of the area (Kraenzel calls this the Sutland after the Sutler who was a supply agent for the army). Away from the Sutland are the in-between areas, generally without the major transportation and public services found in the Sutland. There the towns, which Kraenzel identifies as Yonland, are smaller with more limited services and facilities. The theme he develops is that the Yonland does not have the population base needed to maintain a full range of institutional services and facilities, but services are organized on a limited area basis as a part of the cultural holdover from eastern settlement. At the same time, the Yonland is subject to exploitation by the Sutland; Kraenzel sees a need to establish a proper division of labor between the two types of areas. He advocates integrating the services of the Yonland with those of the Sutland headquarters in a mutually accommodating form (41, pp. 357–58).

Another suggestion in the same vein is by Fox, who recommends the organization of communities into larger units he calls Functional Economic Areas (FEAs) (20). These are areal delineations around centers with a minimum size of 25,000 population (perhaps smaller in sparsely populated areas) which would provide the services and employment opportunities for people within the area; FEAs would be multicentered, but services would be organized for the entire area. Advocates of FEAs claim that such areas represent the logical expansion of the service community from the horse-and-buggy to the rapid transportation age. Further, Fox emphasizes that FEAs are comprised of both rural and urban populations and that this is a more realistic representation of the structure of American society than are the concepts of autonomous rural and urban populations. He believes that a major impediment to sound economic and social policy is our institutionalized belief that a separate rural society exists and can be manipulated successfully apart from the society as a whole (19). These changes have profound implications for the location and delivery of services including health services.

RURAL HEALTH CARE SYSTEM. The focus of organization of the health care system is outside rural areas. Medical centers and other complex organizations are the location of specialized services; training of physicians and other health personnel takes place in complex training institutions; and policy and financing are matters involving federal and state governments, insurance companies, and professional organizations.

The regular medical profession is almost universally accepted as authoritative in matters of health. Even among groups which might be expected to adopt alternative healing philosophy and techniques, the pervasiveness of "scientific medicine" is apparent (17). The general characteristics of rural society, however, are reflected to some extent in the organization of rural medical practice. The most apparent unique quality of rural practice is its simple organizational form and its domination by general practitioners. Rural practice is predominantly office-based—solo practice or limited groups. Characteristically physicians form informal colleaguial networks which serve as information and referral systems (26, 47).

The character of the organization of rural medical practice can perhaps best be understood in terms of its historical development. The location of doctors followed the service-center community. It was necessary for the physician to be close to the homes of his patients, not only because transportation was difficult but also because the bed of illness was in the home. Medical knowledge was relatively limited, and the tools of the trade could be carried in a "little black bag." The "old doctor" was like every other doctor of his time—perhaps more or less competent and possibly possessing special cures, but surely a general practitioner of the "art" of healing. The relationship between doctor and patient was highly personalized, and confidence was placed in the individual practitioner rather than the medical profession as a whole.

The modern rural doctor practices in a different context. He has been educated in a standard curriculum and at a high level of concentration. He has the powerful scientific tools of his trade; complex diagnostic apparatus; and treatment that requires the office, the clinic, and the hospital together with a large number of auxiliary personnel. Home calls are no longer common, for the physician is more efficient if he remains at his work station, and the bed of treated illness is not in the home but in the hospital. Rural doctors tend to establish practices in places where there are hospitals; and Bible's national sample of nonmetropolitan physicians indicates that the presence of a hospital is an important consideration in choice of location (12). This process has tended to concentrate physicians in fewer places servicing rural areas—a trend that is consonant with other services in rural areas and consequently in agreement with the characteristics of the organization of communities.

As a consequence of the process of concentration of doctors in places with hospitals and secondarily by the increase in group practice, there has been a steady erosion of the location of physicians in smaller places. In Missouri there were 197 places that had medical doctors in 1952 but were without an MD in 1967 (29); Fahs and Peterson reported a similar kind of loss in the upper Midwest (Minnesota, North Dakota, South Dakota, and Montana) between 1921 and 1965 (16). The loss of doctors in the smallest places does not result so much from a movement of doctors out of these places as it does from a failure to replace those who have died or retired (28). These losses may be expected to continue because older doctors are overrepresented in the smallest places.

Because of the limited mobility of rural doctors, however, location of physicians may partially reflect a situation of 40 years earlier when the doctor began his career. In Missouri situations have been observed where physicians have spent their entire careers in a single place and in the end have outlived the town in which they began practice (28).

Another development apparent in the health care system is the increase in specialization of physicians. Most recent graduates of medical schools specialize in some area. The location process has selectively drawn specialists to urban areas and concentrated general practitioners in rural areas. In the ratio of GPs to population the various residential areas are quite similar; difference in total physician/population ratios is accounted for almost entirely by concentration of specialists in urban and metropolitan areas.

Since rural medical services are an integral part of the larger health system, the concentration of general practitioners in rural areas suggests that rural populations depend on outside physicians (and their related facilities) for specialized services. The questions of how the system is articulated and how continuity of services is provided are of major concern.

PATHWAYS TO MEDICAL SERVICES. Consumers of health care show certain behavior patterns as they make decisions about illness and use of health services. These patterns are pathways to medical services, and like other paths they may be circuitous.

Illness as a Social Phenomenon. Perhaps no sociological concept has been more influential in organizing thought about health behavior than the sick-role (58). As stated by Parsons, the sick-role has four components:

1. The sick person is exempted from normal social obligations.
2. The sick person is not held personally responsible for his condition.
3. There is an obligation by the sick person to want to get well.
4. There is an obligation by the sick person to seek competent help except for minor illnesses.

The sick person is exempted from normal duties such as going to work or attending school and is not stigmatized for being ill.[1] At the same time he is expected to want to get well and to seek appropriate help in doing so. Thus the incumbent of the sick-role makes a deal with society to remove himself as quickly as possible from a status

1. A major distinction between illness and delinquency as forms of deviant behavior is that in the first instance the person is not held responsible for his condition, whereas in the second he is. The change from viewing alcoholism as a crime to viewing it as an illness has largely eliminated blame for the condition.

that society regards as socially debilitating or deviant in exchange for special privileges and use of resources. Given such major privileges and dispensation of obligations, it should be expected that the community would pay close attention to the process of assuming the sick-role.

As the sick-role has been explicated, it has become apparent that it does not represent a single set of role expectations. Parsons defines it as a cultural artifact of middle-class American society. Precisely because this segment of the society influences behavior and outlook to such a high degree, this version of the sick-role is useful in understanding illness behavior. Subsequent conceptualization and research, however, have emphasized variability among people in assuming the sick-role, the different meaning illness has for different groups, and the effect of types of illness (i.e., acute, chronic) (22, 25, 38). Gordon develops the variation in the sick-role by considering its meaning for different socioeconomic groups and by considering different characteristics (seriousness and certainty of prognosis) of the illness itself. On the basis of a study of 808 persons in New York City, he confirmed his hypothesis that the sick-role represented a multidimensional relationship. An additional finding was that socioeconomic group identity was more closely related to assuming the sick-role than to behavior after the condition of illness had been established (25, p. 99).

Suchman further elaborates the sick-role as one of the stages in an illness career: (1) symptom experience stage, (2) sick-role stage, (3) medical contact stage, (4) dependent-patient stage, and (5) recovery or rehabilitation stage (68). The first three stages pertain to behavior and decisions which may be interpreted as pathways to medical services. Once the person assumes the sick-role and enters the medical-care system, the decision-making process is more likely to be taken out of his hands (although there is always the possible decision to leave the medical care system).

Health Utilization Process. The delineation of the sick-role suggests a sociological analysis of illness behavior. It has been common to consider single social-cultural factors such as socioeconomic status, attitudes and orientation, ethnic group identity, and numerous other factors either individually or serially as they relate to utilization of health services. This mode of analysis has increasingly come into critical review. McKinlay comments: "Any further research concerning relationships between rates of utilization and various attributes of social status—such as occupation, income level, education, and residential location—could add very little to what is already known in this regard." He calls for new theoretical insights and research strategies that will enable researchers to determine some of the influential intervening mechanisms between these crude sociodemographic variables and the specific behavior under examination (46). Addressing the same problem Odin Anderson says, "Further research on utilization of services—that is, hospital and physicians' services—should be conducted in well-defined operating situations. Otherwise, we will simply continue to accumulate more interesting data that are difficult to relate to specific contexts" (5).

The interaction of variables using a processual framework is one way of overcoming deficiencies of single-factor analyses. A processual model, developed from the work of a number of researchers, now appears quite standard (2, 13). It involves the interaction of: (1) need factors, (2) predisposing factors, and (3) enabling factors (see outline below). Andersen has employed this model in one of the more comprehensive studies of utilization of services. A general finding from this research is that need, predisposing factors, and enabling factors combine in different ways for utilization of different types of services (physician visits, dental visits, and hospitalization). For example, all three factors were related to use of physicians, whereas the need factor was not strongly related to the use of dentists, and the enabling component was not strongly related to the use of hospitals (2).

In a research bibliography, Aday uses the following detailed breakdown of the health utilization process to form categories for organizing some 200 studies (1). The outline indicates the type of variables considered under each of the components of processual models. Empirical studies were found to represent each of the subcategories in the outline.

    I. Predisposing variables
        A. sociodemographic
            1. age
            2. sex
            3. education
            4. marital status
            5. family size and composition
            6. race and ethnicity
            7. religious preference
        B. social-psychological
            1. general health care attitudes
               a. health beliefs and medical orientation
               b. perceived availability of care
               c. tendency to use services of a physician
               d. skepticism of medical care and physicians
            2. knowledge and source of health care information
            3. situation-specific stresses
               a. perceived susceptibility
               b. perceived seriousness

        c. perceived chance of recovery
        d. psychological readiness
    4. generalized stresses
        a. psychological
           (1) upsetting events, crises, chronic stress
           (2) fear, worry, anxiety, etc.
        b. structural
           (1) social isolation—powerlessness, anomie
           (2) broken or intact family
    5. patient-physician interaction
    6. previous health behavior

II. Enabling variables
    A. economic
        1. socioeconomic status and occupation
        2. income
        3. price of medical services
        4. method of financing
           a. third-party payers
              (1) voluntary insurance
              (2) medicare, medicaid, welfare
           b. type of coverage—indemnity, Blue Cross/Blue Shield, major medical, etc.
           c. method of payment—fee-for-service, prepayment, etc.
    B. organizational
        1. alternative organizational forms
           a. prepaid group practices
           b. prepaid dentist plans
           c. solo fee-for-service plans
           d. comprehensive health care plans for low-income enrollees
        2. type of practice—solo or group
    C. availability of service
        1. region
        2. residence (rural-urban)
        3. distance
        4. supply of medical personnel and facilities
           a. physician/population ratio
           b. hospital bed/population ratio
        5. regular source of care

III. Need
    A. health and mobility status
    B. perceived symptoms of illness
    C. physician-rated urgency
    D. chronic activity limitation status
    E. disability days
    F. diagnosis

As can be seen, the predisposing factors heavily emphasize beliefs, attitudes, and perception; the enabling factors tend to be economic or organizational. Rural-urban residence is regarded as an enabling variable reflecting the availability of services. As research continues on utilization of health services, the complexity of both the independent and dependent variables becomes more apparent.

Sociocultural Factors. Specific relationships exist between sociocultural factors and the use of health services. Here we consider beliefs, social structure in the form of networks of primary group interaction, and specific mechanisms of contacts with the health care system. Beliefs could be considered as predisposing variables, social networks as enabling variables, and contacts as the linkages between the lay system and the medical care system.

BELIEFS ABOUT ILLNESS AND HEALTH SERVICES. It seems obvious that beliefs about health services would be closely related to health service utilization. Relatively early in the research on health behavior, a conceptualization that related social-psychological factors to use of health services was formulated, and it continues to be a common research strategy. In a study reported in 1958 Hochbaum found three cognitive factors to be associated with participation in a tuberculosis x-ray screening program: belief by the person in the possibility of contracting the disease, belief by the person that he might have the disease without knowing it, and belief that early diagnosis would be beneficial (35). In a more generalized form Rosenstock identified "readiness factors" as: perceived susceptibility, perceived seriousness, and perceived benefits of taking action (63). These or similar cognitions have been utilized in research of polio immunization (64), Asian flu immunization (62), rheumatic fever prophylaxis (34), and use of dental services (39). In these studies the advantage of combinations over single cognitions is stressed.

In spite of the reasonableness of the expected relationship between cognitions in the form of perception of illness and orientation to medical and other health practitioners to use of health services, the relationships tend to be weak and the findings ambiguous. In Andersen's study health beliefs as measured by seven indices were insignificantly related to hospitalization and showed insignificant or low correlations with use of physicians and dental services (2, p. 44). Battistella found that readiness factors were relatively unimportant as predictors of delay by older people in getting medical services. This led him to reexamine readiness factors in other research with the conclusion that, even though significant relationships were found in a number of studies between readiness cognitions and use of health services, the strength of the relationships was such that they had little explanatory power (7). In a more general review on the evidence Bice, Eichhorn, and Fox concluded that there is little support for the existence of a relationship between such factors as values, attitudes, and beliefs and use of health services (13, pp. 267–68).

There is contrary research evidence, however, which needs to be considered. Suchman examined the relationship of types of personal health orientations to health behavior for a sample of persons who had experienced relatively serious illness during a two-month period. Indices of knowledge about disease, skepticism of medical care, and dependency in illness were constructed on the basis of which two types of health orientation (popular and scientific) were identified (67, p. 100). Generally Suchman found differences in health behavior to exist on the basis of popular and scientific health orientations. For example, those with a scientific health orientation were more likely than those with a popular health orientation to take symptoms seriously, less likely to delay seeing a doctor upon experiencing symptoms, and less likely to feel dependent on others in an illness (67, pp. 101–2).

An additional finding of the Suchman study is that health orientation is closely related to the degree of integration of the person into the primary group structure including ethnic groups, friendship groups, and families (67, p. 103). This suggests that statements of beliefs may have different effects for health behavior on the basis of whether or not they find support in primary group relationships. As a corollary, the expression of beliefs may outlive the particular primary group structure in which they originated. The latter may account for Nall's finding that "folk beliefs" were not related to health behavior while integration into the primary group was. Specifically he found that among a Mexican-American sample, folk beliefs such as *mal ojo* (bad eye), *mal de susto* (illness of fright), and witchcraft were fairly common; such beliefs, however, were not related to accepting and following a treatment regimen for tuberculosis (50, p. 303). He did find, however, that strong integration into family, locality, and ethnic group was associated with rejection of the regimen (50, p. 306). The principle involved is that beliefs are useful in predicting the direction of behavior if such beliefs are in conformity with those of other members of the primary group and the person is committed to the primary group. (Ethnic identity is not the same as strong identification with the group.) Without such group supports, beliefs may have little predictive value. Therefore, beliefs should be examined in the context of primary group structure.

There appears to be good reason to expect that primary groups should affect health behavior. The status of being ill (incumbent in the sick-role) depends in part on validation of the illness condition by significant others—often family, friends and neighbors, and peer groups (60). Primary groups not only affect beliefs about health and illness but also serve as situational facilitators or constrainors in seeking health services. In specific situations primary groups provide a context of decision-making in which support and resources can be made available to facilitate use of services, or in which discouragement and alternatives (to professional care) provided by the group can act to constrain use of professional services.

SOCIAL NETWORKS. The most sustained effort to understand the effects of lay networks on behavior is found in the work of rural sociologists on the diffusion of information and adoption of innovations in agricultural technology (37, 43, 61). This type of research might be applicable to the use of health services (10, 15, 46).

The diffusion literature as it has developed in rural sociology encompasses two quite separate components: (1) the communication system and (2) the adoption process. The communication system includes the interconnection of mass media and local interpersonal channels which follow the community organizational structure. Characteristically information reaches the individual via a two-step process in which mass-media messages are received by certain community members (cosmopolites) and relayed through the "natural" interpersonal network. In the "natural community" not all persons are equally involved in the network; some are isolates while others are the focal point of intersecting lines of communication. Furthermore, some individuals are sought out as sources of information, and such influentials serve a function of validating practices. Much of the diffusion research is devoted to delineating community organizational structures (neighborhoods, peer groups, class divisions), charting the flow of information through these channels, and identifying and describing the socioeconomic characteristics of various functionaries (innovators, opinion leaders, etc.) in the communication networks.

The adoption process is a step-wise decision-making model of the adoption of a given practice (56). A five-stage model has become quite standard: (1) awareness of an innovation, (2) interest (in which more information is obtained), (3) evaluation, (4) trial, and (5) adoption. In the adoption process, consideration is given to the *characteristics of the innovation* (compatibility with existing practices, divisibility—degree to which innovation can be tried on a limited basis, simplicity, and relative advantage); *characteristics of the potential adopter* (age, education, financial resources, competency, social status, social participation, communicative behavior, cosmopoliteness); and *characteristics of the social milieu* (community values and norms, social isolation, presence of special functionaries—innovators, opinion leaders, influentials, membership in groups, programs of planned change) (27).

Further analysis considers adoption of innovations over time—identifying early, middle, and late adopters. The validating stages (two and three) of the adoption process tend to utilize interpersonal sources of information (friends and neighbors), while the first stage relies more heavily on mass media.

In developing a rationale of the relationship of lay networks for the utilization of health services, Freidson suggests that seeking health services is related on the one hand to acceptance of professional health services as being legitimate and on the other hand to extent and strength of a person's lay network. Lay referral networks consist of consultants—potential or actual—running from the intimate and most informal confines of the nuclear family through successively more select, distant, and authoritative persons until the professional is reached (21).

There is ample evidence that definitions of illness and behavior associated with being ill vary among identifiable groups. In a classic study Zborowski found that different ethnic groups responded differently to pain, presumably as a result of differential socialization (75); Zola found that complaints presented at a public health clinic were substantially different for different ethnic groups (77). Similarly social class position is associated with definitions of illness and pathways to services. Koos reported, for example, that lower-class people exhibited different health behavior than middle- and upper-class people (40); Hollingshead and Redlich demonstrated the relationship of social class to the type and extent of treatment in mental illness (36). Suchman pointed out that it was during the assumption of the sick-role stage that the lay referral structure was of greatest importance.

> How the individual's lay consultants react to his symptoms and their acceptance of any interference with his social functioning will do much to determine the individual's ability to enter the sick-role. The sick person will seek confirmation, advice, reassurance, and finally a form of "provisional validation" which temporarily excuses him from his normal obligations and activities (68, p. 115).

In his study of persons with relatively serious illnesses Suchman found that almost all respondents had discussed symptoms with someone before seeking medical care. Most discussions, however, were limited to one other person; only 5 percent reported speaking to three or more other persons. Furthermore, discussions were most likely to be with relatives (84 percent), usually the person's spouse (68, p. 119).

In another analysis from this same sample (utilizing both sick and well respondents) Suchman examined the relationship between a person's perception of being in a cohesive primary group network (ethnic group exclusivity, friendship-group solidarity, and family orientation of tradition and authority) and reported dependent behavior during illness. Significant and consistent relationships were found between illness dependency and cohesiveness of primary group networks irrespective of the particular ethnic group to which the person belonged.

> Regardless of ethnic-group membership, it would seem that the degree of support one seeks and secures from one's social group is influenced by the degree of social integration of the group. The more cohesive the group, the greater the dependency of the individual upon it for support during illness (69).

In a study of a sample of 503 persons in Windsor, Canada, Battistella had expected to find greater delay in seeking health services among socially isolated middle-aged and elderly people. His reasoning was that family members, neighbors, friends, and co-workers may be important influences in helping individuals interpret the significance of the symptoms and in encouraging early initiation of physicians' care. The data did not support the hypothesis but rather suggested the opposite. He offers the following ex post facto explanation:

> Isolated persons may delay less because of feelings of apprehension, insecurity, and helplessness, which lead them to seek reassurance and emotional support from physicians. In contrast the non-isolated may have more self-confidence and feel more self-reliant in interpreting the significance of symptoms. Relatives and friends may act to alleviate anxiety for individuals complaining of illness by defining symptoms in nonserious and commonplace terms (6).

Booth and Babchuk used a diffusion model in attempting to understand the use of new health resources.[2] Twenty-four percent of a sample of 800 noninstitutionalized adults 45 years and over from Omaha and Lincoln, Nebraska, had used a new health resource during the year preceding the interviews. For the vast majority (93 percent) it was a physician. The researchers posed five questions about the process that led to the selection and use of new resources.

1. How persuasive are interpersonal transactions in decisions of clients to use a health service . . . relative to the use of the other sources of information?

2. Indicator of use of a new health resource was a positive response to the question: "During the past twelve months have you consulted a doctor you have never seen before, or utilized some medical service—like the ones on this list?" On the list were the following services: doctor, hospital, nursing home program, meals-on-wheels, mental health or psychiatric clinic, service for the visually impaired, homemaker service, rehabilitation service, and alcohol treatment center (15, p. 91).

2. What situations prompt individuals to engage in such exchanges?

3. What are the characteristics of those consulted?

4. What is the nature of the interaction that characterizes decision-related exchanges?

5. What effect do the interpersonal exchanges have on the decisions clients ultimately make?

The findings are presented here in terms of the five questions:

1. Compared with mass communication, the use of personal contacts played a major role in decisions to use new health resources. Seventy-eight percent of the respondents indicated that interpersonal relationships were instrumental in their decision (15, p. 93). Of considerable interest was the finding that most respondents only remembered talking to one other person before taking action which raises a question about a network of *informants* (a finding consistent with that of Suchman).

2. Two factors were especially associated with decisions to seek advice about health services. One was the severity of the illness; the other, interpersonal resources at the individual's disposal. With regard to the latter factor, those reporting extended kin and friend relationships were more likely to use consultants in making decisions about use of health resources (15, p. 94).

3. Physicians were not used frequently as advisors in the use of new health services, nor were other professional counselors such as ministers and lawyers. Kin were consulted most frequently; among kin one's spouse was most likely to be the advisor, followed by an adult daughter and an adult son (15, p. 94). Shifts in patterns of advisors were observed by age; for example, middle-aged men were more likely to seek advice from friends, while elderly men were more likely to seek advice from family members—a change which corresponded to disassociation from employment (15, p. 95).

4. The writers sought to determine if the relationship were instrumental (cope with the external environment) or expressive (supportive or involved in tension management). They found that most of the conversations with friends and neighbors were instrumental in nature while those with family members were more likely to be expressive.

5. Respondents judged that two-thirds of the advisors were very influential in decisions to use a new health service, and in most cases the very influential advisors were thought to be more knowledgeable than the respondent (15, p. 96).

We can interpret the studies cited in this section as showing the importance of primary groups as validators of the sick-role and as advisors in seeking medical services. It is not clear, however, what the exact effect of lay networks is on the level of use of service. Freidson regards them as a resource which facilitates obtaining professional services (if the lay and professional cultures are congruent). Booth and Babchuk found that those with fewer interpersonal resources were more likely to delay in seeking new services. This is inconsistent with McKinlay's finding that location of the individual in a strong lay network reduced the amount of services obtained in clinic settings and with Battistella's and Suchman's research, which supported the idea that lay advisors tended to reduce or delay medical services.

A problem in understanding the relationship of social networks to access to health services in rural areas is that few studies of the effects of primary groups on seeking medical care are based on rural population samples. Sheldon Lowry et al. considered participation and other variables in relationship to an index of health practices somewhat in the tradition of diffusion studies (45); a number of studies have considered group effects on preventive practices, especially immunization and family planning, which are tangential to our central concern (61).

We can, however, extrapolate from our earlier characterization of rural society as being based on organizations of relatively limited scale and with greater emphasis on primary group relationships and advance the following propositions as guides to research.

1. The effects of primary group networks will be greater in rural areas than in urban areas. Therefore, the findings of the importance of primary groups as validators of the sick-role should be accentuated for rural populations.

2. Primary group networks operate as factors to reduce use of services:

    a. by denying the status of illness to some individuals;

    b. by suggesting alternatives such as home treatment and by offering support which otherwise might be sought from professionals.

3. For serious and emergency illness, primary group networks may increase use of services by serving as resources.

4. Lay networks may be especially critical for rural people in seeking extralocal health services.

National survey data are not inconsistent with these propositions in that rural people tend to make fewer physician visits (55), which conforms to expectations from the second proposition, and to utilize hospitals to as great an extent as the urban population, which conforms to the third proposition (54). Also in support of the third proposition is the fact that differences in use of physicians between rural and urban populations is greatest in the childhood years when many illnesses are not severe and home treatment may be acceptable. While these propositions and data in conformity with them are not tests of hypotheses, they indicate that group structure explanations for differences in rural and urban use of services may be as important as cultural (belief) explanations.

CONTACTS WITH HEALTH CARE SYSTEM. If professional health care is to be received, contact must be made with the health care system. As the system is now organized, initiative rests with clients who have considerable latitude and some alternatives in the services sought. Components of the health care system have their own requirements for entrance and style of relationships.

Each encounter with the health care system does not require establishing new relationships; many contacts between client and provider are based on past experience. Thus characteristic patterns of decision-making are established in the family, symptoms that need attention are commonly recognized, and the places to get health services are known.

The health care system in rural areas is commonly represented by private practitioners in solo practice or in association with a small number of other doctors. But these services represent only the initial contact points which may eventually lead to a vast medical care system with other units in the communities (such as hospitals) and extend outside the community to specialty centers.

To enter the medical care system, the client is expected to seek out a physician, who in turn has access to the various services. In this way the physician serves as a gatekeeper to the medical care system. There is a certain amount of routinization of the doctor-patient relationship. A common form is establishing a continuing and anticipatory relationship with a single practitioner commonly referred to as the family-doctor relationship. Mutual obligations on the part of the physician and client are implied. For the client this involves consulting the family doctor first in an illness and following his advice in regard to treatment or referral to other physicians or services. For the physician the obligation is to provide continuity of care for the family and to facilitate access to the complex health care system. In rural surveys the proportion of families reporting a family doctor usually exceeds 80 percent (30, p. 29; 33; 65).

In a Missouri study the reasons given for having a family doctor were those associated with establishing a relationship in anticipation of a need. These included the desirability of having someone available in emergency situations, the assurance of services for more common ailments including chronic illness, and the convenience of having a regular doctor. Another set of responses involved the usefulness of an established relationship in providing better care because the doctor knew the patient's history and maintained records. Relatively less important were responses that indicated the family-doctor relationship is primarily one based on personal loyalty, friendship, or faith in the individual practitioner (31).

The actual family-doctor relationship may be too fragile to support the pivotal role attributed to it. Even while acknowledging a family-doctor relationship, clients often bypass the family doctor in seeking specialty services for self-diagnosed ailments, depending on lay referral in place of that from the family doctor (30, pp. 31–37). The family doctor for his part may not have contact with relevant parts of the health care system and be less than willing to refer patients to specialists he may regard as competitors. Since he has no monopoly to entrance to the complex health care system, the family doctor may not be in an ideal gatekeeper role. In spite of the limitations of the family-doctor relationship, it is presently the most universally regularized contact between client and the health care system.

While the family-doctor relationship is our main example of routinization of behavior, it is not the only situation in which behavior is routinized. The widespread use of hospital emergency rooms and clinics as the primary source of medical care by many families becomes routine behavior. This has led some to refer to the emergency room as the family doctor of the poor. To this point, however, it should be noted that rural areas have fewer such facilities.

Other behavior of the family in getting services for their members is also regularized—decisions about when illness is serious enough to require outside intervention and what personal procedures to follow. Such routines provide the basis for the organization of behavior that should yield to research; it is within this context that beliefs and other cognitions as well as lay consultants probably can best be studied as contributors to behavior.

CONCLUSIONS. Demographic, normative, and organizational diversity persists in American rural society. On the macro level there appears to be little support for the hypothesis that rural-urban differences in values and beliefs account for rural-urban differences in selection and utilization of health services. Belief and value differences may in fact be greater within rural areas than between rural and urban areas, although evidence is piecemeal and inferential. A well-designed and conceptually focused study is needed to test the hypothesis on a broad scale. Such research needs to be conducted and reported in such a manner that it gains widespread attention of the public and policymakers; otherwise the idea will continue to persist and be acted upon that rural and urban populations have basically different beliefs and values about health and health care.

Instead of expecting some general rural-urban value differences to support differences in health behavior, it seems more useful to consider the organization of rural health services and the processes of seeking and getting health services within the context of community situations. Research should focus on more sophisticated conceptual models which place health and illness behavior within the context of existing group patterns and detail the processes of access to health services as sociological phenomena. Such a strategy should be sensitive to rural organization situations. We cannot expect easy understanding of rural health access problems on the basis of gross rural-urban differences. If we are really serious about understanding health consumer behavior, we must look closely and carefully at the processes of deciding, organizing, and doing.

The strategy I favor is to regard illness as a social phenomenon and develop sociological analyses of the processes involved in utilizing health services. The concept, sick-role, has the advantage of placing illness in the realm of social behavior. One cannot take this concept seriously without soon concluding that both illness and health behavior as dependent variables and their associated independent variables are complex. The idea of illness behavior as a process, with the implicit or explicit conceptualization of illness stages or an illness career, appears to be useful.

By taking this approach, beliefs, primary group structure, and patterns or routines of behavior (among other concepts) can be incorporated into coherent conceptual models. Beliefs appear to be most useful as predictors of health behavior when viewed within the context of primary group relationships. In other words, beliefs are part of the ongoing social process that finds definition and support in primary group interaction. The effects of primary group relations in the form of lay referral systems are extended to the routines for gaining access to the medical care system. In this approach we can incorporate the rich theory and substantive information on group processes and community behavior. As an example, the research on diffusion of information and the adoption process may be usefully applied to health behavior.

The rural situation may accentuate the effects of primary groups on health behavior. Special problems of access may exist on the basis of disjunctures of local communities and urban-based health care systems. In such a context lay consultants may have added impact on decisions and may be especially important as resources of access. The strength of primary group relations in rural areas may in fact account for more of the differences between rural and urban health care utilization than availability of services or differences in values. This is only a conjecture, but it suggests the possibility of payoff in this line of research.

CHAPTER ELEVEN

COMPREHENSIVE HEALTH PLANNING ISSUES FOR RURAL HEALTH RESEARCHERS

IVAN R. HANSON

ECONOMISTS rely heavily on the existence of a market for allocating scarce resources, but markets do not exist, or function badly, in many areas of community services, including health. The maldistribution of doctors might be one example of inadequate market operation resulting in misallocation of resources. To correct such difficulties, planning has long been recognized as an alternative to a functioning market.

Health planning is not a completely new activity, as Roemer has pointed out (24). But comprehensive planning, now the main thrust of the health field, is comparatively new; prior to 1966 most planning was single-purpose.

The difference between rural and urban health planning is not distinct. The problems of rural areas—transportation, specialty service linkages, emergency services, and others—are important; but the principles, processes, and organizations of rural health planning aimed at solving them are not notably distinguishable from urban health planning.

COMPREHENSIVE HEALTH PLANNING. Although there is extensive project, program, and other single-purpose planning in the health field, the comprehensive health planning (CHP) efforts now under way are the most far-reaching and are the focal point of health planning for both rural and urban America.

IVAN R. HANSON is Associate Professor, Department of Health Administration, Health Sciences Center, University of Oklahoma, Oklahoma City.

The author wishes to acknowledge the counsel of Charles M. Cameron, Larry Fowler, and Nan Stout, University of Oklahoma.

Objectives. Comprehensive health planning originated with federal legislation passed in 1966 which created the mechanism for planning at state and local levels. The expectations for revamping the health delivery mechanisms are best noted directly from the act.

> Comprehensive health planning is viewed as a process that will enable rational decision-making about the use of public and private resources to meet health needs. Its concern encompasses physical, mental, and environmental health; the facilities, services, and manpower required to meet all health needs; and the development and coordination of public, voluntary, and private resources to meet these needs (22).

Perhaps the most salient feature about CHP that distinguishes it from other health planning is its orientation toward people and everything that affects their health rather than toward facilities or technology. This does not mean that there should be no specialized or program planning, but that all planning must be coordinated. It is a pluralistic endeavor, recognizing that different population groups or geographic areas will have different needs and that the physical, mental, or environmental impacts on the total health of the population must be addressed by planners (13). The anticipations for "promoting and assuring the highest level of health attainable" (22) have not been reached. Some writers have criticized the legislation for having goals that are too nebulous, but perhaps they confuse specific objectives with broader goals. It does appear that the legislation designers were overly ambitious in attempting to restructure the health delivery mechanism through an underfunded, essentially voluntary network of local organizations.

Structure and Mechanisms. To carry out this enormous task, Congress authorized funding for state and local planning agencies.

Statewide health planning agencies (called A agencies because they were created by Section 314(a) of the Public Health Services Act of 1966) are concerned chiefly with matters of broad policy that affect the whole state or at least certain whole classes of institutions, activities, or resources. These agencies function in a wide variety of ways to influence the establishment of facilities and services throughout their states as well as state government health policies and programs. An A agency now exists in each of the 50 states, District of Columbia, and Puerto Rico.

Areawide health planning agencies (called B agencies because they were created by Section 314(b) of the Public Health Services Act of 1966) are responsible for bringing together people in local communities to define their specific health problems and for dealing with particular institutions, activities, or resources in the area. In most parts of the country the B agencies are multicounty units that coexist with the Economic Development Districts or with the councils of government in metropolitan areas. About 200 B agencies have been created in the United States and cover more than 80 percent of the population (8).

Since the health planning field of the magnitude and comprehensiveness currently being attempted is so new, there are relatively few qualified, specially trained people capable of performing the wide variety of tasks required of health planners. Training grants were given to colleges and universities but were terminated at the end of fiscal year 1974. Funds for training and technical assistance now go directly to the state and areawide agencies.

Organizations have been created at both state and local levels which combine professional staffing with volunteer councils and committees. Most of the agencies have had to rely on minimal professional planning staffs; often rural communities have had only one- or two-person staffs to coordinate the planning in multicounty organizations.

The strength of the A and B agencies was intended to rest with the many local citizens who serve on the governing councils and on the multitude of committees. Most significantly the federal legislation stipulated that the majority of members on local boards must be consumers, which would theoretically wrest absolute control of decision-making about local health affairs away from the providers (mainly doctors and hospital boards). Following this shift in power, it was reasoned, the health care system would also shift from being provider-oriented to being consumer-oriented. In reality it is not clear that such a shift in power has taken place. Nevertheless, anecdotes float through the health planning world about the surprising strength of consumer blocs in unexpected situations.

Funding for local health planning was a combination of federal and state funds. The federal government provided matching grants on a 50–50 or sometimes 75–25 basis. It was the responsibility of the A and B agencies to assemble the local matching funds, sometimes through tax money but most often through donations from local health agencies and institutions. This sometimes created a potential conflict of interest when local hospitals who were asked to contribute might subsequently have their actions subjected to close scrutiny or criticism by the planning organization.

Thus since 1966 between 200 and 300 CHP organizations were created throughout the United States with ill-defined objectives, inadequate organizations, and unstable financing. The sanguine expectations were for a reorganization of the health care delivery system, a shift in the balance of power for health resources decision-making from providers to consumers, and an overall sense of communitywide determinism about improving the status of local health conditions and expenditure patterns.

Since no unique health planning techniques existed, the most frequently verbalized model was one that searched for a "community of solution" (2, 4, 27). It was based on rather idealistic notions of how a major industry in the nation could be restructured through grass-roots action committees. Most planning staff effort was devoted to data collection and persuasive tactics as a catalyst for change; little effort was spent on developing formal plans.

Beginning in 1972 the author had teaching contact with several hundred health planners from throughout the nation at a series of continuing education short courses at the University of Oklahoma which were financed by a grant from HEW. Through successive sessions the disenchantment with the "community of solution" approach became more apparent, and planners began to argue for "more teeth" in the planning process.

Teeth eventually came in three ways—through certificate-of-need legislation, A-95 review and comment procedures, and eventually Section 1122 review and approval. Certificate-of-need legislation for hospitals and/or nursing homes now exists in 21 states (12). Briefly, any group wishing to construct or enlarge a hospital or nursing home must present a case to the designated reviewers as to why this facility is needed in that location and what services it will perform to meet community needs. As an illustration, Oklahoma has certificate-of-need legislation for nursing homes (pending for hospitals) which gives the State Commission of Health the authority to approve or deny licensing for the proposed facility. The A and B CHP agencies have input into this process and make recommendations to the State Commission.

"Review and comment" procedures through Circular A-95 require that applications for federal funds in the health field must be reviewed and commented on by state and local groups who have been officially delegated the authority to do so (19, 20). Many A and B agencies have this responsibility since they are the relevant planning agency. It gives these agencies an opportunity to consult with local groups proposing a project and may result in having a beneficial influence in the initial design of the project. This process does not give absolute power, however, and the federal grant may be approved over the objections of the A and B agencies. It should be noted that some groups have review and comment responsibilities not related to A-95; some federal programs not covered in A-95 and some third-party payers may also request additional review and comment.

The stronger, controversial "review and approval" powers came through the 1972 amendments to the Social Security Act commonly referred to as Section 1122 (23). This federal legislation gave certain designated state planning agencies the power to approve or reject proposals to expand specified services or facilities. The capital expenditures reviewed include: (1) those which exceed $100,000, (2) those which change the bed capacity of the facility, and (3) those which change the services of the facility. If the designated planning agency rejects the proposal of the applicant and the applicant proceeds with the project, the federal government may deny certain reimbursements for Maternal and Child Health programs (Title V), Medicare (Title XVIII), and Medicaid (Title XIX). The reimbursement denied would not be for all charges incurred on behalf of the patient but would exclude only those which resulted from increases due to debt service charges for the denied project. Criteria for the review and approval are based on need, manpower availability, economic feasibility, and cost containment.

Because this legislation has been in effect such a short time and expansion plans already under way were "grandfathered" in, the impact of this procedure on developing a more orderly growth and development in the health care system has yet to be measured.

Current Status. New programs such as CHP frequently have growing pains—exhibiting confusion, drawing criticism, and stimulating discussion about what they are trying to do and how they are doing it. Four landmarks changed CHP through the early 1970s. The first was the creation of the Expectations Study Group in 1972 to develop a series of statements about what should be expected of CHP in the future and paths of actions for achieving these expectations. The significance of this was the recognition that CHP seemed to be foundering and needed greater direction. The group's report dealt with four issues: (1) CHP purpose and principles, (2) operational expectations, (3) actions needed to achieve expectations, and (4) competencies and skills available to the agency.

The Expectations Study Group reaffirmed the broad, comprehensive principles stated in the 1966 legislation and reliance on the democratic process of voluntary planning at the community level. Also reaffirmed was the requirement that more than half the council members should be consumers in order to balance the provider-dominated medical industry. The group defined in considerable detail 16 specific activities which constitute health planning (6). These activities have since been condensed into eight: agency management, community organization, planning coordination, plan development, data management, special studies, project review, and public issue involvement (3).

The results of this work in defining more clearly the direction and actions of health planning had scarcely begun to be diffused throughout the agencies when the second significant event took place. The Comprehensive Health Planning Service in Washington directed that a "technical assessment" be made of each A and B agency in the country. After pilot studies were done to develop a format for conducting the assessment, teams of volunteer and professional health planners were organized and trained to evaluate their peers. The final results of data thus generated have not been fully analyzed, but the preliminary findings seem mixed. Some agencies appeared to have had an impact on the health care system in their communities; others had not (10). The preliminary findings did spur the movement toward massive inputs into developing plan documents. This is perhaps the most significant impact of the technical assessment, because it changed the focus of planning from "come let us reason together" to development of formal plan documents.

The third major decision greatly affecting the CHP movement was the passage of certificate-of-need and the capital expenditures review legislation (Section 1122). This gave agencies the teeth they had desired, but it also severely strained the staff capabilities of agencies. Reviews became very time-consuming and often were extremely burdensome for the staff. More importantly, they reinforced the need for a formally developed plan against which review decisions could be made, documented, and defended.

The fourth landmark was the effort mounted for new legislation in the 93rd Congress to replace P.L. 89-749. The statutory authorization and funding for CHP was to have expired in 1975. Congress debated through much of 1974 about how planning should be organized in the future. There seemed to be a consensus about disenchantment with the outcomes of CHP efforts under the excessively broad guidelines and organizational structure set forth by the 1966 legislation. Simultaneously it seemed that two other federally sponsored programs—Regional Medical Program and Hill-Burton—ought to be more closely allied with CHP, since they were financing facilities and programs (sometimes independently) that would influence the structure of the health industry for which CHP was trying to plan.

Several bills were introduced in both the House and Senate to transform the existing agencies into a new coalition. Legislators hoped that the old problems of too few resources, insufficient and untrained staff and volunteers, uncertain mandate for power, and competition among federally supported programs would not be repeated with creation of the new organization.

RESEARCH FOR PLANNING. Seven areas of research that would be of benefit to planners are: (1) effect of national health policy on planning, (2) research on health issues, (3) health information systems, (4) improved evaluation techniques, (5) economic impacts of planning, (6) financing comprehensive health planning, and (7) research in social and behavioral change. Some of these issues deal with the "stuff" of planning, generating the data planners would use in carrying out their work. Others are more oriented toward evaluating the planning process itself. Both are needed.

National Health Policy and Planning. National health policy in the mid-1970s seems to be moving toward a regulated health care system in order to contain costs (9, 21). The health planning organizations are part of the mechanism for enforcing this regulation. McClure has suggested this would be disastrous for planning because, carried to the ultimate, planning organizations could take on the configuration of something like the Civil Aeronautics Board which would transform local areawide agencies into enforcement bureaus for national policy and leave little time for planning (16). The move toward regulation could be enhanced depending on the way national health insurance is enacted. If it is channeled through private insurance companies, as with medicare and medicaid, the regulatory burden may not be as great as if it is done exclusively through the governmental bureaucracy.

Another possibility in national policy for containing costs and assuring some level of health care as a right is to restructure the health care delivery system by encouraging health maintenance organizations and other alternative configurations to the fee-for-service system. McClure suggested that planning agencies, rather than being the regulatory authority and financial managers of the health care system, would be free to identify problems and propose options and would limit their regulatory activities to keeping the market open and fair and providing some consumer protection regarding quality assurance and additional protection through adequate information similar to truth-in-lending (16).

Research on Health Issues. In addition to the traditional demand and supply analysis and projections, we need evaluation studies on experimental projects now under way. Neighborhood health centers, family health centers, experimental health centers, and other mutations in the search for new delivery organizations are being tested throughout the country. We do not yet see any widely published work on the community impacts of these experiments which can be generalized and interpreted by health planners and decision-makers in other areas.

It is apparent that many of these experimental projects have not thoroughly planned their post-project evaluation before the project started so that there could be effective analysis. Their economic portions particularly could be improved. Local health planners can match researchers with projects to the potential benefit of both.

One aspect of the problems and techniques that is frequently overlooked is the level on which data are available. Much of the information available on the national level that deals with economic aspects of health is not readily usable by planners for local or multi-county analyses. It is hoped that disaggregation problems can be solved at least partly by an improved information system.

Health Information Systems. Some statisticians have wondered if CHP activities would utilize statistical data (11). Several early efforts were made at designing information systems for health planning in the years immediately following the passage of P.L. 89-749 (5, 17, 26).

The need for data collection, analysis, and dissemination was examined by the Study Committee of the Public Health Conference on Records and Statistics. Their work resulted in a book that discusses information systems and data sources for the areas of health services, health facilities, health manpower, environmental health, and demographic and socioeconomic data (14). This work coincides with the independent development of some state health information systems, and the decision by the federal government to try some experimental project systems is being funded by the federal government (18). Research money is available, and it is badly needed. It is all too easy to get caught up in the hardware aspects of the system, but the biggest research needs are in the users of data generated. Who will use them and in what form? Local administrators and county public health officials are growing increasingly weary of the data requirements placed on them, and few see any direct use for them. A well-organized CHP staff should be able to work with local and county officials to develop projections for the counties from these data, but it is not yet very likely in rural areas.

Research to be done here is frequently cooperative with the A agencies and universities, so there is plenty of opportunity for research involvement.

Improved Evaluation Techniques. Evaluation is needed to ascertain the effectiveness (both qualitative and quantitative) of investments, experiments, and innovations in the field of health care delivery. Equally important is improvement in the adaptation of evaluation techniques to the health field so they can be used by small planning staffs. Progress is being made at adapting techniques to the health planning field, but more work needs to be done on cost-benefit and cost effectiveness techniques for example. At the present time many are too complex to be used except by experts who have adequate computer facilities readily available.

Not unrelated are the data problems of quantifying benefits in health. Most of the benefits now are expressed in terms of early deaths prevented and time lost from work. More needs to be done on the benefits of absence from pain and anxiety and productivity impacts of underemployment due to minor or chronic illness.

Researchers have a great contribution to make here, not only in acquiring the information but also in seeing that the information reaches the planners. Maybe what is needed is a Cooperative Extension Service in the Department of Health, Education and Welfare.

Economic Impacts of Planning. Planning is an alternative to a market, but at what price? Market structure analysis looks at the size of administrative and promotion costs as one measure of performance in an industry. Could it not also be said that planning costs are a similar cost, and that the amount of money spent on planning enters into the performance measures of the health industry?

Money is being spent on planning every year (and more is likely), but is it achieving benefits greater than the costs? Some local planners feel they save the community money through better coordination, but no widely published work has demonstrated that planning is the cost-effective way of achieving savings. Rosenfeld reported more than 50 percent of the B agencies responding to a questionnaire indicated that construction, expansion, and renovation had occurred in their area without their approval, which indicates that project review effectiveness may be limited (25). May also reported preliminary work indicating there is no evidence that planning has had an impact on the hospital system in places with areawide planning agencies compared with those that did not have them (15). Frequently discussed specific activities of planners that could be evaluated are: shared services, institutional mergers, and training programs established for subprofessionals.

What effect if any has planning had on the following major health issues?

1. Escalating hospital and medical costs
2. Inadequate and badly distributed primary health professionals
3. Lack of mechanisms for redistributing resources to health-deficient populations
4. Presence of gross inequities in health care stemming from badly fragmented financing, insurance, delivery, control and policy direction

Answers to these questions get at the very essence of the role of planning in the health care sector. Does planning really have any impact on the services, or could this restructuring be brought about by a well-designed federal financing system?

Financing CHP. To date we have seen no research on financing planning as an aspect of community government comparable to the monumental work of Harold Groves and others who worked in taxation and government financing a few decades ago.

Accurate annual expenditures for CHP were not available, but some estimates were made. In fiscal year 1972 the federal appropriations for CHP were $27 million for the following categories:

314(a)	$ 7.675 million
314(b)	13.200 million
314(c)	4.125 million
federal level	2.000 million
	$27.000 million (8)

Federal grants to A and B agencies totaled about $21 million and were matched on either a 50–50 or 75–25 basis, which would put the state contributions at something less than the maximum possible of an additional $21 million. The total annual direct expenditure for CHP would be something less than $50 million.

This amount is considerably less than the forecasted cost of fully implementing CHP. The Expectations Study Group made some estimates for B agencies if the entire country were to be included under an agency jurisdiction. The sizes of staffs for these agencies were estimated based on population, scope of the CHP mandate, and multiplicity of skills needed for carrying out this mandate. The group of experts determined that a minimum staff of ten professionals for a population of 600,000 people would be needed, but that such an optimum level would not always be reached in areas where population distribution and substate planning regions dictate otherwise. Currently the median size agency is three professionals. A total of 301 B agencies was projected, compared with 172 then in existence. Employment forecasted was 3,798 professionals and 2,532 supporting and clerical staff for a total of 6,330 people. The total annual cost of this employment would be $145,590,000. The cost per employee was estimated at $23,000, the federal government average expenditure per employee. The effects of population growth and inflation were not taken into account in determining how this would change in the future (7).

Raising financing of this sort would take a drastically different source of revenues than the current panhandling techniques used to raise local matching funds. The Expectations Study Group proposed that a fixed percentage of all health dollars expended in an area be allocated to CHP agencies or subcontracted to specialized planning agencies. Also the cost of performing certificate-of-need review procedures could be financed either through state appropriations or fees. (HEW does reimburse Designated Planning Agencies for Section 1122 reviews.)

In any event, careful consideration must be made for determining (1) whether planning is an effective use of these funds and (2) how this revenue can be raised at state and local levels.

Research in Social and Behavioral Change. Many people—both rural and urban—resent the planning process, view it as socialistic, and do not recognize the need of a complex society for rational choice mechanisms. More research as well as better adaptation of existing research on motivation, awareness, and other behavioral and communication factors involved in planned change is needed. Economists frequently are not interested in this kind of research, but it is fundamental to the problem of valuing in estimating costs and benefits. Research results in this area might help planners make better choices about which planning model to use in their area and how to deal with conflict resolution, for example. Making planning more appropriate and effective might also serve to keep it in the area of voluntarism rather than moving toward absolute control.

EPILOGUE. After the major portion of this chapter was written, Congress passed new health planning legislation. President Ford signed the bill into law only hours before a pocket veto would have occurred on January 4, 1975. This legislation—The National Health Planning and Resources Development Act of 1974 (P.L. 93-641)—consolidates some of the planning and regulatory agencies in the health field. The CHP A and B agencies plus Regional Medical Programs and Hill-Burton programs will be combined into Health Systems Agencies.

Several issues are arising as a consequence of this legislation:

1. The geographic areas to be included in the required health service areas are a source of conflict. The law specifies they shall have a minimum population of 500,000 but may go to less than 200,000 in "highly unusual circumstances." Again the familiar issue is raised as to what is an appropriate planning area. Certainly more research is needed on how to make rational decisions that account for distance, density, and politics.

2. The state agency in addition to planning must serve as the 1122 review agency and administer the certificate-of-need program. All states must pass certificate-of-need legislation by a deadline if they do not already have it. Every five years the agency must also review all institutional health services offered in the state and make public the findings on their appropriateness. An important issue here is that much greater public accountability for health services is being mandated. The consequences seem to draw the health industry toward a publicly regulated industry. The alternative actions and their impacts under a regulated system have not been explored and need to be researched.

3. By mid-1976 the Secretary of HEW must issue guidelines concerning health policy—including standards on appropriate supply, distribution, and organization of health resources and a statement of national health goals. Considering the paucity of available data to set such standards, much research needs to be done in a short time.

While this recent legislation has changed the structure of health planning from what was described in the text of this chapter, the topics on which research is needed to benefit planners are reinforced. It is imperative that research be done to augment the decision-making under an increasingly regulated system in the health industry.

CHAPTER TWELVE

SOLVING HEALTH CARE PROBLEMS WITH THE SIMULATION APPROACH

GLENN L. JOHNSON

SIMULATION RESEARCH is a promising approach for studying the problems of the health care industries, whether the problems occur at project, program, or policy levels. Simulation permits both public and private researchers and decision-makers to better ascertain the consequences of alternative courses of action for solving problems, and it is useful in designing and selecting solutions.

DEFINITION OF SIMULATION. In this chapter we will be dealing with "generalized, computerized, systems-science" simulation.
   Such simulations are not specialized with respect to type or source of data, technique, discipline, or philosophy. They are adapted to utilize modern, high-speed, electronic computers and hence can be referred to as computerized. They also deal with the structure of systems and the activities that go on within such systems; hence the approach of systems scientists is advantageous, and simulations involv-ing their work can be referred to as systems-science simulations. Though systems scientists made their name in the aerospace industry originally, the systems-science approach is applicable to any system including environmental or ecological systems; economic, social, and political systems; and medical and health care delivery systems.

   The two essentials of simulation are that the system represent (or be thought to represent) at least some aspects of a real world system

GLENN L. JOHNSON is Professor of Agricultural Economics, Michigan State University.

Prepared under Michigan State University Agricultural Experiment Station Project No. MICL01079 and under contract with the Department of Health, Ed-ucation and Welfare, Washington, D.C.

200

and that it be capable of operating through time. Examples include ship-testing basins and pilot plants as well as mathematical representations of operating systems such as universities, hospitals, and agricultural sectors. Models also can be expressed in the common language rather than in mathematics and still be representative of real world systems at points of time and through *time*.

PURPOSE OF SIMULATION. When asked the question, Why simulate? the experienced simulator is likely to answer, "Because decisions concerning practical problems are almost always based on knowledge concerning: (1) the structural nature of an existing or newly designed system about which a decision is being made and (2) how it would operate through time." Such an answer indicates that simulation is not a new thing dependent on recent advances in mathematics, various subject-matter disciplines, and computer technology. It recognizes that down through the ages it has been important for decision-makers to understand the structure of the systems they are trying to modify and to envision how the system's behavior would be affected by their decisions. Even before the advent of the written word, it is likely that the family, governmental, and military decision-makers who attained the greatest successes were those who did a superior job of envisioning the system in which they existed—including how it would operate through time if various modifications were made in it.

There is a need to maintain flexibility in modeling the structures and operations of real world systems. Generalized, computerized, systems-science simulation models have been more successful than the more specialized approaches in maintaining the flexibility of traditional projections while exploiting the computation efficiency of the modern electronic computer and utilizing such specialized techniques as linear programming and econometric estimation of parameters of simultaneous equations; thus, part of the answer to the question of Why simulate? is that simulation can maintain the flexibility of the more creditable, traditional ad hoc projections with respect to sources of data, kinds of information, disciplines, and specific techniques without being constrained to specific types and sources of information, specialized techniques, or a single philosophic point of view. Furthermore, simulation can deal with criterion variables that are normative as well as with positive variables without necessarily maximizing or assuming maximization. Like the old seat-of-the-pants projections, simulation can permit creative, inventive, and original interactions with decision-makers.[1]

The generalized, systems-science simulation approach is not to be compared with such specialized techniques as linear programming, simultaneous econometric equations, cost/benefit analysis, input-output analysis, etc. It is not a specialized technique; instead it is an *approach*. As an approach, it utilizes any such specialized technique that may be appropriate; the approach could concentrate entirely on a particular technique or merely model some small component of the system under consideration. In many instances the investigation reveals that it is not advantageous to use certain specialized techniques such as linear programming, simultaneous econometric equations, or cost/benefit computations.

APPLICATION OF SIMULATION. The building of a simulation model is much like building a working model of a ship or airplane. One does not attempt to model the abstract; instead, one models some *thing*. The system involved in the solution of the practical problem of concern is modeled in practical, problem-solving work.

The systems we are interested in modeling and simulating here are medical and health care systems. Which subsystem within the medical and health care industry we should be concerned with is determined by the practical problem with which we wish to work. In some instances we may be concerned with simple models such as the *process* of admitting persons to hospitals, because problems are occurring at that point. In other instances the problems may involve a community health care *project,* so a larger subsystem would have to be modeled. In still other instances the problem may involve medical or health care *programs* involving substantial numbers of projects, in which case still larger subsystems have to be modeled. Or the focus may be on medical and health care *policy* problems. Generally speaking, policy problems involve the operation of very large subsystems of the health care industry involving numerous programs and projects. At this point it is sufficient to make the point that the particular part of reality to be modeled and simulated depends on the practical problem we face. Practical problems are defined in terms of the *value* of conditions, situations, and things being sought and/or avoided in real world situations. Information about values is normative.

1. Readers interested in the details of simulation model construction are referred to simulation models that have been developed for the agricultural economies of Nigeria and Korea (5, 6), which are available in publication form from the Department of Agricultural Economics, Michigan State University, East Lansing.

Normative information accumulates throughout the problem-solving process. At the beginning of a simulation project it is usually not clear what all the relevant values are. As the project progresses and as the model develops, normative information is accumulated as to what is more and what is less important than originally thought; thus the problem and the system to be modeled and simulated change as a simulation study of a problem progresses from beginning to conclusion.

PROCESS. Simulation is an iterative, problem-solving process which involves problem formulation, mathematical modeling, refinement and testing of the resulting model by creative design, and execution of experiments intended to provide answers to the questions posed. We conceptualize the process as shown in Figure 12.1. As the arrows indicate, the general movement of the process is from definition of the problem toward model application, but the reverse arrows indicate that the process is iterative or "learning" in nature. Prior stages often have to be repeated on the basis of feedback information acquired during a subsequent stage. In this manner changes in model structure, parameters, etc. are introduced which lead to a better model. The output of a simulation is a set of system *performance* variables associated with each set of policies and/or strategies.

The first step in solving a practical problem is problem definition. Problems involve failures to attain as much as possible of the conditions, situations, and things that are valued positively and/or encountering more conditions, situations, and things that are valued negatively than is necessary in the existing situation. A problematic situation cannot be fully understood until it is described in nonnormative terms as well as normative terms of what conditions, situations, and things are valued positively and negatively. The situation for which the problem exists must be known before a decision-maker can identify the problem as one for which solutions may be attainable.

The relevant values are both pecuniary and nonpecuniary: the latter involves the values studied in consumption and welfare economics; sociology, psychology, and medicine study both pecuniary and nonpecuniary values. Eventually, selection of the *best* among alternative courses of action as the solution of a problem requires a single normative common denominator among the *goods* and *bads* involved. Interactions between investigators and decision-makers are important in learning about these trade-offs. The long laborious process of learning normatively about these trade-offs cannot be shortened by immediate premature recourse to the maximization computations of economists without paying the costs of irrelevant maximization. Those costs include justifiable rejection of results by decision-makers.

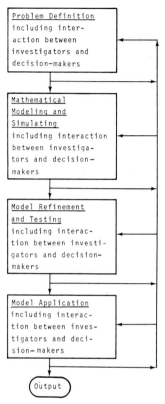

FIG. 12.1. Model formulation as an iterative, problem-investigating process.

It seems inappropriate to regard the simulators as dealing only with the positive or nonnormative while leaving answers to normative questions wholly up to the decision-makers, because: (1) decision-makers help in making normative observations and analyses, and (2) the staff members must know what is important before they can tell what kind of nonnormative information they should use in constructing the simulation model.

After the simulator is given responsibility for helping to solve a defined problem, the second step is to develop a mathematical model capable of simulating the performance of the system through time in response to decisions that may be made concerning projects, programs, and policies to solve the problem.

The third step for the simulator attempting to assist decision-makers is to refine and test his model. In building, refining, and testing the model, it is extremely important for the simulator to have contact with decision-makers. Such contact often permits them to see how the model operates and to point out the shortcomings of the model for the purposes of reaching decisions on the specific problem. Initial simulations of the future consequences of proposed solutions will often result in a redefinition of the problem. Such redefinitions make it necessary to simulate a different system, which in turn makes it necessary to change the mathematical models developed in the second step. Model testing involves application of the usual statistical tests of significance and choices among hypotheses where such tests and choices are appropriate. However, since the simulation approach is a very flexible one using information from a wide variety of sources, the rather specialized, positivistic tests of statisticians are not adequate to handle the subtle questions of validation and verification involved in testing models dealing with the normative as well as the positive and leading eventually to prescriptions to solve problems at hand. Our verification and validation techniques are highly specialized on the positivistic content of our work with little attention to problems of verifying and validating the normative information and prescriptive conclusions. The credibility which a simulation attains, however, depends importantly on the validity and veracity of its normative and prescriptive contents. Before decision-makers will actually use the results of a simulation model in making decisions concerning alternative courses of action, they must have faith in the model. Faith in a simulation model is increased by seeing the model modified to meet objections raised by decision-makers to the model itself. Thus the interaction between simulators and decision-makers is extremely important. Each application of the model becomes a test of the validity and veracity of the model.

In most cases the construction of a simulation model is a multi-disciplinary task. Problems define the system to be modeled, and problems are no respecters of the disciplinary boundaries of university organization charts. Ernest Nesuis, director of the University of Kentucky's Agricultural Extension service, has observed; "Universities have departments; farmers have problems." Attempts to develop simulation models of medical and health care delivery systems are bound to involve far more than economics. In fact, economics is likely to be unable to furnish more than a fraction of the concepts and descriptive information required to simulate that part of a medical and health care delivery system involved in any particular practical problem. The medical discipline itself will be required to furnish substantial amounts of information and concepts concerning the production, utilization, and values of medical and health care services. Engineers and architects may be involved in developing physical facilities important in many health care delivery systems. Sociologists may have important contributions, as will the administrators of hospitals, projects, and programs. Nurses and technicians also may have information, concepts, and ideas to contribute, depending on the problem and the particular subsystem under investigation. It is important to note that typically the information required from many disciplines to model a system cannot be supplied by "interdisciplinarians"—i.e., investigators who purport to know enough about a large number of disciplines to study any particular subsystem found to be relevant to the solution of a particular practical problem. More than superficial knowledge of many different disciplines and areas is usually required; in-depth knowledge of such subjects as the different phases of medicine, pharmacy, economics, civil engineering, hospital architecture, statistics, nursing and biochemistry is necessary. Thus simulation work becomes a multidisciplinary team effort involving substantial (if not always lengthy) contributions from a large number of people with very great competence in their respective disciplines.

Necessary characteristics of the members of a problem-solving team are an interest in working on practical problems and a willingness to join others in cooperative efforts to bring their highly specialized, in-depth knowledge of a particular area to bear on the problem in concert with similar knowledge from equally competent people from other disciplines.

MODEL FOR A HEALTH CARE SYSTEM. In the case of medical and health care delivery problems, the thing to be modeled is the system in which the problem under investigation is located. The medical industry of Michigan's Grand Traverse area has been studied in considerable detail but not enough to develop detailed models of the different subsystems of the medical industry which would be relevant for various problems (1, 2). I will discuss in a very tentative way what would be involved in studying a subsystem of the area's medical industry that would be relevant for solving a particular problem.

Specifying the Problem. The problem with which I will deal is that of an inadequate health care delivery system for aged commercial farmers of the Grand Traverse area. While the residents are not extremely wealthy, they have average incomes for a northern state. The farming of the area is mixed but includes a substantial number of fruit farmers who are well-to-do. The problem of health care for the aged, well-to-do, commercial farmers is mainly one of organizing facilities to serve them and not one of inadequate private resources with which to provide health care during retirement. However, there are other farmers in the poverty class with inadequate resources to provide health care in their old age regardless of how well the health care delivery system is organized to serve the needs of elderly people. The problem then is twofold, involving the development of a superior organization for delivering health care to the rural aged—both those who have adequate resources and those who do not. Thus a rather large subsystem of both well-to-do and poor farmers is involved.

Solving this problem requires organized knowledge of the present as well as knowledge as to how the system would operate over time if modified in various ways. A simulation model for such a system needs to be flexible enough to permit modification to account for and estimate the consequences through time of modifying the system in accordance with possible project, program, and policy decisions resulting from the creative and imaginative efforts to build a better system to care for the area's rural aged.

Existing Situation. An initial step in the simulation process is to examine the components of the subsystem to be modeled. Undoubtedly a careful investigation will indicate the existence of a wide variety of arrangements to care for the aged. A large number of the aged provide their own housing and transportation services and have incomes and resources with which to buy assistance from the area's hospitals, public service agencies, doctors, dentists, and osteopaths. Those well-to-do persons with less physical capacity are in the area's nursing homes and hospital facilities. Also substantial numbers are living with their children. The existing situation includes a relatively high proportion of retired people with the physical capacity to deliver health care services to incapacitated older people. Few of the retired, however, provide health care services to others except on an informal, private basis within families where retired couples look after each other and occasionally a brother or sister looks after his or her brother or sister.

To know the existing situation requires knowledge of the financial reserves of the aged. These reserves take the form of savings accounts, income, paid-up insurance policies, Social Security claims, medicare arrangements, real estate, other real property, and other forms of personal property.

Generally speaking, the Grand Traverse area is a high-wage-rate area with expensive common and skilled labor for looking after the aged. Thus it might be desirable to develop both public and private organizations to facilitate the production of health care services by the aged for the aged. The area presently has no such public facilities. Such organizations should involve both rural and urban aged in order to include a better mix of skills and capacities.

The relevant subsystem also includes the existing public and private agencies that provide medical and health care services to the aged. Generally speaking, the Grand Traverse area is well endowed with hospitals, clinics, and medical practitioners.

There is a substantial number of rest homes, and the hospitals of the area have a rather high proportion of their facilities devoted to geriatrics. To my knowledge there are no "retirement communities" designed to provide a changing pattern of services to persons passing from retirement at age 65 through the remaining years of their lives.

The area is in a rather heavy snow belt in the northern part of Michigan's lower peninsula. In some parts of the region the expected snowfall is more than 100 inches per year. This means substantial transportation problems for isolated, aged, rural residents. Despite this, many persons retire into the area because of the beautiful scenery and the pleasant four seasons which characterize the region. Thus the proportion of aged persons in the region is higher than normal and the problem of providing health care services for them in the winter is greater than in many other regions of the United States. This means that the simulation model will have to be spatially as well as time oriented and that it will have transportation components involving possibly the minimization of transportation costs.

Construction. A simulation model of the part of the Grand Traverse medical industry that serves the rural aged would have to model the existing resources, facilities, populations of the aged, the destination of their health care expenditures, the production of health care services, the provision of medicines, and the provision of equipment and building services. Once a model is constructed, it would have to be examined to ascertain if it has sufficient flexibility to project the consequences of changing the system institutionally, technically, and/or humanistically to better serve the aged. Since the rural aged are not adequately cared for, whether rich or poor, a considerable amount of flexibility will be required to estimate the consequences through time of the various proposals that may be advanced for improving the system. Though not much work has been done systematically on how the present system could be modified, a research effort devoted to modeling and improving the present system would probably lead to a wide range of proposals on the part of creative, imaginative people. These proposals will have to take into account the high wage rates of the area, the area's climate, and the skills and capability of the aged themselves as well as their medical condition and age. Because the skills of the aged are considerable at age 65, innovative problem-solvers are likely to seek ways of utilizing some of these skills, particularly if they are held by the aged poor. Some 65-

year-old persons might like to work for a few years to pile up credits in the system for the years in which they will be unable to work. However, the mixture of skills held by retired commercial farmers and their wives is not adequate to care for the aged. Thus proposals should not be confined to rural residents alone; larger groupings of people are needed with wider ranges of skills. In addition to the cooking, nursing, and handyman skills likely to be prevalent among rural residents, urban skills are needed—those of nurses, lawyers, carpenters, plumbers, electricians, MDs, dentists, eye specialists—along with a wide variety of other skills that can be used to provide facilities and health care services to the aged.

Perceptive problem-solvers studying the problems of the aged in the Grand Traverse area are likely to see the need for new institutional arrangements in which to account for the contributions of the aged to the care of other aged people as well as the need for physical facilities in which it is possible for some of the aged to look after others of the aged.

The Grand Traverse area includes many villages and small communities on excellent all-season roads and highways. Many of these communities need additional industry. Some of them would make excellent locations for new facilities for the aged. Again, inventive problem-solvers are likely to conceive of facilities in addition to but not excluding nursing homes. Some of these small villages and communities have churches, grocery stores, nursing homes, and other facilities providing the services the aged need in a general environment far superior to the urban areas in which many nursing homes are located. One wonders about the possibility of establishing facilities in such communities including separate houses and apartments for the aged as well as clinics and nursing homes for persons requiring supervision, bed care, and eventually complete hospitalization. Such villages and communities could be utilized as retirement communities without being devoted entirely to the aged. Such arrangements would provide a more desirable mix of ages than commonly found in rest homes and could provide a capable older person with productive employment for additional years in providing services not now produced and distributed to the aged. The institutional arrangements would have to involve some sort of central organization or association with (1) a central accounting system, and (2) a system for controlling the utilization of the aged in order to avoid exploitation of some of the aged by the aged and to eliminate the incompetent from the service group.

A model of the system described above would necessarily involve a demographic component for persons from 40 to 95 years of age. Such a distribution of ages would permit the demographic components of the model to make projections 25 years ahead without running out of people below 65 years of age. The demographic components would have to be specific with respect to wealth, incomes, and physical capacities as well as to age. The model would also need components that would deal with the utilization of resources to produce and distribute medical and health care facilities for the aged. These components would have to be built in a flexible, detailed way so they could be modified on the basis of projects, programs, and policies that might be considered to solve the problems of health care for the rural aged of the Grand Traverse area. The model would also have to keep track of monetary flows *from* the people being cared for, from governmental agencies, and from voluntary agencies *to* the suppliers (including some of the aged) of health care services.

DISADVANTAGES OF SIMULATION. One of the first criticisms to be leveled against the simulation approach involves the **GIGO** principle—Garbage In, Garbage Out. Modeling such systems requires a large amount of information and data about the existing structure and how the structure would perform in the future, and poor information produces poor models of existing situations and systems. However, the data and information required to solve a problem do not change as a result of computerizing the computations or of expressing the model systematically in mathematical form. Essentially the same data and information are required for paper-and-pencil, desk calculator projections as are needed to make projections on the computer, provided the same problem and hence the same system is under consideration. The advantage in describing the situation mathematically and running the computations on the computer lies in the greater efficiency of the electronic computer; this efficiency makes it economic to operate the model with various assumptions about the data. If the model is operated with certain variables or parameters at their highest possible value and at their lowest possible value without significantly affecting the results, we can be relatively confident our information about the variable or parameter has sufficient accuracy. On the other hand, variables thought to be reliable may prove unreliable when the model is operated with them inserted at their highest and lowest possible values. This process of investigating the consequences of inaccuracies in data is referred to as sensitivity analysis. Sensitivity analysis tells us a great deal about the adequacy of our knowledge and where we need to improve our data. With paper-and-pencil projections it is simply not practical to carry out sensitivity analysis because of the high costs of computations.

Another question about the simulation approach arises when

simulation models are used to project the consequences of institutional, technological, and humanistic innovations that have never been used in the past and for which there is no relevant history to use in validating and verifying the model and its projections. The tests for the validity of such models are: (1) logical consistency, (2) consistency with such related experiences as we have had in the past with similar components of the model, and (3) clarity. Models must be definite and clearly enough stated to be understandable for decision-makers using them before they will be regarded as valid. The first real empirical test of any newly designed system occurs when it is used to solve the problem for which it was designed. At that time the model and its projections pass or flunk the pragmatic *test of workability*.

The more general question of validation and verification is further complicated by differences in the philosophical underpinnings of various builders and users. For instance a positivistic modeler or user believes that only the nonnormative content of the model can be validated or verified; he believes metaphysically that it is impossible to verify the normative content of the model and the prescriptions to which the model may lead, since prescriptions are based on the normative as well as the nonnormative or positivistic content of the model. By contrast, pragmatists (of which there are many in colleges of education and in institutional economics) hold metaphysically that normative and positive knowledge do not exist independently of each other; thus pragmatists reject the possibility of independent validation or verification of either the normative or positive content of the model and concentrate almost entirely on validating or verifying the prescriptive content. To the pragmatist the most important test for validating or verifying a prescription is the test of workability. It is when the model is used to produce a prescription which is then applied that the model is judged for validity. Validation by the test of workability occurs problem by problem, because both the normative and positive concepts that go into the model are presumed dependent on each other within the context of the problem under investigation. Simulation models used in a problem-solving context should not be constrained by the metaphysical presuppositions of different philosophies.

Because general, computerized, systems-science simulation models are quantitative, questions are often raised about how nonquantifiable information can be used in them. This question is not as serious as it appears to be. Not all quantification must be cardinal—some of it can be ordinal. Still other forms of quantification involve no more than counting the occurrences of certain events, which may or may not be quantitative. A situation that often arises occurs when someone such as a sociologist, psychologist, or political scientist says that there is *something* in the environment that defies quantitative simulation in the sense of being measurable cardinally or ordinally, or even count-able. My own experience in such situations leads me to conclude that if the person raising the objection really knows something about that something, it can be incorporated in a quantified simulation model; however, it must be admitted that a quantified model cannot handle that which the psychologist, political scientist, or sociologist *does not know* but only asserts *may* exist.

Simulation models are flexible with respect to sources of informa-tion and specific techniques. One component of the model may employ a specialized technique such as recursive linear programming; another may be an input/output analysis, a third a complicated factorial analysis, a fourth a cost/benefit analysis, and a fifth a spec-tral analysis. However, many of the components will be simple, con-sisting of strings of differential questions collapsible into single equa-tions linked to other equations through various "accounting" identi-ties. Because such flexible overall simulation models containing such a wide variety of components become large and complex, they are not easy to describe in the tidy, elegant ways used for specialized compo-nents involving, say, recursive linear programming or systems of simul-taneous equations with probabilistic parameters estimated by well-known econometric techniques from time series data. Users of such general simulation models must recognize that the advantage of having flexibility with respect to types of information and research techniques involves the cost of greater complexity.

Another problem is that general, computerized, systems-science simulation suffers from and is often "tarred" with the brush of the credibility gap which has developed among decision-makers and ad-ministrators as a result of their experiences with inappropriately used, more specialized models. Among the specialized models inappropri-ately used by researchers and decision-makers are models involving systems of simultaneous equations with parameters probabilistically estimated from time series data. Other types of specialized models that have developed credibility gaps with decision-makers and administra-tors are: (1) linear programming models that maximize prematurely, (2) input/output analyses that ignore relevant details within sub-sectors of the economy, (3) cost/benefit ratios that assume common denominators among "goods" being sought and "bads" being avoid-ed when such common denominators do not exist, and (4) oversimpli-fied models of agricultural development concentrating on such single factors as land tenure, education, creation of human capital, tech-nological advance, underemployment, and distribution of resource ownership. Much of the overspecialization on research techniques re-sults from attempts to handle practical problems with the concepts and techniques of a single discipline rather than recognizing that practical problems require information and techniques from many different disciplines for their solutions. Simulators have to avoid specialization by discipline, technique, and philosophy if they are to escape the justifiable complaints leveled at specialized studies.

CHAPTER THIRTEEN

AN ANALYTICAL MODEL FOR MULTICOUNTY HEALTH PLANNING AREAS

MARVIN R. DUNCAN

REPORTED IN THIS chapter is a linear programming application to planning for hospital services delivery, developed as part of a project in which the Center for Agricultural and Rural Development, Iowa State University, provided research support to an Iowa multicounty health planning council. The council's need was for an analytic tool to support the decision-making process relative to formal proposals the council had received from hospitals that wanted to change service capability and capacity.

Linear programming techniques have been applied to support decision-making in other settings, and several researchers have used them to examine aspects of health care systems. Feldstein used the technique to study health resource allocations in developing countries (6). Gurfield applied the techniques to eliminate bottlenecks and determine staffing patterns (8). Revelle and Feldmann used linear programming to balance tuberculosis control activities in developing countries (19). Navarro discussed the application of systems analysis to planning health services delivery (14). Dowling used a linear programming approach to investigate the form and specification of hospital production functions (5). Feldstein applied the technique to planning for an optimum mix of hospital cases (7). But researchers have not applied programming techniques to situations in which

MARVIN R. DUNCAN is an agricultural economist with the Kansas City Federal Reserve Bank.

The research this chapter reports was done while the author was a research associate with the Center for Agricultural and Rural Development, Iowa State University. The author gratefully acknowledges the assistance and counsel of Robert W. Crown, Farm and Rural Development Division, Agriculture Canada, Ottawa.

hospitals are already in place and where planners need to make decisions or marginal changes in capacity, which is precisely what health planning councils are asked to do. Important decisions on capacity and access changes in the hospital services structure are currently being made with a minimum of objective data or without knowing how those decisions affect other hospitals in the planning area. Use of a linear programming model in such situations can provide very important and useful information for area health planners.

UTILIZATION AND COST. A characteristic phenomenon plaguing hospitals in nonmetropolitan America is underutilization of facilities. In other words, more hospital beds have been constructed than the present population can utilize fully enough to approach the minimum point on a hospital's cost curve. In 1971 average occupancy in non-SMSA (Standard Metropolitan Statistical Area) hospitals was 71.1 percent compared to 79.4 percent for hospitals located in SMSAs (18). The true measure of excess capacity may be masked with what some researchers suggest is a tendency for *supply* to create its own *demand*.[1]

Empty hospital beds cost about two-thirds as much to maintain as full hospital beds. A high fixed cost is evidenced. In the 10-county North Iowa Health Planning Area, for example, there were 760 acute care hospital beds utilized at an occupancy rate of 65 percent in 1972. Since then an additional 90 acute care hospital beds have been planned for construction. With no viable means for attracting new patients from outside the planning area and prospects poor for a significant increase in the area's population, the unavoidable conclusion is that utilization rates will fall when the additional beds are placed in service. This is in addition to a trend toward shorter hospital stays, resulting in part from professional accountability in hospital utilization, which in itself tends to reduce occupancy rates. The trend toward shorter average lengths of stay is evidenced nationally by an increase in the turnover rate (number of annual admissions per bed) of 18.8 in 1967 to 23.3 in 1971 for all hospitals (18).

Hospital administration consultants recommend minimum occupancy rates of 75 percent for smaller hospitals and 85 percent for larger hospitals. At these rates the $54,000 cost per new hospital bed can be amortized without unduly affecting the per patient-day cost of hospital care (11).

1. Newell has suggested that "the supply of beds itself modifies demand. In an area with few beds, the patients, practitioners, and consultants are accustomed to few admissions and short durations of stay. In an area with many beds, the 'threshold' of admissions may be lower and cases who have passed over that threshold may be retained for longer than necessary" (15).

The health care industry is experiencing rapid cost escalation relative to the cost rises for goods included in the consumer price index. In 1950 total health care expenditures in the United States were $12 billion or $78 per capita. This represented 4.6 percent of the gross national product (13). By 1972 costs had risen to $83.4 billion, or $394 per capita, representing 7.6 percent of the gross national product (17). Hospital per diem costs rose at an annual rate of 6.9 percent from 1960 to 1965 and 13.9 percent from 1966 to 1970. Estimates of expected cost escalation from 1970 to 1974 range up to 20 percent. Hospitals in the North Iowa Health Planning Area experienced a 25–30 percent increase from 1972 to 1974 alone.

HEALTH PLANNING LEGISLATION. A federal-state partnership in planning health care delivery was formed under the Comprehensive Health Planning and Public Health Services Act of 1966 and the Partnership for Health Amendments of 1967 (3). At state and substate levels health planning councils (three-fourths federally and one-fourth state funded) were created and were to have 51 percent consumer representation.

Section 1122 of the Social Security Amendment of 1972 and subsequent amendments in 1973 sharply strengthened the review authority of state and substate level health planning councils (2). The federal legislation required that all capital expenditures planned by health providers which (1) involved an excess of $100,000, (2) changed the total bed capacity, or (3) resulted in substantial change in service in which federal reimbursements were anticipated for depreciation and interest (such as medicare, medicaid, and maternal and child health payments) fall under such review procedures. Hill-Burton applications also required such a review. (In Iowa, for example, a minimum of 40–45 percent of any acute care hospital's patients involve some federal reimbursement.) Though a negative recommendation could not stop a building project, it could prevent the institution from receiving federal reimbursement for interest and depreciation. Implicit in the legislation is the need to investigate the cost effectiveness of proposed changes in health care delivery.

Iowa's Experience. Iowa's experience in developing procedures to implement federal health planning legislation is typical of most states. The Iowa Office of Comprehensive Health Planning established, as a result of federal legislation, minimum levels of utilization guidelines (16). These vary from a low of 40 percent for a five-bed hospital[2] to 90 percent for hospitals at or greater than 130-bed size. Such a range of minimum utilization levels takes into account the need to accommodate unexpectedly high levels of utilization, such as might result from an influenza outbreak, while at the same time assuring efficient levels of utilization of any new hospital bed construction. Similar minimum-use-level policies are in effect or being considered by health planning bodies across the nation. These minimum occupancy levels follow from an assumption that the demand for hospital services takes the shape of a Poisson distribution[3] (20). Though the assumption may not be tenable for a given hospital, it is commonly used by hospital industry groups and may be applicable for an entire planning region (12).

Decision-Making Setting. Health planning councils at state and sub-state levels are faced with numerous proposals for building and remodeling projects. Each proposal is stated in terms and data most favorable to its own purpose. Supporting analysis, if any, for these projects is often a micro type of analysis and is related only to the effects of the projected changes on the institution presenting the proposal. Furthermore, certain expansive liberties are commonly taken in estimating potential trade areas and effective demand for the proposed services. Frequently, conflicting proposals by competing institutions are presented to the health planning councils. A high degree of political sensitivity is involved in the decisions made by the health planning councils.

The councils must make decisions within a planning framework. The objective function they wish to maximize is a complex one. The effect of changes in one part of the hospital care system on other hospitals in the area and on accessibility to services must be weighed. Councils are not afforded the luxury of deciding where to approve new services as though none presently existed; decisions must be made within a framework in which substantial previous capital investment has taken place in health care facilities. Trade patterns and community habits have adapted over the years to the existing facility capabilities, or perhaps the existing facility capabilities have adapted to trade patterns and community habits. These facilities will not disap-

2. In practice a five-bed hospital would be extremely rare, although a clinic with five inpatient beds would come under the requirements of minimum utilization levels.
3. The Poisson distribution is a discrete frequency distribution of the number of times a rare event occurs:

$$f(x) = \frac{e^{-\lambda}\lambda^x}{x!} \text{ where } \lambda > 0; \ x = 0, 1, 2 \ldots.$$

pear because a new facility is approved or even built; unneeded facilities can only be phased out over a long planning horizon. Capital recapture and physical, use, and locational obsolescence must occur before such facilities, even though severely underutilized, can be phased out of use. Additionally, proposals presented are more usually in support of an addition to or change in service capability of an existing institution.

The questions to which the health planning councils must have answers are:

1. What effect will changes in service capability in one hospital have on the utilization of not only that facility but other facilities in the area?

2. What effect will relaxing or tightening manpower constraints on part or all of the hospital system have on utilization in any hospital or subset of hospitals in the planning area?

3. What effect will such changes have on the cost of a patient-day of care (transportation included) or on the total cost of delivering hospital care in the area?

4. What changes can be made in existing facility service capabilities to minimize the per patient-day cost to area residents—subject to a variety of access constraints?

PROGRAMMING MODEL. The model develops an optimal cost-minimizing solution by allocating patient-days of service demand to the hospitals in such a way that the summation of patient-day service costs and transportation costs is minimized. Trade-offs in patient allocation, resource use, and cost levels are explored. The model deals with marginal redistribution of service utilization among five major services extended by hospitals in a geographic planning area: (1) medical-surgical, (2) obstetrics, (3) pediatrics, (4) intensive care, and (5) psychiatric. Not every hospital would necessarily have all five services. Figure 13.1 illustrates the linkages among hospitals, services, and population by age category.

Components. The model is composed of a set of production activities (hospital services) and patient-day demand-generating activities for each of the 35 service demand sectors (geographical subareas). These are linked together by a transportation matrix that moves patient-days of service demanded to the appropriate service in a hospital in such a way as to minimize the value of the objective function (cost of service delivery and transportation).

To be of maximum usefulness to health planning councils, it was

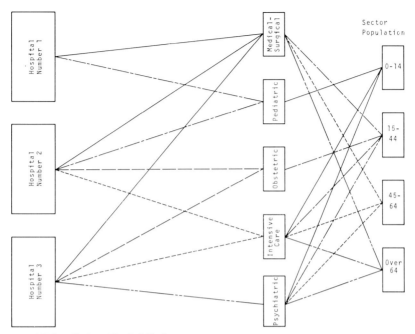

FIG. 13.1. Model linkages.

necessary to develop a technique that was parsimonious in its data requirements and could use available data (data are from one time period). If cross-section data could provide a sufficient base for reliable analysis, the task of data collection and analysis would be substantially lightened. This model assumed the adequacy of cross-section data.

Data requirements had to be limited to those available from hospital administrators and public sources, and overall operating costs of such a model needed to be modest.

Data Needs. Two major classes of data were developed: one class related to the utilization of hospital services and the origin of patients utilizing those services; the other related to the service capability, resource base of hospitals, and the cost of providing that service. Data for input into the programming model were collected by survey form from each hospital in the planning region. Data requested were readily available in hospital records and financial reports.

UTILIZATION. Utilization measured by patient-days of service extended in each of the five service categories for a fiscal year was collected. Utilization was further classified within each service by age categories. In the model these age categories were: 0–14, 15–44, 45–64, and over 64. When cross-sectional utilization data did not adequately represent recent historical patterns, data were gathered for each hospital for the previous three fiscal years. Average lengths of stay in each service for each hospital were collected, as were maximum potential patient-days of each service (beds in service × 365).

PATIENT ORIGIN. Patient origin data were collected from each hospital indicating the town from which each patient had come and the number of patients originating from each town. The data were available from admission records or community relations departments of hospitals.

RESOURCE REQUIREMENTS. Full-time equivalents of human resources available to each hospital were collected by the following categories:

1. General practitioners (including family practice specialty)
2. Specialists (medical doctors and doctors of osteopathy having a recognized medical specialty and being either board-qualified or board-approved). These first two categories included all physicians having active staff relationship to hospitals. Consultants were not included.
3. Registered nurses (including all staff personnel who were RNs)
4. An LPN category (licensed practical nurses, nurse's aides, and orderlies)
5. Specialized medical personnel (all those not previously categorized who had medically oriented specialties such as anesthetist, pharmacist, radiology technologist, medical technologist, speech pathologist)
6. Other personnel (all other employees of each hospital such as clerical, housekeeping, janitorial, administrative)

HOSPITAL COST. A survey form was developed to collect hospital cost data in which data were categorized by service subcategories that could be assigned in whole or on a proportionate use basis to one of the five major service categories. Expense in each service subcategory was disaggregated by salaries, supplies, fees, and miscellaneous or other. Thirty-two service subcategories were identified. These included such items as operating room, anesthesiology, laboratory. Fiscal services expense including administration, depreciation, debt servicing, and equipment rentals were identified and allocated to services on the basis of utilization as fixed and administrative expenses. The total cost assigned to each major service category provided by the hospital was then divided by the total patient-days of utilization of that service to identify a patient-day cost for each service in each hospital.

ASSUMPTIONS. Our experience in data gathering using the described format was that hospital administrators were able to provide data in the format requested and to indicate the service cost subcategories attributable to delivery of a given service. Thus, within the data set developed, reliable comparability of data among hospitals was achieved.

Certain assumptions were made in constructing the model.

1. Cross-section data reasonably represented patient origin patterns and utilization rates for each hospital, not only for the year for which it was collected but also over recent past and future time periods.

2. The cost data collected fairly represented both absolute patient-day cost for a hospital service and one hospital's costs relative to the same service in other hospitals in the area.

3. The cost of a patient-day of care was adequately reflected by the cost allocated by the hospital and a transportation cost that was a function of distance and elapsed travel time both for the patient and for family and friends visiting patients.

4. Individuals electing to seek hospital care made their selection of the hospital providing the needed service based on an effort to minimize the summation of hospital incurred cost per patient-day and transportation costs. Both costs were composed of additive parts and were together additive. Careful interpretation of program results and some relaxing of the assumption were in fact necessary.

5. For changes in utilization of a hospital service within rather broad ranges, the resource demand coefficients for service production were invariant. This was not unreasonable, since manpower numbers were usually adjusted to permit efficient utilization of such manpower.

6. Average demand for services coefficients by age cohort for the planning areas equally well represented patient demand for services of age cohorts within each demand sector in the planning area.

7. Travel distance for every patient-day of service in a demand sector was calculated from a central point in the sector, i.e., a central city.

8. The planning area was essentially a closed system, with as many persons leaving the area for service as coming into the area for service. Therefore, excess capacity in a hospital in the model could have been filled only by patient demand presently being serviced at another area hospital. This assumption could have been easily relaxed by adding a set of service activities to represent a composite of

all out-of-region hospital services. Further, demand sectors could have been created for out-of-region areas that generated patient demand for in-region hospital services.

Formulation. The linear programming model developed for a multi-county health planning council in northern Iowa could quite easily have been adapted to more hospital services, more or fewer demand sectors, and a different sized transportation matrix (9, 10). The model incorporated an interhospital service comparative advantage production sector, a transportation network, and 35 service demand sectors subdivided by age grouping into 140 service demand activities generating hospital services demand. Production costs, transportation costs, and hospital services demand represented that experienced in the year 1972.

COST MINIMIZATION. The programming model minimized the cost of satisfying hospital service demand and transporting that demand from a demand sector[4] to the hospital service at which the demand was satisfied (i.e., where the patient received care). This model had 38 hospital service activities tied to service demand-generating activities[5] by 551 transportation activities.

HOSPITAL SERVICES. Each hospital service related to 3–6 demand sector activities. Each demand sector was linked via a transportation activity to every hospital service that data indicated it had related to or logically could have been expected to relate to.

Demand for hospital service was for a specific service rather than simply for services of a hospital. Logically defensible, this approach meant that patients did not go to a hospital for services that hospital did not deliver. Consider that patients may have demanded medical-surgical services from a hospital that did not deliver obstetrics service and demanded from another hospital obstetrics services. A further refinement of this reasoning might have resulted in services being defined as to whether they were of a primary, secondary, or tertiary care level. For example, a given hospital might have delivered primary level care in medical-surgical services and also delivered secondary level care. Thus that hospital would have had two medical-surgical services activities differentiated as to service level. Although the model did not utilize this particular refinement, it could have been added.

4. The demand sectors were geographic units constructed from subcounty census reporting districts.
5. Service demand-generating activities were column vectors that created patient-days of service demand based on both the population of the age category in the activity and the coefficients that indicated patient-days of each service demanded per person in the age category.

PATIENT DEMAND SECTORS. Patient demand sectors consisted of multiples of subcounty census reporting districts. In Iowa these contained only one township. In many other states they were composed of from two to many townships. Demand sectors were built of subcounty census reporting districts that had these characteristics:

1. People uniformly related to one or more hospitals for satisfaction of hospital services demand as evidenced by hospital utilization data
2. A demand sector tied together by a transportation network
3. A demand sector with a central city
4. Demand sectors constructed of contiguous subcounty census reporting districts

Based on these criteria, demand sectors were of different geographic sizes and different population sizes. Figure 13.2 illustrates demand sectors identified for the North Iowa model.

DEMAND ACTIVITIES. Each of the 35 demand sectors generated four service demand activities.[6] These were segmented by age: activity 1 comprised the 0–14 age population, activity 2 the 15–44 population, activity 3 the 45–64 population, and activity 4 the over-64 population of that demand sector.

Each demand activity had a fixed bound or limit at the level of the population of that age category in the demand sector. Patient-days of demand for each of the five hospital services were derived from demand activities. The volume of patient-days of demand was determined by the size of patient demand-generating coefficients in the demand activity.

DEMAND COEFFICIENTS. Coefficients were developed for each of the services demanded. The model used coefficients defined by dividing the patient-days of a service utilized by an age category by the total population of that age category within the planning region:

$$d_{ij} = S_{ij}/P_j$$

where: d_{ij} = demand coefficient for service i from age category j;
S_{ij} = patient-days of service i utilized by age category j;
P_j = planning region population of age category j.

6. It is important to remember that the hospital service activities provided services to patients, and service demand activities generated patient-days of demand that utilized those hospital services provided.

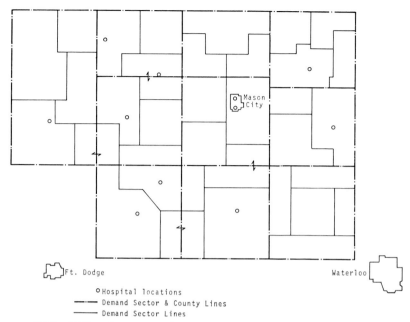

FIG. 13.2. Consumer demand sectors in the North Iowa Health Planning Area.

Not all services were demanded by each age grouping. For example pediatrics were demanded only by activity 1; obstetrics services were demanded only by activity 2. The demand coefficient for obstetric services in that category reflects only the demand by females of course.

Refinements in patient demand-generating coefficients could have been achieved through use of time series data and regression techniques. Use of coefficients generated in that way could have been readily incorporated into the model. Coefficients developed for an entire state or multistate region from time series data or cross-section data might have had more validity than those developed from cross-section data from only one planning area. Unfortunately data gaps difficult to resolve were confronted when attempting to secure such state or regional data.[7] Consequently cross-section coefficients for the planning area in question were a reasonable approximation of those that could have been developed using more sophisticated techniques.

7. Third-party payers of hospital costs had such data but were reluctant to release it to researchers. A few data-processing firms could have developed approximations of uncertain reliability but at a relatively high cost. Unfortunately the American Hospital Association did not have data from which such coefficients could be developed.

TRANSPORTATION NETWORK. Transportation activities were defined in
the row section of the programming model as equality rows. Thus
every patient-day of demand that entered a transportation activity
was transported to the hospital services activity related to that transportation activity for service demand satisfaction. No patient-days of
demand could get lost in the transportation matrix.

Statement. The model had 279 rows and 1,089 real variables; those
real variables were hospital service provision, transportation, and
demand-generating activities. The model, though of considerable
size, solved quickly and inexpensively.

Figure 13.3 contains an abbreviated picture of the linear programming matrix. The interested reader could trace patient-days of demand through the model from demand-generating activities through
the transportation network to the hospital service that provided care
for the patient-days of demand.

The model was a cost minimization model where the cost minimized was a summation of patient-day costs and transportation costs
(1). Algebraically the objective was to find a set of Xs such that
$f(c) = cX$ was a minimum subject to these restraints:

$$AX \leqq b; \ X \geqq 0$$

where: c = objective function value;
    X = column vector of hospital services, transportation, and
        demand-generating activities;
    A = matrix of transformation coefficients;
    b = column vector of resource restraints.

TRANSFORMATION COEFFICIENTS. The resources used to produce hospital services were those human resources previously identified.

The transformation coefficients for a hospital were determined on
the basis of resources used in that hospital to produce hospital services.
Since competition was among services of different hospitals and not
within a hospital, characteristically each service competing for a unit
of patient demand would have had a different set of transformation
coefficients. Here one might have inserted engineering coefficients if
a new facility were contemplated and its impact on existing facilities
were to be determined. Hospital service activities were upper bound-
ed at the maximum patient-day capacity of the service.

Objective Function

PATIENT-DAY COST. The objective function for a hospital service was
the patient-day cost of delivering that service at the level of utilization of the service during the relevant data period. Patient-day

	Hospital Services Activities								Transportation Activities								Demand-Generating Activities					
	MS0001	PED001	OB0001	MS0010	PED010	OB0010	IC0010	PSYC10	MS00101	PED0101	OB00101	MS00110	PED0110	OB00110	IC00110	PSYC110	0101 AGE	0201 AGE	0301 AGE	0401 AGE	
GP001	X	X	X																		≤ b
SP001	X	X	X																		≤ b
RN001	X	X	X																		≤ b
LPN01	X	X	X																		≤ b
MPS01	X	X	X																		≤ b
OPS01	X	X	X																		≤ b
GP010				X	X	X	X	X													≤ b
SP010				X	X	X	X	X													≤ b
RN010				X	X	X	X	X													≤ b
LPN10				X	X	X	X	X													≤ b
MPS10				X	X	X	X	X													≤ b
OPS10				X	X	X	X	X													≤ b
MS0001	-1								1												=
PED001		-1								1											=
OB0001			-1								1										=
MS0010				-1								1									=
PED010					-1								1								=
OB0010						-1								1							=
IC0010							-1								1						=
PSYC10								-1								1					=
MS00R01									-1			-1					X	X	X		=
PEDOR01										-1			-1				X				=
OBOOR01											-1			-1				X			=
IC00R01															-1		X	X	X	X	=
PSYCR01																-1	X	X	X	X	=
Bounds	Up	Up	Up	Up	Up	Up	Up	Up									Fx	Fx	Fx	Fx	
Obj. fctn.	X	X	X	X	X	X	X	X	X	X	X	X	X	X	X	X					N

FIG. 13.3. *Programming tableau. The columns represent model activities: hospital services, transportation, and demand-generating functions (MS, medical-surgical; PED, pediatric; OB, obstetric; IC, intensive care; PSYC, psychiatric). Service activities from two hospitals are represented; for example, MS0001 is medical-surgical from hospital 1, and MS0010 is from hospital 10. Transportation activities transfer patient-days of service demand from demand-generating activities to hospital services; for example, MS00101 transfers demand from demand sector 1 to hospital 1. Each demand sector has four demand-generating activities categorized by age; for example, AGE0101 generates demand from the 0–14 age group for pediatrics, intensive care, and psychiatric services. Rows GP001 through OPS01 are human resources available to hospital 1; GP010 through OPS10 are human resources available to hospital 10. Resources are in terms of man-years (GP, general practitioners; SP, medical specialists; RN, registered nurses; LPN, licensed practical nurses, nurse's aides, and orderlies; MPS, medically oriented specialties such as laboratory technicians; and OPS, all other personnel ranging from housekeeping to administrative duties). Rows MS001 through PSYC10 are transfer rows related to hospital services activities. Rows MS00R01 through PSYCR01 are transfer rows related to demand-generating activities in demand sector 1.*

cost was a summation of professional salaries, supplies, fees, miscellany, and administrative and fixed expense used in a particular hospital to deliver the historical level of patient-days of the service under consideration.

Cost subcategories were assigned to a service or prorated among services based on utilization, as was the administrative and fixed cost subcategory. The patient-day cost was based on utilization during the data period. Hospital administrators with whom we had consulted supported the methodology used in determining patient-day costs by service. Since the model was primarily concerned with marginal changes in utilization, the assumption of constant patient-day costs over a limited range of utilization was not unreasonable.

TRANSPORTATION COST. Transportation activities contributed to the objective function whenever the level of movement in any given activity was greater than zero. Transportation cost was determined to be a function of time and distance for the patient demanding hospital services as well as time and distance for persons who visited the patient in the hospital:

$$TC = F_1\ (T_1) + F_2\ (D_1) + F_3\ (T_2) + F_4\ (D_2)$$

where: TC = transportation cost;
T_1 = time expended by patient in round trip to hospital of choice;
D_1 = distance traveled by patient in round trip to hospital of choice;
T_2 = time expended by visitors traveling round trip to hospital;
D_2 = distance traveled by those visiting hospital patient.[8]

The equation used to determine transportation costs for each transportation activity was:

$$TC = [(2D/45) \times 2.10]/ALS + 2CD/ALS + [(2D/45) \times 1.79E \times 2.10]$$
$$+ (1.79C \times 2D)$$

where: TC = transportation cost, objective function for the activity;
ALS = average length of stay in a particular hospital service;

8. F_1 (T_1) was the round-trip distance to the hospital service used divided by an average speed of travel times a time charge (federal minimum wage) and divided by average length of stay in the hospital service. F_2 (D_1) was the round-trip distance times a mileage charge and divided by the average length of stay in the hospital service. F_3 (T_2) was round-trip distance to the hospital divided by an average speed of travel times number of visits per day times number of visitors per visit times a time charge. F_4 (D_2) was round-trip distance times number of visits per inpatient day times a mileage charge.

$D =$ miles from demand sector to hospital service;

$E =$ number of visitors per visitor trip;

$45 =$ miles per hour speed (assumed to be reasonable for the planning area);

$1.79 =$ patient visits per inpatient day verified by consultation with panel of experts;

$C =$ cost per mile for transportation (15¢);

$\$2.10 =$ federal minimum wage.

INSTITUTIONAL CONSTRAINTS. It was recognized that certain institutional constraints inhibited the movement of patient demand to the service offering least cost satisfaction. Such constraints included the hospital service preference of the admitting physician (based on his preference function and very important in determining utilization patterns), the patient's subjective evaluation of service quality in a hospital relative to quality in other hospital services in the planning area, and trade patterns for other goods and services. Since such institutional constraints could not be accurately specified, the hospital service activities were constrained to fall within 70–130 percent of historical utilization patterns. Historical utilization patterns were assumed to reflect such institutional constraints in addition to patient-day cost of the service and transportation costs.

MODEL OUTPUT. The model, then, allocated differentiated patient demand to appropriate hospital services through a transportation network. The allocation was a cost-minimizing decision subject to hospital resource constraints and service capacity. All demand generated in the model had to be satisfied by a hospital service.

Output of the programming model was used to provide data for the location of hospital service demand satisfaction. Various changes in service capacity, manpower constraints, demand sector population, and demand coefficients were imposed on the model to determine the costs of providing hospital services in a planning region under different utilization patterns. Trade-offs in utilization levels among hospital services were determined. Shadow prices on limiting resources and capacities were developed in the model solution.

Results. The model was useful in answering a number of questions. In the North Iowa Health Planning Area it was used to determine the impact on the area's hospital utilization patterns of consecutive decreases in manpower availability in area hospitals. As the manpower resource constraint was tightened in a hospital, the redistribution of patient-days of service demand among the remaining hospitals was determined. The impact on utilization patterns in the area hospitals resulting from deletion of a service capability in a particular hospital or deletion of an entire hospital was tested. Population projections were incorporated into the model, enabling planners to determine probable utilization patterns in area hospitals at some future point in time. Changes in patient-day cost resulting from new construction were also incorporated into the model objective function, as could have been changes in transportation costs.

The complete model could have been used to simulate the effects on the hospital services system of various changes in costs, resource use coefficients, resource and capacity constraints, and population changes or demand coefficient changes. Planners could have adjusted demand coefficients to reflect a lack of transportation or inability to pay for health care services. The probable impact on part or all of the area hospital services system could have been observed.

The model was constructed to utilize readily available data and provide problem solution inexpensively. It was devised for use by multicounty health planning groups, but with some adaptation it could be used at a multiplanning area or statewide level.

As with all programming models, care was necessary in interpretation of model results in order not to exceed the validity of the data on which the model depended. For the limited (albeit highly useful) objectives established for this model, solution results appeared to be valid within the context of the model objectives. Planning groups using this model would need to rely on professional persons to assist in generating the model and in the interpretation of model solutions.

CHAPTER FOURTEEN

INTRODUCTION OF HEALTH CARE SYSTEMS TO RURAL COMMUNITIES

ARTHUR D. NELSON, MD

WE CAN POINT with pride to the excellent medical centers in our cities and their suburbs, but unfortunately modern medicine is less available and accessible to those who live in rural America. Almost by definition, "cottage" industries prevail in rural areas, and the health delivery system is no exception. Most often this situation stems from inadequate concentration of population to support institutions of the size and complexity required to deliver a full range of services. Manpower is a part of this deficiency. Senator Edward Kennedy has said:

> One of the most difficult and intransigent problems in America's health care crisis is that of attracting health professionals into rural . . . areas of our nation. For decades, health care professionals have increasingly gravitated toward urban centers and the surrounding suburbs. . . . The result is that more and more rural communities have no physicians at all, and thousands of rural communities have critical shortages of health manpower (11).

In fact, 140 counties do not have a single doctor.

In reminding physicians of their responsibilities, Dr. Merlin K. DuVal, former Assistant Secretary of Health, Education and Welfare (HEW), has said:

> We are living in a society that has chosen to declare certain rights for itself; having provided most of the resources that helped make us successful, society has now enunciated its own expectations in the field of health. The challenge is to solve the inequitable distribution of health services in such a way that the rights of both the patient and the physician can be respected and accommodated (3).

ARTHUR D. NELSON, MD, is director, Family Practice Center, Scottsdale Memorial Hospital, Scottsdale, Arizona.

Some people ascribe our problems to a surfeit of success. We have done so well as to raise society's expectations above our capacity to deliver. Dr. DuVal explains rural shortages by arguing that the concentration of physicians and resources in urban and suburban settings is merely the result of freedom of choice exercised by physicians and health care institutions. This is the same freedom of choice that has resulted in the remarkable progress in medical care and the development of the outstanding capabilities we have. Unfortunately, despite the fact that nationally we are placing heavy bets on enlarging medical schools, there is no evidence to suggest that producing more physicians or even creating more facilities could change this present imbalance.

The so-called voluntary nonprofit system has generally failed to improve the distribution picture. Although many rural villages and towns have mustered funds to create clinics or small hospitals as free-standing isolated entities, such units tend to be low in quality or efficiency (24). Some lie fallow for lack of manpower.

Those rural citizens who suffer most are ethnic groups, the poor (4), migrant workers, and the aged, who not only require more service (1) but have difficulty gaining access to sources of care. Rural families tend to have a lower average level of education and may not appreciate the need for early and adequate care (2). They also tend to have less health insurance than their urban counterparts.

Our federal health establishment has usually taken the categorical approach to solving perceived health problems in the nation. We have programs for migrant farm workers and for children and mothers; we have programs for heart disease, cancer, and stroke. We support comprehensive health planning and services, and through PL 89-749 we support neighborhood health centers and networks. In fact, we could go on for some time listing other categorical activities. However, as former Secretary of HEW Finch has said, "[Categorical programs] now threaten entirely the basic reasons for most of the programs: the delivery of services" (5).

Financing mechanisms have also failed to enhance the development of rural health delivery resources. Blue Cross and Blue Shield and private insurance have been operational for decades. More recently medicare and medicaid have emerged. None of these third-party payment mechanisms nor the direct payment fee-for-service approach has resulted in any stampede of physicians or hospitals to areas of deprivation and need. The happy expectations we had for medicaid have not come to fruition. Based on our experience since 1966, it is patently clear that the infusion of large amounts of money into an inelastic and relatively inexpansible system results in increased costs, not more care. In 1970 the nation spent $63 billion for health care, and millions of people were underserved. The figure rose to $75 billion in 1971—7.4 percent of the GNP—and millions were underserved. The figure for 1975 exceeded $104 billion, with millions of citizens still underserved. Thus money alone is not the answer to the problem of maldistribution of health delivery services.

How we spend money is as important as how much money is spent. For example, medicare and medicaid and, in many instances, Blue Cross reimburse institutions at cost. This approach does nothing to encourage management efficiency. Rather it deprives institutions of surplus or profit with which to maintain, expand, or improve their services. In many instances also it fosters the use of the most expensive modalities of care, namely hospitals, rather than the less costly but not covered ambulatory care.

PRIMARY CARE. In rural areas access to the system is the greatest problem of all. Citizens sorely miss the genial country doctor who used to provide for their primary needs. Where has he gone? Why has he not been replaced? What can be done about it? These are issues that cannot be answered easily, but some significant features of the problem can be outlined.

Where has he gone?

In all too many instances he has died an untimely death from overwork and frustration, and he has not been replaced. Long hours, low pay, high overhead, professional isolation, and lack of facilities have all contributed to the unattractiveness of rural practice. The general practitioner of yesteryear, once the workhorse of American medicine, has been declining in numbers, as his prestige and income have declined relative to the specialists in the profession. The public must share the blame. They ask: "Are you a specialist, Doctor, or *just* a GP?" They revere and reward the surgeon who operates on them in a crisis and deprecate the services of the physician trying to keep them healthy. The relative value fee scales now accepted nationally also influence the career choices of young physicians. They quickly realize that the money flows to the surgical specialists and subspecialists, not to the primary care physicians.

Why has he not been replaced?

Here too the answers are multiple. The medical educational establishment, with recent exceptions, has stopped training physicians to meet the practice needs of the country. This does not imply an insidious plot. On the contrary the situation has developed as a result of a series of public actions taken over the years. In the early 1900s the revolution in medical education stimulated by the Flexner report provided a scientific basis for medical practice. The explosion of medical knowledge resulted in specialization. When medical schools were denied direct federal financing in the late 1940s, they received indirect sources of support through research and training grants from the National Institutes of Health. As a consequence they have produced at least two generations of research-oriented specialists whose training process has changed the classical dialogue between physician and patient from "What can I do to help you?" to "What can you do to help me?" Medical school emphasis on entrepreneurial grantsmanship has displaced the "people-oriented" physician. Practitioners, particularly generalists, have almost disappeared from the average faculty. Of those remaining, the "in" faculty take care of inpatients and the "out" faculty take care of outpatients. Patients have been transformed into "teaching material." Those with ordinary illnesses are sometimes crudely brushed aside on the grounds that service should not dilute teaching activities. Small wonder that graduating medical students have not been attracted to primary care!

What can be done about it?

Happily changes have been made, and more should follow. General practice has found a new lease on life by its conversion to family practice. Family physicians can be tested and certified as specialists, when appropriate, by the American Board of Family Practice, established in 1969. Two hundred fifty residency training programs have been approved to prepare young physicians for this specialty. Group practices are recognizing the utility and appeal of the family physician and are attracting him with salaries commensurate with those paid other specialists. The institutionalization of medicine (16) is providing the family doctor with facilities, resources, and access to hospitals on the same basis as other specialists (9). Finally, medical schools seem to have gotten the message and are beginning to concern themselves with family practice, community medicine, and other areas of public need. Thus there is some reason to be optimistic about the future.

ESTABLISHING HEALTH DELIVERY SYSTEMS. Frequently heard these days is the call for the development of more effective systems to provide health services. Listed below are some examples of progress to date and future trends.

Some of the outstanding clinics and group practices in this country are located in rural areas. Examples include the Geisinger Medical Center in Danville, Pennsylvania; the Guthrie Clinic in Sayre, Pennsylvania; the Marshfield Clinic in Marshfield, Wisconsin; and the Mayo Clinic in Rochester, Minnesota. In each instance the clinics have grown by attracting patients from a multicounty, and sometimes a multistate, referral system which has been developed in response to their demonstrated quality and capacity to serve. As competition has developed, some of these clinics have established satellite centers within their catchment areas in order to compete with others who offer more accessible care. Such primary units also maintain the flow of referral patients to the base center.

Early hospital system development also has tended to encompass rural institutions. Robert Toomey has developed a pioneer hospital system based at Greenville, North Carolina (25). Stephen Morris has provided the leadership for the Samaritan Health System, extending outward from Phoenix, Arizona. He has taken positive action compatible with his own observation: "There is general and growing realization that the health care system of this country is in need of repair" (13, 17, 18). Anne Somers has long advocated a leadership role for the hospital: "It is the one institution with the potential for providing *or assuming responsibility for* [italics mine] the provision of the full range of comprehensive health services—prevention, treatment, rehabilitation, and aftercare" (22).

Some of the organizations mentioned above include prepaid, closed panel, group practices. As outstanding examples of that approach we should also consider the three largest: Kaiser, the Health Insurance Plan of New York, and Group Health Association of Washington, D.C. Sytematization underlies and supports the activities of each. By virtue of their size and ability to supply primary, secondary, and tertiary care, they can extend high-quality, reasonably priced care to both rural and urban patients (14). Unfortunately, legal obstacles to the formation of prepaid group practice plans still exist in some states (6).

Satellite developments are emerging as a few universities attempt to extend their services to rural areas. Leaders here include the University of Florida, the University of New Mexico, Stanford University, and the University of California, Davis, with other medical schools beginning to follow suit. Such institutions as Lancaster General Hospital in Pennsylvania and the Hunterdon Medical Center in Flemington, New Jersey, have also developed ambulatory centers at a distance from their major facilities.

Another excellent example of regional support for a rural institution is the arrangement in Washington between the Virginia Mason Hospital of Seattle and the much smaller and formerly isolated Willapa Harbor Hospital in South Bend. Through transfer of management, professional, and back-up services, the larger unit has supported efforts by the smaller to maintain quality services (21).

Where earlier our problems seemed insurmountable, these new patterns of success help us to draw certain conclusions:

· If laissez-faire has not worked, perhaps the time has come to
  introduce planning and management.
· If traditional and categorical approaches have not been successful, innovation and cooperation would appear to be needed.
· If pouring money into the existing system has merely increased
  the cost of services rendered without improving the amount
  or quality, perhaps it is time to consider austerity as a reasonable strategy. Nothing heretofore stated would lead us to
  undertake a revolutionary restructuring of a system which
  assuredly has its strengths; rather experience would lead us to
  believe that we must selectively build upon the best of what
  exists.

SYSTEMS SPECIFICATIONS. If we are to extend health systems
to rural areas, we must develop specifications for what we are
trying to achieve. Criteria for rural systems must meet the legitimate requirements of the several groups affected.

Patients are crying out for accessible, acceptable, available, comprehensive, considerate, effective care (8). It would appear that access,
cost, and convenience are more important than choice. As Dr. Borne-
meier of the American Medical Association has observed, the traditional cry is "Is there a doctor in the house?"—not "Are there two
doctors in the house?" Patients want quality assurance and hope
their expenses will be budgetable and controllable. The fact that a
number of health facility bond issues have recently been approved by
voters indicates that the public accepts the principle of communitywide sharing of capital costs. More and more the public is demanding
a voice in how the system works. They are frightened by its cost and
fragmentation. They no longer rely on health professionals alone to
make the system responsive. Now in town-meeting style they reaffirm
their belief that the system is theirs, is designed to serve them, and
must be more responsive to their needs than it has been in the past.
Congress has declared that health care is a human right. The public
says "Don't just talk about it, deliver it!"

Health professionals also have their requirements. Laws can be
changed overnight, but the doctors we have today are the only ones
who will be practicing tomorrow. Therefore, any changes made must
be attractive to some of our present supply of physicians under *their*
conditions. Under existing circumstances they will not change location or habit patterns unless their requirements are met. These
include:

1. Adequate facilities and resources with which to practice at the highest level of the state of the art

2. Interaction with other professionals to maintain the stimulus needed for continuing education and to develop the opportunity for professional advancement, recognition, and reward

3. Professional challenge

4. Security

No one seems satisfied with a terminal activity, however comfortable or lucrative. Physicians, like others, seem to desire opportunities for promotion and/or movement. They might be willing to spend a few years in some areas if such service clearly leads to improved professional and living conditions through later assignment elsewhere. This confirms the need for systems and organizations within which successive challenges at a variety of locations can be offered as part of an individual's career development. Any hospital or health center can function only if it can attract and retain a staff adequate to supply the professional needs of the patient population to be served. Conversely, staff members can justify their existence only if patients are served and if facility resources and referral outlets can be mobilized in support of patient needs. Obviously there also must be adequate, predictable financial support for both institution and staff.

It would appear that the viability of many institutions without linkages and regionalization is uncertain. Planning, management, resources, and training programs might be shared between institutions to enhance the effectiveness of each.

Institutions may also have to assume responsibility for a broader spectrum of patient care activities than has been their traditional function. Hospitals that have captured most of the health care resources of an area must accept the responsibility for deploying them to meet the medical needs of their communities (22).

EXPERIMENTAL DELIVERY SYSTEMS (26). Public Law 91-515 amended the Public Health Service Act by authorizing "projects for research, experiments, or demonstrations dealing with the effective combination or coordination of public, private, or combined public-private methods or systems for the delivery of personal health services at regional, state, or local levels" (20). To this end in 1971 the Health Services and Mental Health Administration created the Experimental Health Services Planning and Delivery Systems Program. This program presumes that those who know the problems best can find the best solutions, out in the communities where the problems exist.

The experimental systems approach builds on what is already available—a voluntary, pluralistic system with admixtures of catgorical federal programs. It expects to use a community management structure for purposes of expanding the capacity and efficacy of the system through improved access, greater efficiency, and assured quality. This may be a desperate last-gasp effort to work out solutions through the voluntary system. The Experimental Health Services Delivery Systems Program suggests that providers, third-party payors, the public, and political officeholders be brought together in a governing body to manage the system. This board is to be autonomous and problem-oriented and not geared to the vested interests of members of the board. Using the regional concept recommended long ago by Dr. Joseph Mountin, the experimental systems are designed to serve well-defined medical trade or catchment areas, integrating and expanding on existing health care resources (19).

All of the Experimental Health Services Delivery Systems Programs have been encouraged to develop an action plan through systems analysis. Community surveys and evaluation of existing data are to be used to describe problems affecting the region as a whole. Priorities must be established to determine which problems, if solved, would have the most beneficial effect on the health and health care of the population. The systems approach should identify resources available and establish a management plan for attacking problems on a priority basis, using existing and available resources. Naturally, an evaluation of the results would follow to determine utility and cost effectiveness.

In recognition of the identifiable problems facing almost every region in the country today, the experimental systems approach will emphasize development of primary care resources.

To provide staffing for delivery systems, new kinds and better distribution of health manpower are mandated. Significant support in this area can be expected to result from federal contracts and grants awarded by the Bureau of Health Manpower Education to train physicians' assistants. Their effective utilization will require better manpower resources distribution. Interrelationships among educational programs within areawide health education centers will assuredly be needed (10). Public demands for quality assessment must be met. To this end it will be necessary to collect data for evaluation and definition of further action steps needed. The program will encourage interinstitutional arrangements or mergers to improve economy or effectiveness of all health care resources in the community. To maintain ongoing support, stable financing mechanisms are absolutely essential. Finally, health services data systems will be required to document performance and evaluate results. The ultimate goal of the program is the establishment of a viable, acceptable, integrated communitywide delivery system.

Problems. Inasmuch as a basic purpose of the experimental systems
program is to provide a learning opportunity, it is appropriate to
consider some of the problems encountered and some of the
lessons learned in the early years of the program. We realize now how
difficult it is to get a system organized. Time is needed to establish
a management corporation and to teach its membership to focus on
regional, not parochial, goals. Surprisingly it seems to be a new
idea in health administration to manage primarily in the public
interest. It will take time to sell the concept.

It also takes time to establish credibility for the new corporation. Participants must be reassured that the purposes of the program are evolutionary, not revolutionary. Trade-offs must be considered and made. The cash-flow pattern must be identified, plotted,
and analyzed, and the corporation tied in. None of the programs
has yet managed to capture or reinvest dollars saved through systemization. A whole new philosophy is needed to turn the system from
producing the very best for *some* citizens to doing the most possible
good for the *most* people.

Physicians and administrators in the existing system do not
seem to realize that maintenance of the status quo is not an option.
Already controls are being imposed inexorably on the so-called free
system.

No one knows when Congress will get over its love affair with
the categorical approach and move to an integrated system approach.
The transition will be difficult because it will require our lawmakers
to relinquish some of their traditional prerogatives in favor of delegating authority to lower echelons of government and the voluntary
sector. When Senator Kennedy can refer to "the commitment Congress and all Americans have for local community control over those
services which are designed to serve the people," it would appear the
lawmakers are getting ready to do just this (12).

Progress. Already there is evidence to suggest the experimental systems
approach may work. The state of Arkansas has developed a program management plan, illustrated in Figure 14.1, that was
designed to cope with the gut-wrenching issues of how best to manage
a health delivery system. Arkansas has begun to assess problems, design
solutions, and effect change in the existing order. The state is concentrating a great deal of energy in nursing home cost analysis and
consideration of prospective reimbursement, which has led to an attempt to establish a common accounting system across all nursing
homes in the state. If successful, Arkansas will be able to perform a
fund flow analysis in this area at least.

Arkansas also is focusing on emergency medical systems and

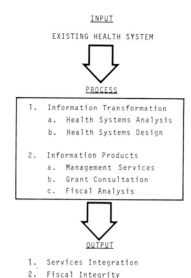

INPUT

EXISTING HEALTH SYSTEM

PROCESS

1. Information Transformation
    a. Health Systems Analysis
    b. Health Systems Design

2. Information Products
    a. Management Services
    b. Grant Consultation
    c. Fiscal Analysis

OUTPUT

1. Services Integration
2. Fiscal Integrity
3. Communication Clarification
4. Evaluation

FIG. 14.1.   Arkansas experimental health services delivery system.

studying urban ambulatory care programs and rural systems models. To guide the decision-making process, an early effort is being made to collect hard data through a federal-state-local data system.

The Arkansas program is secure to the extent that it was designated by former Governor Bumpers as the conduit for revenue sharing. Their board is becoming, for all practical purposes, a health authority for the state.

In the five-county area surrounding Binghamton, New York, the NY-Penn Health Management Corporation also is in pursuit of an integrated system (7). It has established a representative board and has tied into a number of ongoing federal projects, including regional medical programs, primary nurse practitioners, emergency medical services, and experimental medical care review organizations. It has also brought National Health Service Corps physicians into the area, thus winning the grateful appreciation of rural constituents. It is now focusing on primary care centers; gerontology; and problems in drug abuse, alcoholism, and manpower.

Indianapolis, Indiana, and Marion County form a city-county complex which also is well on the way toward systems integration. The basic philosophy, directed toward an urban problem complex, is nonetheless applicable to rural problems as well. They began by describing what it is, informing and educating people, and assessing where money comes from and where it goes in the health field. They already know that $1,000/family is spent on health services in the area. They postulate that the community ought to get more back in the way of services.

The Mon Valley project in Monessen, Pennsylvania, attacking essentially rural problems, has managed to effect consolidation of two hospitals and other health care activities in their area. The project has a functioning board and corporation which—through research, community organization, and program development—have begun to stimulate citizens of the area to action.

ALTERNATIVE MODELS FOR RURAL HEALTH SYSTEMS

Rural Cooperatives. Historical precedents for rural cooperative endeavors already exist in areas such as credit, equipment sharing, marketing, and even health. Some of the early community health cooperatives, stemming from the Farm Security Administration days, are still in existence. Cooperative efforts in health also are exemplified by union activities such as those of the United Auto Workers, the International Ladies' and Mens' Garment Workers' Unions, and the Meat Cutters Union. Although primarily addressed to urban problems, the unions' approach could be applied to rural areas as well. Despite the formidable opposition of medical societies and voluntary hospitals, unions have been able to enter into arms-length transactions with professionals and institutions to improve health services for their constituents.

Health Care Corporations. The service potential of voluntary hospitals is limited by the reluctance of patients to pay for education, charity, and hospital expansion. Further resistance results from hospital domination by medical staff and conservative trustees, whose orientation has been toward in-house rather than communitywide health care activities. Some believe changes will have to be made— probably in the direction of converting voluntary, private, nonprofit institutions into publicly financed, publicly accountable aggregations of institutions. The American Hospital Association proposes that these be called Health Care Corporations. Not only two-way public-hospital communication and education but also public representation on hospital boards will be required to raise hospitals' goals and objectives to levels required by this franchising approach, which has been named "Ameriplan" by the American Hospital Association (23). There would be three essential requirements for the Health Care Corporation to be successful:

1. A group of provider hospitals would have to reorganize, using the systems approach, to provide a total health care package. This could be financed on a prepaid capitation or HMO approach.

2. The federal government would have to assume the financial burden for about half the load—the aged, poor, and near poor. The other half would come from employer-employee coverage.

3. Standards and controls would be prescribed at the federal level and implemented at the state level to ensure even quality and full public accountability for both financing and operations.

Under sponsorship of Representative Al Ullman, the Ameriplan was introduced into Congress as one approach to national health insurance. To date there is no evidence that it will ever become law. The current mood of Congress seems to favor support, regulation, and control of the existing system rather than the creation of new systems with new incentives.

County Models. In Maricopa County, Arizona, and Alameda County, California, the public sector has given us examples of the systems approach to the delivery of health care. Using integrated departments of health services which offer a full range of facilities from hospitals to outpatient centers, they emphasize ambulatory care in particular. Because their physicians are salaried, these systems offer no incentives to overutilization of acute hospital beds. On the contrary, they encourage the alternative use of nursing homes and home health services in addition to outpatient services. Their fiscal operations are budgetable and controllable, an observation never made of medicare and medicaid programs.

Their tax-based support requires that these county systems be responsive to the public through elected officials and through boards of health acting in the public interest. Capital funding using bond issues voted on at public elections spreads the cost of these community resources over the entire area. Unless the voters view proposed capital commitments as being in the public interest, they will not pass them. The Maricopa and Alameda county systems of health care offer an attractive model to other communities and illustrate the value of regionalization and system coordination.

State Health Authorities. An alternative to experimental systems or health care corporations may well be the state health authority. Rhode Island, Delaware, and New Jersey have been experimenting with this model. Many medical leaders are pessimistic about voluntary cooperative arrangements. By involving the office of governor and assigning line responsibility for systems management and operation, it is possible to introduce the "clout" essential to change.

Consideration of the authority model will bring into focus issues of
local self-determination (and taxation) vs federal taxation and income
sharing. At some point the taxpayer must decide for himself whether
he prefers to send money to Washington and hope that some filters
back for useful application to problems that concern him or pay taxes
to local or state government where he can monitor use of such monies.
The success of state authorities depends partly on control being re-
linquished at federal and regional levels and on competence being developed at local levels. It may be some time before this model can
be tested and demonstrated to be effective.

CONCLUSIONS. Deficiencies in rural health care delivery exist, and
   will continue, unless systems elements can be introduced and
   expanded. Such innovations will have to be attractive to the
public, to professionals, and to institutions and must demonstrate
their effectiveness by solving problems of access, cost, and quality for
rural health services. A number of systems approaches can be considered. These include expansion of primary services, group practice
arrangements, hospital systems development, satellite extensions, comprehensive systems development, health care corporations, county
health agencies, and state health authorities.

Systems evaluation methodology must be built into any such
demonstrations to help us identify the "better way" we all seek. Long
before we achieve the sought-for improvements, we will have to find
the ways, through sociobehavioral research, to educate the public to a
need for change, and to persuade the involved provider professionals
and institutions to relinquish territoriality and the status quo to accept change. Finally, we will have to refine our tools of outcome
analysis to permit us to compare results and tailor future rural health
delivery systems to the exact needs of the public they must serve.

CHAPTER 15

CONSUMER INVOLVEMENT IN THE DELIVERY OF HEALTH SERVICES

JOHN HATCH AND JO ANNE EARP

IN HEALTH efforts undertaken in and by rural communities, the initiative of the individual community must be captured by health planners through the active involvement of the community's residents. Most planners believe in and operate on the premise that the "rural . . . community constitutes the key to improvement of rural health conditions" (8, p. 105), but there is often little agreement as to the definition of community and even less about what role health "change agents" and community members play in this effort.

Agreement appears necessary because those familiar with efforts to improve health conditions in rural areas continue to believe that the most effective approach is through mobilizing the resources of the community itself. Success in community action depends on understanding what community members value and place greater priority on. The development of effective health services in our society, however, must also take into consideration the professional and technical services rendered in health care and the problems of organizing and implementing health programs.

It follows from this argument that health planners must develop more self-reliant, self-aware communities—communities that are conscious of their health needs and able to identify their problems and then, through their own strength, solve the problems. Thus the objective is for professional health workers in rural communities to engage in a joint effort with community members in order to increase the consciousness of the population, bolster its ability to make the best

JOHN W. HATCH is Associate Professor, Department of Health Education, School of Public Health, University of North Carolina. JO ANNE EARP is Assistant Professor, Department of Health Education, School of Public Health, University of North Carolina.

use of technical resources and professional services available from the health sector, and generally "enlist [the people's] active participation and involvement in measures to solve their own health problems" (8, p. 108). As Geiger has said, plans for the long-term survival and growth of rural health efforts, plans which intend to be more than stopgap measures, must concentrate on the development of viable, effective, community-based institutions (1). Such an approach is beneficial not only for the laymen of the community but also for the professionals. To the extent that professionals are involved in the self-assessment process, they become familiar with the unmet needs of the community. This supplements their inadequate training in understanding the rural community.

While spectacular initial gains in the health sector can sometimes be made without a great involvement on the part of the community *if* there is no scarcity of resources, effective long-run changes must utilize community resources. A preventive orientation is demanded, and environmental, social, and attitudinal change is the focal point of such efforts. Health professionals working in rural areas must train themselves away from the diagnostic, pathological, curative orientation they learned in school and retrain themselves to view health programs as fitting into existing strong local social institutions. This means they should specifically look for nonhealth-directed systems that function well as possible models for health systems. The goal is to shift the locus of orientation from middle-class professional expectations and customs for the delivery of *medical* care to the identification of the cultural, social, and familial strengths present in the target community for the provision of *health* care. Before the inherent strengths of the social system can be used as keystones in program designs for delivering health care, however, professionals must determine specifically what makes these systems or organizations work well in the particular situation.

The case history of the Tufts-Delta health project in the rural communities of Bolivar County, Mississippi, provides an example of how new programs can be shaped so that they either duplicate underlying aspects of viable community social structures (in this case, the Baptist church) or build health-specific objectives into existing non-health-oriented social structures. The greatest barrier to social change in health areas may be the problem of developing a compatible relationship between those who possess technical competence and those in need of it; the most effective method for inducing such change is surely a collaborative one, in which the expertise of the professional reinforces or supplements the efforts of the people to be served.

TUFTS-DELTA HEALTH CENTER. The Tufts-Delta health project, begun in 1966 in Bolivar County, Mississippi (a rural area 100 miles south of Memphis and 20 miles east of the Mississippi River), was among the first rural health projects sponsored by the Office of Economic Opportunity (OEO). Tufts University of Boston, the project's initiator, attempted from the beginning, in what was largely a successful effort, to involve the community both in setting program priorities and carrying out the project. Though providing health services to the poor in this area was not a new concept, the use of community development practices and principles to meet the health care needs of poverty populations and effecting social change was. Thus, while the concept of a health center for the very poor of Bolivar County did not arise *de novo,* the use to which it was put was new in Mississippi in the middle 1960s.

In 1940 the Knights and Daughters of Tabor opened a 40-bed hospital in Mound Bayou, Mississippi. At the time the average income of member families of the fraternal order was less than $400 annually, and many adult members were not able to read or write. Unlike most rural efforts up to that time, the project was not dependent on the expertise or backing of a health professional for either its impetus or implementation. It survived—indeed flourished—for several years for a number of reasons: the fraternal order had successfully managed a previous organized activity (a burial association) since its founding shortly after the Civil War; a well-organized grass-roots structure, reinforced by an interlocking church membership and an extended family-kinship system, provided easy access to clique networks; a black women's college society had carried out a public health–oriented summer service program five years prior to the establishment of the hospital.

When the Tufts-Delta Health Center began its community organizing efforts in 1967 among these 20,000 people, 90 percent of whom were black and among the poorest in the nation (average annual family income—$900), they followed the earlier example of the fraternal order and built on the strength and natural organizational structure of the Baptist church. This was consonant with the theoretical beliefs of community organizers that local cultural patterns and social systems provided a better foundation for building new institutions than did reliance on other models perhaps more alien to the cultural norms and expectations of the area. From a practical standpoint it was also an obvious strategy, because (1) 90 percent of the health center's target population had no other organizational affiliation apart from the church and (2) 86 percent of the black population in Bolivar County were Baptist church members. The community and whatever organizations were eventually established there could not have been understood apart from an appreciation of the role played by the church in the lives of its black members, nor could new organizations have endured without building in part on the church structure.

The churches in the area were not large units, seldom over 150 people in membership. They were, however, both ubiquitous and influential. Functioning in much the same way as a clan, they offered each of their members—who were often related by either blood or marriage—the opportunity of holding a status-conferring formalized position: (a) within the church, (b) in the denomination's regionalized structure, and (c) in the community itself. These positions or roles had a set of assignments or tasks associated with them. In return for performing those duties or obligations, role-occupants could expect to enjoy status rewards in this very highly structured social system.

Hence the black Baptist church was able to confer status and dignity on its members. The church gained in the exchange, maintaining itself as the most—indeed the only—influential social structure (formal or informal) outside the family in the lives of these very poor rural people. As such, the church often served as a primary resource for intervention in familial groups or kinship networks in times of crisis. As both the most influential institution and the acknowledged source and initiator of practical instructions on daily problems, it helped set the established code of conduct for people's daily lives and enforced sanctions against those who violated that code. Finally it acted as the communication center for all the affairs taking place in the community and served to legitimate the aims of and methods used by newcomers or outsiders wishing to "organize" or otherwise intrude in community affairs. Thus the church structure was an important model as well as a participator in the successful initiation and operation of any community organizational effort in Mound Bayou. The style and structure of the North Bolivar County Health Council, which later developed as the overall coordinating agency for the comprehensive health center plus other community development efforts, was closely patterned on the organization of the Baptist church.

The earliest actions of the OEO-Tufts staff in 1967 were the recruitment and training of a local community organization staff of 12 persons. These outreach workers were employed to make home visits to as many families in the target area as possible. This was a community that had been decimated by many factors, the most potent being the fantastic advances in agricultural science and technology. For example, as a result of the changes in farming and the production of cotton, 60 percent of the labor force had become technologically obsolete by 1965; a mechanical harvester could pick an amount of cotton equal to 140 men a day. Selective migration had resulted in a community almost bereft of its better-educated younger males. The median age of the community was 15 years; the average age of male heads of household was 57 years. Furthermore, the median education level among those 25 years and older was 4.5 years. This was also a community in which there were three females for every two males among adults over 21.

The locally recruited community organization staff had several objectives: getting acquainted with the people and their problems as well as the social and physical environment that gave rise to them; orienting the population to the project's existence, potential, and facilities; and providing the health professionals, who went along on these early visits to the community members, with a rare opportunity for meeting their prospective clients on the latter's own turf—in situations more familiar to the recipient than to the provider. This last objective, an obvious reversal of the traditional approach, was deliberately arranged in order to establish a basis of trust for future contacts. The use of courtesy titles—Mr. and Mrs.—for those not used to being so addressed by those not used to being addressed in any other way— Dr.—was an example of this initial trust-building activity. While not an original objective of these first visits, another consequence was an occasional arrangement for providing crisis medical care to those persons who needed such care.

Following the home visits, the next step in the development of the project was a series of small group meetings tailored, almost on the spot, to the interests of those who assembled for them. These meetings provided insight for nonnative health center employees into friendship, kinship, and church networks, while concomitantly revealing special interest groups and influence clusters in each of the several target communities. The meetings also gave center officials an idea of what the most pressing concerns of the people were, what their health and medical needs were, how these two coincided or even if they coincided, what the community understood was meant by comprehensive community health care, and how closely those expectations paralleled the professionals' or center's understanding and expectations. As might be expected, a gap often existed between what was desired and what the plans intended to provide. In addition, the range of concerns expressed by the people always exceeded those the professional and health center were prepared to handle. Food, clothing, shelter, employment, and justice always topped the list. Health had a low priority except for the provision of crisis medical care. Thus the meetings, like the visits before them, oriented and educated the professionals as much or more than they did the community.

These early meetings produced a clear consensus among the

health center people that the top priority of the target population was adequate nourishment and that malnutrition (due to either insufficient numbers of calories or the erroneous allocation of these among sources of nutrients) was the most pressing problem. In a meeting in Rosedale this was poignantly demonstrated when, following presentations by the center staff, a mother of nine hesitantly rose to her feet and made the following observation: "I thank God, the Government and the Office of Economic Opportunity for what they say they gonna do. It's nice to have a doctor when you're sick and know that a nurse will visit. All the other stuff you talk about sounds nice too, but if you folk could help us get some food I don't think we'd be sick so much. Please can't you help us?" The challenge—and need—was clear. Prevention of hunger, of malnutrition, was the most obvious point of entry to other health-directed activities of the future. And in the sense that an adequate response to the demand for food required the provision of other services, it was a natural for fulfilling other needs—for example, the need for employment—as well.

When a series of meetings was arranged to discuss the possibility of backyard vegetable gardens, the response was so overwhelming (1,000 people indicated an interest) that the project in that form had to be abandoned. Instead a food cooperative—organized, administered, and operated along Baptist church organizational lines—was begun and continues to thrive today. The food cooperative became a farm cooperative geared to the nutritional and employment demands of the community. It became a self-supporting, profit-producing, independent enterprise with a board of delegates chosen by 12 separate clubs representing thousands of members. While the board determined and implemented policy, it remained strongly committed to the involvement of consumers (who were also the producers) in the determination of cooperative policy as well as in the provision and distribution of cooperative-related services.

The health professional's backing for the food cooperative and his direct and indirect experience with getting goods, services, and technical assistance from a distant bureaucracy (the Department of Agriculture) were valuable not only in directly attacking a major etiologic factor (diet) in many of the medical problems presented but also indirectly in demonstrating a willingness to understand and respond to the people's needs, priorities, and ways of doing things. As a result they trusted his judgment later on when he wanted them to undertake unfamiliar and seemingly unnecessary health-related activities. Besides providing expertise and building confidence, the health professional's initial support for and participation in the food project also helped develop a membership list which was later of use in more traditionally health-directed aspects of the center's program.

After this initial project was undertaken, the center's staff and community organizers began to expand their focus as well as their manpower; on the basis of the identification of social clusters and situational priorities, the health center formed several working committees. As a result of expansion, the center became an unwieldy planning vehicle, and its centralized nature was a drawback as an implementing force. Subsequently in 1968 each of the informal community groups that formed the core of the project selected five members to serve on a central planning committee—an umbrella organization serving all of northern Bolivar County. The result was the North Bolivar County Health and Civic Improvement Council, Inc., which was composed of 10 semiautonomous health and civic improvement associations, each with its own committees (technical resources, by-laws, planning, mother and child, home and community improvement, elderly, sick, youth, program, complaint) and each sending three delegates to the council's board of directors. By 1970 the council had a membership of nearly 5,000 persons and had been successful in initiating a number of projects not usually included even in a broad definition of health care delivery and utilization. Among these, apart from the farm cooperative, were a legal services unit; a nutrition, recreation, and health education service for the elderly; and a system of locally owned and controlled service and activity centers (8, pp. 157–67).

While the council's activities went beyond the provision of health care services, the health center continued to focus specifically on health-directed activities. It too expanded so that by 1970 it employed more than 200 people, most of them indigenous to Bolivar County, and had 6,000 patient or resident encounters a month in all its divisions. Its effectiveness as well as its effort also showed a notable change. By 1970, five years after the initial exploratory efforts of the Tufts-OEO workers, the infant mortality rate for the target population of 20,000 people had declined from 60 to 21 per thousand.

The center and the council are still highly interdependent, although the center's board remains autonomous to the extent that it is composed of five individuals from Tufts University (until recently) as well as five members of the county who are selected by the North Bolivar County Health Council. The day-to-day operations of the center's staff are coordinated with the council and the 10 health associations, and these groups have control over the center through their veto on the latter's staff positions. The council is really the representative voice of the community as well as the coordinating mechanism of the individual service agencies. It also operates the patient transportation system and pays the expense of the 10 part-time health association staff workers. The center is essentially structured to deal with problems related to health, but it remains very much in contact with the community and hence able to respond to its felt needs. Approximately 60 percent of the staff is field-based.

While the community's needs were paid attention to and their wishes usually respected with regard to the manner in which projects were carried out, felt needs were neither the sole nor often the most important criteria guiding the health center in setting its program priorities. Though initially the recipients' and providers' perceptions of the most pressing concern coincided (the alleviation of food problems), felt needs and expert judgment did not mesh so well with regard to the second project—digging wells and building privies. It took an examination and review of mortality statistics and morbidity patterns to validate the area most appropriate in cost/benefit terms for the next major concentrated effort. Such a review revealed that infant mortality had risen in the Mound Bayou area (to somewhat greater than twice the national average in 1967), a fact that none of the residents was aware of. The precipitating cause in many of these infant deaths was acute diarrhea, and the etiologic agent was waterborne bacteria. Hence the health center made environmental sanitation objectives its next campaign, with a focus on changing people's attitudes and habits about securing, storing, and preparing water.

Although fortunate, it was not simply fortuitous that community perceptions and professional expertise paralleled one another in defining the alleviation of hunger as the first priority for a health campaign. As others (4, 9) have pointed out, there is a natural hierarchy to the health problems plaguing underdeveloped countries as well as poverty communities. Hence the initial campaign against nutritional-malnourishment problems was both predictable and appropriate.

Although rural and poor, the community's understanding of what was meant by health care (and thus the approach it expected the professionals to take) did not differ greatly from the understanding and approach of a middle-class or urban population; that is, they were crisis-oriented and had a bias for the provision of curative medical care to the very sick. The health center's approach was more a public health orientation with an emphasis on prevention among people who were not yet sick. Their method was primarily the creation of a psychosocial, as well as physical and physiological, environment which would provide future immunity from potentially disabling diseases. Hence, in order to reduce the infant mortality rate at the same time as substituting a preventive health orientation for a curative one, several types of health education campaigns were needed.

First, health workers had to establish the direct, visible causal chain between a long-term habit (use of certain well water) and an undesirable statistical outcome (higher infant mortality). This required the redefinition of a harmless tradition into its components, including the presence of a harmful etiologic agent (which could not be seen) and a general practice that was selectively dangerous. It also demanded the understanding, or at least acceptance, of a seeming paradox: that something cool, tasty, clear, and readily available was "bad" and something that tasted inferior and was difficult to obtain was "good." Secondly, the environmental sanitarians and other professionals had to translate such information, understanding, redefinition, and acceptance into behavioral terms—and hard labor ones at that (i.e., well-digging, often 40 feet down before safe water was reached).

While none of the health education campaigns in Bolivar County produced instantaneous victories, none was more difficult than this one. Neither did any demonstrate so well the validity of the classic behavioral science tenets: i.e., presenting the "correct" information does not automatically change either attitudes or behaviors; decisions are made on the basis of preferences and nonhealth criteria rather than on the basis of a desire or concern for improving health; new ideas are difficult to instill as well as to accept and new habits most difficult of all to induce, especially when they require replacing old, prescribed behaviors with new actions whose effectiveness cannot be empirically demonstrated immediately and thus must be taken on faith. However, as with the mitigation of hunger, a large measure of success was attained. Wells were dug all over the county, and new water and new habits replaced the old. Other campaigns followed (e.g., extermination of rats and insects, the digging of privies) but none so quickly rewarding as the alleviation of hunger.

Each of the health campaigns, as well as those only marginally health-related, encountered resistance to a greater or lesser degree. All required a reliance on behavioral change and community development strategies; all demanded an awareness of psychosocial dynamics, a knowledge of health principles, and a highly developed talent for spontaneous ingenuity. For example, inducing the "granny" midwives, who had delivered most of the people in the county, to bring their skills and wisdom within the walls of the health center required all of these ingredients. At first the midwives were suspicious and defensive at the imagined or implied criticism of their work and were protective of their power. Their ability to counteract the effectiveness of the maternal and infant care project was clear, as was the strength of their influence if it could be used in a cooperative effort for the advancement of the infant mortality project. The "grannies" were finally persuaded to bring their expertise inside the center and work with, if not for, the project. But as in the case of the wells, this undertaking required considerable finesse and skill. A similar situation developed with the use of home remedies and faith healers; allaying suspicions about the use of injections (or sometimes the failure of health workers to give injections) was another example.

Many points might be made and many aspects emphasized in this case history of the Tufts-Delta health project. In the health campaigns as well as the initiation and establishment of the center itself, an unanticipated consequence—and at the same time a causal determinant—was the degree of participation elicited from the community member-recipients. Although the professional's and the client's points of view did not always coincide, and there were other problems as a result, the community's involvement was considered a major asset as well as outcome of the project. The center staff had the wisdom and patience to understand the benefits accruing from *their* joining in the community's perceptions and pursuits, rather than narrowing the health center's focus to specifically health-directed activities "for the community" and defined "by the center."

For people neglected or betrayed in a systematic fashion over many years—whose verbal skills, power, and influence are less than adequate when confronted with the middle-class value system in which health care delivery in this country is embedded—community outreach, awareness, involvement, and at times control may be the only means of getting past the mistrust and hostility which often are greater barriers to change than is ignorance. There may be flaws in a position that embraces without question *community control* as necessary to the provision of health care, but we endorse a variant of that concept within the context or limitations described in the Mound Bayou case history. Without community participation, a major constraint on the verbally superior, resource-heavy professional is lacking; and a major mechanism for absorbing the needs, desires, and fears of the client-population is frivolously (some would say immorally) overlooked.

The encouragement of maximum, real participation by the community has several benefits—some already explicitly pointed out, others implicit in the example of the Tufts-Delta health project. To mention only one, it prevents a misallocation or imbalance of resources to segments of the community that are the most vocal or visible. Usually such groups are the most resource-laden, although not the most in need. Thus community outreach, home visits, open meetings, and the other techniques detailed above are more likely to produce an even more accurate representation of the community than is reliance on either community control or the solo practitioner sitting in his office awaiting the visits of his patients; such methods also tend to prevent overreaction to any one of the community's usually interdependent problems or inequitable attention to the demands of a particularly resource-heavy subgroup.

Describing the benefits of endorsing in practice a conceptually "good" idea (consumer involvement) does not address itself either to the weaknesses or failures of that concept or to the pragmatic realities of how a traditionally silent, often mistrusting or hostile majority is encouraged to appear, speak, and act in their own behalf. Others have addressed themselves to both these issues. It may be somewhat dishonest not to discuss some of the stress factors seen today in Mound Bayou, after the center's successful establishment and operation.

Smooth and mutually beneficial relationships were never established between the OEO-sponsored Community Hospital[1] and the health center; instead an uneasy truce and an underlying jealousy pervaded this association. The sponsors of two locally based hospital insurance programs rightly perceived the new "free" service to the poor as competitive and extremely threatening to their survival, and whatever benefits had accrued from this source in the past had to be foregone by the center's enrollees. The flow of new resources outside the control of the existing community elites (both black and white) posed a threat to their privileged position and resulted in trouble at times. From the other side, community control was considered to be compromised by the presence of both "outsiders" and "professionals" in decision-making positions.

As a result of these stress factors as well as a natural progression over time, Tufts's relationship with the project was terminated in 1972. This left control vested in a relatively small and not as widely representative group of persons closely tied to the town's mayor and political patronage system. However, faced with a choice between no health service and less than representative service, the community selected the only rational alternative. In addition, the *quality* of health care did not play a part in any of the major funding, controlling, or delivery system decisions described above.

It would be erroneous to view these final comments as a sad and inevitable epilogue to a spectacular success and failure story. The center flourishes today, and the concept of community participation in the delivery of rural health services remains very much alive. Much that was thought is no longer thought, and much that was learned remains viable and has been implemented. Growth as well as decay has resulted, and this rural, poor county is different—statistically as well as ideologically—than it was before the community health effort was undertaken.

1. This hospital was created as a result of the merger of two fraternal order–sponsored, physician-controlled hospitals which went bankrupt.

It is not the concept of community participation on which the Mound Bayou Health Center foundered, although this principle is not without its critics, nor are their criticisms without validity. Giving "power to the people" may be necessary but not a sufficient means for solving the health problems of poor rural communities. Technological, structural, political, epidemiologic, attitudinal factors and provider-consumer determinants are all implicated in the rural dweller's failure to receive adequate medical care. Furthermore, in the most neglected communities—those not necessarily hardest to reach because of poverty, racial factors, or illiteracy but neglected because of sociocultural value differences and normative isolation—creative ways must be found to encourage and support these groups attempting to deal with the health hazards from which they are at greatest risk. Obviously the most effective solutions are multifactorial in nature.

THE QUESTION OF CONSUMER INVOLVEMENT. Community participation alone cannot succeed in bringing about changes needed in relatively isolated and poor communities. Professional expertise, organizational know-how, and resources are needed from the outside, and these outside factors must be integrated into the existing social structure in a joint effort in which the community members are honestly involved.

A rural community—even a poor, isolated, and semiliterate rural community—may well be able to support and benefit from a citizen participation approach to health care delivery, as the Mound Bayou example illustrates. Few studies exist, however, that examine the correlation between types or degrees of consumer participation and health outcomes. In a descriptive study of a successful health program carried out in an isolated rural area of Florida, Reynolds found that community cooperation on the delivery of health care did coincide with citizen responsibility and consumer participation (6). However, there was no discussion of health outcomes.

In a study of 49 OEO-sponsored health centers, Schwartz found varying degrees of community involvement from local control to no participation at all (7). There seemed to be general agreement among professionals in the centers studied that the citizen participation was an asset; among other things it helped the professional staff gain insight into the felt needs of the community. The rationale for *community control* often seemed to be a moral one rather than one based on political or strategic considerations. Much of the observed conflict centered around concerns not specifically related to health issues but instead having to do with perceived "invasions" of the community's prerogative to determine what would happen on its own turf. Schwartz concluded that while local residents of poor communities did not have the power to control, they clearly possessed the power of negation (7)

There is general agreement among most community development people that consumer participation in some form is desirable and hence will continue to receive the support of those "in the field" (although not perhaps of those "behind the desks" with control over the budget); the form of participation may be something other than representation on boards of trustees. The test is in the effectiveness of community representation in achieving the real goals of consumers— whether these objectives are limited to gains in the health sphere, embrace larger social changes, or have influence or control over policy-making as their desired outcome. Probably too much reliance has been placed in the past on consumer participation in the abstract as the be-all and end-all solution for attaining both health outcomes and general social change.

Even employed as a method for inducing an already aroused and informed community to take direct social action on health issues, the vision and dynamism of the consumer responsibility concept cannot succeed without expert legal, technical, and administrative skillls to back it up. The latter may not be sufficient for making changes, but they would seem to be a necessary component for success. Furthermore, simple realism suggests that continued federal support for a meaning-ful consumer role will be needed. Without federal funds, expertise, and the governmental ability to remove (as well as impose) constraints, rural community health efforts *with or without consumer involvement* will not succeed. Without professional input and lacking operational indicators of program effectiveness, the federal presence will not be forthcoming. The benefits of relying on professionals and/or pro-viders, as well as the doubts about a total commitment to consumer participation, are not all pragmatic ones, however.

The history of consumer participation in the development and administration of health care systems did not begin with the civil rights movement of the 1960s or the consumer movement of the 1970s. Citizens as individuals, and even more as union members, have been setting and implementing health policy for decades (2). However, these earlier groups are not really participatory precursors for the OEO health center consumers or prototypes for rural community health program citizens who now demand a fuller, more meaningful type of involvement or representation in the delivery of their health care. The members of these more recent health movements differ from their predecessors in the following ways: (1) they are not organized around a sharply defined, tangibly threatening issue (building a dam); (2) they are not bound together by a formally structured group (a union) or the urgency of an informal, emotionally intense cohesiveness (diabetics); (3) they lack prior experience in dealing with survival issues as an organized force; (4) they are usually poor and therefore have little of value to exchange or to "pay their way" with; (5) they are often inexperienced in dealing with both the bureaucracy and professionals; and (6) they are constrained by political boundaries as well as physical handicaps (hunger). Furthermore, just because they share the same geographically defined catchment area does not mean they form a community of similar attitudes or underlying values (toward volunteerism or participation).

This last constraint has a wider implication. In addition to not sharing similar attitudes and values, often a community has very dissimilar needs when it is simply defined as a political subdivision or catchment area. Often the total need of the community is a diverse as well as an abstract concept—even if rural communities are more alike than they are like urban ones. Within a community area are special interest groups—farmers, the elderly, accident victims, or medicaid recipients—who have not only their individual vested interests but their particular (and often narrow) focus on "what the community really needs." Thus a "felt needs" approach is often a categorical approach rather than a problem-oriented, comprehensive community overview. Professionals (outsiders) can be useful in a situation like this; they are in a position to capture, maximize, and effectively channel such diversity for the community good.

We have argued for the input of and reliance on professionals on several grounds: pragmatically for their use in obtaining federal funding and their familiarity with the norms of both bureaucracies and formal-group participation; realistically for their overall ability to bind together diverse interest groups into the most effective as well as representative totality; and also because it is questionable how strongly consumers want to adopt all aspects of those roles previously performed by others.

There is a final—perhaps the most important—argument for why the health worker, while relying on the community's technical and social expertise, should not place himself in a position of automatically accepting the will of the community (the people's felt needs) when it comes to planning or initiating health action. Often the popular pressure is to concentrate on the provision of medical care to the sick rather than focusing on providing preventive care to the group as a whole. The creation of an *environment* that will ensure immunity against potential disability and disease is a more abstract and more difficult concept for which to create popular support than is the notion of curing the sick in crisis situations. Even if the preventive orientation is accepted as the basis for formulating program objectives, there often is a lack of correspondence between the means health professionals see as necessary for achieving these objectives and the methods urged by the community. In the authors' experience with community boards, few have been able to identify the major causes of morbidity or mortality in their area. Their sense of what constituted a problem often seemed to be based on: (1) a perception of what matters had recently seemed to become worse; (2) a sense of what *should* be, based on an ideal model of uncertain origin; and (3) a comparison of their health status with the known or perceived health status or others viewed as being better served. Professionals who unquestioningly embrace the rubric of "We must start where the people are" or "The people know their problems best and must be listened to" may not identify the basic problems. At least it may be that health workers of this persuasion are copping out on their responsibilities for improving the *health* of the community. Using such a strategy, the wells of Bolivar County might never have been dug.

This does not mean that the health professional should not have high on his priority list the goal of understanding the attitudes and motivations present in the community and the primary objective of using this understanding as a point of departure for teaching and helping those people in need. However, while he must pay careful attention to the people, he must not forget that it is *they* who have health problems and live under the conditions which need changing, that *they* wish assistance from him—not he from them.

Therefore, if by "starting where the people are" means the actual allocation of scarce resources to the community's perception of need, regardless of contrary evidence suggesting the inappropriateness of such a move, that is irresponsibility; if it means drawing on their interests to begin a process of discovery and innovation, that is another matter. The best data available—that which would enable a group to see their need in terms of other groups' needs as well as in comparison to the norms of what is good, bad, or merely happening in other American communities—should be made available to the citizens in language they can understand. We are not suggesting that the right to choose should not ultimately rest with the consumer-recipient; we are suggesting that there is a professional obligation to enable people to gain the best and widest insight possible into the implications of their choices *before* they choose. Otherwise there is the very real likelihood that the community might opt for nonviable, ineffective, unessential programs or—just as detrimental in terms of long-run changes—become co-opted or diverted by those who might be more articulate, powerful, experienced, or militant but not necessarily better informed or any more committed to achieving the community's best interests.

One other factor is possibly responsible for the partial failure of the community participation concept. Much of the professional input into community health boards has unfortunately been dominated by a limited human relations approach to problem solving. Communications between the ranks, participation in decision-making, and support for the virtues of democratic leadership may be desirable as concepts but do not address themselves to the methods usually used by institutions engaged in a fight over scarce resources in an environment dominated by interdependent, interorganizational exchanges with few mechanisms for accountability built into them. While there is evidence that cooperation, communication, and understanding enhance the internal functioning of organizations (5), the demoralizing effect on a community representative of involvement in a functionally castrated decision-making body not only may not result in enhanced interorganizational functioning but may reinforce the debilitating effects of the cycle of poverty (i.e., a sense of hopelessness) instead (3).

Obviously many practical and specific questions about local involvement remain; for instance, how effective will such a program goal be under a nationally based system of profit-making or profit-oriented HMOs or under a national health insurance plan? Even if considerable support for a community role in planning health care and delivering health services were generated and sustained among those with influence and authority, and agreement could be reached about: (a) the specific benefits community participation brings and (b) the degree of participation desirable and appropriate for each particular community, advocates of community involvement must reach agreement on other issues. These include what type of involvement (as employee, employer, board member, trustee, information gatherer, or program recipient) is most effective and most desirable, how community participation fits into the specific objectives of the program, and what community interests should and *would have to* be represented.

The irresolution of these issues within a context such as that which existed in the 1960s (an attitude that professionals had exerted complete dominance over the health delivery system in the past and that consumers must have a greater say and more control over the management and outcomes of such issues in the future) was coupled with a number of other factors operating at that time. These included: OEO's instability (five directors in seven years) and interagency jealousies and disagreements; a fractious, temperamental Congress when it came to health and social issues; a rapidly changing social environment between the 1960s and 1970s; and, perhaps most surreptitiously damaging of all, the poorly developed nature of the theoretical constructs supposedly underlying those terms ("community involvement" and "consumer participation") so often used as rallying cries by their unquestioning advocates.

As a result of these factors, there was no unifying concept, no agreement, on what was meant by the "role" and "responsibility" of the consumer in health care at the very time such rights were being loudly demanded and a political structure not wholly alien to these concepts existed to partly deliver them. It was never clear under what conditions the consumer and the community were most desirous of being involved or even who this consumer was. Furthermore, there was (and still is) very little research of a quantitative and theoretical nature on the sociopolitical correlates or health parameters associated with each of the possible positions community representatives might assume vis-à-vis the provision of their health care. These include: uninvolved, aware and concerned, involved and a recipient-participant, represented on a policy-making level, employee or employer, or in a decision-making controlling position. This situation was largely a product of the fact that "community control" became the goal before either community or control was clearly defined by the funding or coordinating agencies.

In several locations constituents of the programs became almost totally involved in activities they viewed as being best suited to establish local control, without knowledge of or regard for the complexity of environmental forces involved in the "health chain." As a result, a false sense of security was created in the minds of local people by "community participation," and it is possible that health and health care suffered. A more comprehensive knowledge by the organizers and representatives of the social and institutional framework in which health care is delivered and utilized might have avoided this. In some cases the problem lay with the fact that neither OEO nor the health center professionals ever had the degree of control over resources that communities believed them to have. In others the reasons were more complex.

Although we have reservations and precautions, we firmly believe that broad-based local involvement can have several beneficial outcomes: it may facilitate the attainment of program goals or the better deployment of program resources; it may expand the community's perspective and expectations of what it needs as well as what is of greatest benefit or effectiveness; it may educate and ultimately change health providers' attitudes. Finally local involvement is necessary because it is morally imperative; it can give firm, meaningful, unequivocal support to the democratic ethos that people should have the opportunity to participate in the decisions affecting their lives. Local participation is necessary, although not sufficient, because it is an inalienable right of those in a democracy—a right all too often overlooked by those who hold the reins of power or enjoy the privileges of authority.

CHAPTER SIXTEEN

A LOOK AHEAD AT RURAL HEALTH CARE

VERNON E. WILSON, MD

FOUR BASIC areas will continue to challenge health care system planners:

1. The time that elapses from initial need for appropriate health care to its actual delivery
2. The distance that must be traveled by either the patient or the professional and the complexity of designing economical and timely transportation
3. The appropriate handling of personal, social, and medical knowledge so that the professional, the patient, and the supporting organizational structures can each play an informed and proper role
4. The mutual confidence that must exist among those who pay for care, those who receive care, and those who render care

A lack of understanding on the part of planners for the differences between rural and urban social structures surfaces in plans for rural health care systems. The large urban societies are more familiar with and have adjusted to the less-personalized relationships that exist among members of society. This less-personalized relationship is better tolerated in patient-professional contacts. The well-ordered nature of the rural social structure presents both challenge and opportunity. On the challenge side, rural social structures have a higher resistance to change that comes from outside the structure or seeks to force them to give up their internal prerogatives to comply or not comply with decisions made by external groups. This stems largely from rural society's tendency to remain self-sufficient. On the opportunity side, the very nature of the health care system with its

VERNON E. WILSON, MD, is Vice-Chancellor for Medical Affairs, Vanderbilt University.

forced decentralization presents a good chance for use of the responsible and cohesive decision-making process that exists at the community level in rural areas.

In contrast to the ghetto areas, the small rural community tends to be more stable in its social structure. As a result it is more likely to have a widely understood and predictable process for decision-making, and its organizational and operational structure tends to be more overt and less complicated. However, the techniques needed for invoking change in the rural community are common to more complex situations. If one can provide the solution to health care delivery problems in the simpler rural social models, such solutions should provide a basis in principle for resolving the same kinds of problems in the more complex urban system.

NEEDS OF THE TOTAL HEALTH CARE SYSTEM. The idealized health care system should render the right service using modern methods at the right place at the right time. The corollary requirements are that the care be present in adequate amounts, delivered with the greatest possible efficiency in a pleasant setting, and accompanied by a maximum of mutual trust among all parties. Cost per se at the time of a health crisis is rarely if ever a determining factor. Indeed the public is increasingly making its request that cost not be a constraint on the delivery of care. Finally the output should be measurable. The measurement of the delivered service should reveal the quality of the performance, its cost effectiveness, and its accuracy in relationship to need.

Seen in the perspective of the idealized setting, several interesting features of the health care system are worthy of note. First, a very small amount of time in the total health experience of an individual is spent in contact with *any* health care professional compared to the very large amount of time the individual spends in activities that have a positive or a negative effect on his own health. Second, the high (favorable) cost effectiveness of preventive or early diagnostic procedures seems inversely related to the attractiveness of these services for both patients and professionals. Given these two factors, the investment in time and effort by planners on the education of the individual with the goal of preparing him to render more of his own or his family's care is amazingly small.

SOCIOLOGICAL PROBLEMS. It may well be that the sociological barriers to change in patterns of rural health care are far more imposing obstructions than either the maldistribution of health professionals or the complexity of administration. Some selected personal and sociological issues merit special attention in the development of the rural systems of the future without implying that they are necessarily unique to the rural scene.

The Dependent Patient. One of the more interesting aspects of health care, particularly medical care, has been the dependent role assigned to the patient. Much less is demanded of the sick individual, either child or adult, in his role as a contributor to the family or to society. The individual who has a cold or does not feel well is classically excused from the responsibilities of school or work. Many industries have arrangements that allow the pay of the individual to continue even though he is making no direct contribution to his organization. Beyond the point of effectiveness in aiding quicker recovery or public protection, this attitude of dependency extends to the point that passivity is thought to be positively correlated with cure. Only now are we beginning to understand that this is not only untrue but has an inverse correlation with cure. Nevertheless, the public and professional acceptance and support for passivity on the part of the patient is so great that even information about his own state of health has been communicated poorly if at all to him. Indeed, many patients prefer not to accept informational responsibility for their own illness.

Personal Relationships. A second force to be considered is the high emotional content of illness. Because of the high level of anxiety at the time of interaction, credibility of the professional is a particularly important ingredient in the health care system. At present, credibility seems most easily established through personal relationships. The continuing trend toward specialization both by individuals and by institutions has markedly increased the number of sources from which the average individual gets health care. As in almost any other set of contacts, a break in any segment of that system tends to reflect adversely on the entire system, thus increasing the probability of disappointment and lack of faith in the total health care process. At the same time the bonding that comes from continued personal relationships tends to diminish, thus setting the stage for increased discontent. Superimposed on this characteristic—and certainly an economic factor—is the influence of local trade patterns. Individuals might prefer for various reasons to use the professionals in one community for their health care and another community for their shopping needs, but they are partially constrained to use the physicians and professionals in the common trade area. Perhaps of more concern is the reality that the professionals have disproportionately located in the large populated areas. The rural individual must go increasingly long distances to get sophisticated care when, as a matter of fact, the more complicated his illness, the more likely he is to be financially stressed and disinterested in travel or separation from his home surroundings.

VARYING REGIONS. One of the great challenges in the design of health care systems for rural areas has been the definition of a region. The search has too often tended to focus only on a fixed geographic region. From the perspective of comprehensive care, health care regions must be considered as functional regions rather than geographic regions. This can be illustrated by international centers for very complicated heart surgery or very local centers for response to the common cold. As a matter of fact, two types of regions will be required, depending on the function to be discharged. From the standpoint of facilitating access to care, implying outreach, regions need to be geographic and are probably most effective if their limits are coterminous with geopolitical boundaries, particularly at the state level. Prevention, outreach, and improved access to health care all require precise boundary definitions if 100 percent coverage is to be assured. In contrast, attempts to make these regions self-sufficient for comprehensive care must be abandoned as ineffective, inefficient, and at times specifically dangerous; e.g., the use of a local hospital to do complex gall bladder surgery has in too many instances resulted in lifelong discomfort, disability, or even death. This kind of illustration has variations too numerous to elaborate here, but all lend support to warning of the dangers of militant self-sufficiency.

EXPECTATION VERSUS REALIZATION. The definition of crisis given by Eli Ginzberg of Columbia University is of particular use to planners (2); he states that the depth or extent of the crisis is a measure of the distance between that which was expected and that which was realized. The corollary is that any given state of affairs will not itself evoke a crisis if it is accepted. Thus a change in expectation as well as a change in state of affairs may lead to crisis. Perhaps no place in society is that definition of crisis better illustrated than in health care. A substantial part of the population expects and demands the idealized system described earlier, yet few receive the minimum desired level of services because they are too costly and too complex or too inconvenient to deliver. Perhaps more important than cost and complexity may be the unwillingness of the individual to give up his right to select his own physician, the unwillingness of the professional to give up his right to select his practice and living location, and the right of the individual to determine whether or not to accept the ministrations of any given part of the health care system.

COST EFFECTIVENESS. A great deal has been said about public need for more cost effectiveness within the health care industry, as though it were an administrative issue; nevertheless, it is the pressures of society that have defeated most attempts to develop cost effective programs. Cost effectiveness of various health care processes can and should be better analyzed than at present. The problem is that we have no way to determine whether those processes have a positive, negative, or neutral effect on the health of the individual in the aggregate of his life span. Too often we do not know their effect on the cumulative health of the community. Basic to an understanding of this issue is the acceptance of the fact that health care is a service, not a product. Classically service industries are insatiable consumers of resources, since there is no effective limit of the number of services any given individual might desire if available in unlimited supply. Looking at health care specifically, there is no fixed end point against which measurement can be made to assess whether a given investment was justified or not justified. In theory the end point of effective health care—good health—could be defined as the combination of (1) the capacity to function at an expected normal level, (2) possession of a positive attitude on the part of the individual toward that capacity to function, (3) a positive attitude on the part of the community in which he lives toward that function, and (4) the capacity of the individual to function as an integral part of the society to which he belongs. In fact, objective measures of progress toward this goal have been unavailable for either the individual or the community. Attempting to document a state of health in a numerical fashion quickly reveals that much of society is resistant—indeed antagonistic—to the idea that an individual must be required to be a productive member of society. Even if that assumption were allowed, there is even greater resistance to the establishment of criteria by which that productivity could be measured. Lacking this or a similar device, the measurement of "health" remains impossible.

PRIORITIES IN THE SERVICE INDUSTRY. Given the assumptions (1) that it is not possible to saturate the demands for health care, (2) that it is not possible to measure its cost effectiveness, and (3) that resources will always be limited since taxpayers have other concerns besides the financing of health care, the establishment of priorities even though subjectively determined is the only rational basis for allocation of resources. Nevertheless, there seems to be little willingness on the part of health care providers or the consumer public to set priorities on a logical basis. One of the best examples of illogic in recent times was congressional action during the same session to commit billions of dollars to renal dialysis (which is almost totally used by individuals in their later years with a low probability of cure) and to delete a few million dollars to immunize millions of children (with a long life expectancy and a high level of effectiveness). Such apportionment of limited resources is clearly not cost effective. It illustrates even more clearly that we do not currently have but very urgently need a rational operative pattern for the establishment of national priorities in the use of health care resources.

BALANCE BETWEEN QUALITY OF CARE AND EXTENSIVE-NESS OF COVERAGE. One of the most troublesome and obvious imbalances in the system that further impedes the establishment of priorities is inequity between the quality of care rendered to the individual who receives attention and the extensiveness of coverage of the population as a whole. Our professionals and health care institutions tend to measure the quality of their performance in terms of the additive experience they have with patients to whom they are exposed. In a demand system like health care, this can and does result in very expensive and sophisticated care being rendered to individuals who are fortunate enough to get into the system. It also tends to exhaust the limited resources of a health care system in terms of personnel, material, and expenditures before much less sophisticated health care can be rendered to other less fortunate individuals who for whatever reason did not get into the health care system. Thus the quality of the individual medical response to need may be quite high, while the quality of care rendered to the public as a whole is much lower. This quality may be considered either as a numerically oriented average of quality of care rendered to all people or as a percentage estimate of the number of the population who received care which met acceptable minimum standards of quality. Such variations tend to emphasize the distance between what is expected in treatment and what is realized by patients at either end of the range of quality. Given limited resources, the upper level is obviously not fiscally feasible as a goal for a level of health care to be funded for all citizens from public dollars. The British system has been notably successful in striking this balance in use of public funds. Accepting the limit on resources, the British have almost eliminated the "crisis" in health care related to availability of public-supported care to that population. They have done so by simply distributing the resources evenly and regularizing the methods for gaining access to them. This does have a modulating effect on the sophistication of care available to individuals at the upper social economic level insofar as that care is supported by public funds. It also has a very positive effect on the availability of care for those at the lower end of the spectrum. It certainly reduces social unrest related to health care by its evident equity, even though it reduces availability of more sophisticated care of the type we continue to expect in this country. One can devoutly hope that such an answer will not be required within our own health care system, but it must be accepted as having accomplished at least one important purpose for the British system.

COMMUNICATION. Turning to the communication system required to support complex outreach structures, it is even more apparent that rural health care systems may provide the best basis for pilot programs.

In the total health care system at the present time, there is no shared reservoir of knowledge that has mutual credibility for collaborating professionals or institutions. Even worse, the patient does not have even minimal regular access to the records of his own medical care. Thus in the communication system, we have neither a common medical records system recording professional action nor one that provides and analyzes the relationship of such data to the potentially available and related information stored on a national and international scale. Most interesting is the prevalent lack of faith on the part of both patients and professionals in newer data handling systems, even when used for routine information handling. The latter service is clearly more effectively and efficiently provided by the machine.

THE SYSTEM OF THE FUTURE. Given the problems of distance, credibility, and a need for common information, the single most important resource in need of development is a system of coordinated health care data banks. Such banks may initially be quite simple, resembling the central information system currently operated by the USPHS Indian Health Service for the Papago Indian tribe in Arizona. That system in concept provides a centrally maintained simple record of encounter of any individual in the tribe with one of the Indian health service clinics. This information is then immediately available to any other station at the time of the next contact by the patient. It is partially automated and could, if the use warranted, be fully automated. Although limited in the amount of information that can presently be stored and retrieved, the principle is an important harbinger of systems to come. A data bank must contain at the minimum a thumbnail sketch of each contact the individual has with the formal health care system and basic information to guide the actions of the next professional to whom the individual will go. The patient also should have appropriate access to the same records to govern his own actions as a part of the response to the diagnostic and treatment recommendations arising from the visit. Such a trend will make a more objective ambulatory health care data system mandatory, although it can and must be substantially less complex than the Weed Problem Oriented Record for hospital patients. To take maximum advantage of such systems, the information stored should be in numerical form and readily accessible. The "monastaries" of medical record systems and communication systems must be modified so that any individual who has appropriate and legal right to information can get it quickly, in concise form, and conveniently packaged. As an illustration, the patient or professional should have around-the-clock access to records in case he needs information about his tetanus shot, his immunization record, his reaction to penicillin, or his blood dyscrasia. Such information to be useful must be related to information about whether the individual at the last visit had a complication in his disease, treatment of any variety, or the level of his physical progress. These kinds of information should be in the unified record regardless of the location or time of the previous care.

The rural health care system viewed in this light illustrates the fundamental importance of cooperative effort between a great number of presently totally independent operating units. While independence and initiative of such units need not and should not be eliminated, each unit will need to share key information with all other potential service units. This is a problem faced by all health care institutions—rural or urban. However, the problem may be more resolvable in rural areas both because of their present greater need and because of their long and more firmly fixed patterns of independent responsibility and initiative.

To the reader who is concerned about such "information systems" taking over the health care system, this dissertation implies nothing more than "to the machine will be delegated that which is machinable and to the mind that which needs judgment."

Methods to reduce the time required to get information or assistance to individuals have been developed in many forms. No new devices are needed. What is now required is collaborative endeavor among health professionals, engineers, industrial groups, and the communities to effectively use what is available. The radio has certain unique characteristics, the value of which have been demonstrated in Australia. The TV coaxial cable used for cable television has another; it provides two-way visual and audio communication possibilities. The possibility of using this is suggested as an inexpensive medium for daily supervision of elderly or chronically ill individuals in isolated surroundings.

Triage systems for acute care are more familiar and more highly developed. These are best illustrated in emergency medical care systems such as the one in Illinois. Smaller models are available in many communities across the nation. Although they provide much service for emergencies and catastrophes, they tend to be less used in support of ordinary care. The skillful deployment of professionals in accord with their skills and distance has been highly developed by the military. The following suggestions of the application of the principle of triage seem pertinent to rural health care.

The rural triage system of the future will make informed use of all available sources of assistance. The "activated patient," the minimally trained technician, the nurse practitioner, the family physician, and the referral physician in that order will each provide the maximum appropriate service before referral to the next more costly and complex level of health care service.

By definition the future rural health system will require a more complicated and purposefully designed communication and information handling system than any currently in use for community health care. To effect this much change in the life patterns of entire communities is at least a challenge and by some may be viewed as impossible. One of the fine examples of its feasibility as well as a model for approaching the task is to be found in agriculture. Following the passage of the Morrill Act in 1862, the United States became the world's foremost agricultural system through its experiment stations, extension programs, county agent system, and university support. The same type of system can work in health (4). Because of the wide legislative authorities under which the U.S. Department of Agriculture operates, these changes could be introduced using the existing system if there were additional monetary support and congressional interest.

The time of intervention in many crises is more crucial than the level of sophistication of the professional rendering the care. Few communities are without the services of someone who has had a degree in nursing or one of the nursing arts. Each of these individuals has potential for giving and receiving specialized training for new roles if appropriate working relationships and financial incentives are designed. In most instances, appropriate utilization of their skills on the spot will produce a more effective health care response at lower cost than will the use of ambulances, helicopters, and other means of transporting individuals to the more sophisticated medical centers.

In addition to the need for smooth interchanges between levels of a triage system, each level needs careful attention. The potential is great for the development of a variety of support systems designed to make each level of such a system more self-sufficient than it is at present. The principles are simple, and the engineering and administrative techniques are available. Without attempting to deal with this potential comprehensively, a few illustrations may be helpful in clarifying the intent.

A major loss of efficiency in use of both time to make a diagnosis and resources to provide care arises from the widespread duplication in laboratory tests. A diagnostic test done in one office is rarely accepted in another office and almost never by the hospital or even between hospitals. To further compound the difficulties, few of the data collected are routinely checked from the point of view of the need for such new information to improve the logic of the diagnostic process. In engineering studies this latter process is sometimes called the "theory of decision-making." That theory addresses the economy of input into the decision-making process.

The first problem could easily be reduced manyfold by the selection of the tests most frequently run at the key levels of patient contact in the system. A "black box" set of tests could be standardized and codified so that the results are usable and believable at any level in the system within a reasonable time frame. Such a system would make telephone consultation or computer reference search substantially more valid. It would reduce cost both by elimination of needless duplication and by a reduction in unnecessary referrals where laboratory results play a major role in the diagnostic process. In rural health care this can reduce transportation costs and should also reduce the demands for institutional care too often used for the diagnostic workups.

In the second instance, if the theory of decision-making were accepted as a valid process to assess the efficiency of information gathering, the total number of tests run could in all likelihood be reduced by at least half (3).

In both illustrations, the real barrier is not in the validity of the principle or the availability of engineering sophistication but in the credibility of the process with both patients and the professionals. For those who are impatient with the slowness of the acceptance of change, it is well to remember that the system of health care operates on the primary stimulus of anxiety. The patient must be worried before he or she approaches the professional, and the professional must be concerned if he is to give an adequate response. In an anxiety-charged system logic must follow, not precede, credibility. Although logic may be useful at times in cultivating credibility, it cannot induce it per se. Most workers in the field of social change have overtly or covertly recognized and used this fact in activities less anxiety-charged than health care. Planners for health care systems, particularly the loosely knit rural system, will experience success in effecting change in direct proportion to their capacity to accept this fact. It is a particularly important element in effective operation of the necessarily hierarchical triage health care system.

COST CONTAINMENT. The opportunity to cultivate group acceptance of cost containment efforts is no doubt greater in rural communities than in any other segment of society. Rural communities possess the social consciousness that goes with local initiative and the more stable population. The fact that it is a stable mechanism often makes it frustrating for planners who feel that lack of change means lack of decision-making. Quite often the lack of change is the result of positive decisions not to change. The process is important to capture rather than to antagonize. It is in these communities that the first development of the purposeful priorities system for health care is most apt to succeed, although its initial design will be quite crude. Rural communities are accustomed to purposefully making decisions about what they will and will not use in community resources to accomplish tasks. Health care, considered in that system, will simply be another phase of something they are already accustomed to doing. The rural community's relegation of health to a lower status in the use of community resources has distressed many people. The important issue here is that they have used finite public resources and purposely set priority systems. While introduction of change addressed to improvement of health may be slow, it is feasible, it will be social in nature, and it will be retarded by the use of confrontation methodologies.

Given even minimal success in comprehensive health planning activities, rural communities will have some salutary effect on the establishment of priorities. The greatest promise lies in the small rural communities, provided these communities are allowed to operate as responsible social units. Such change, while slow in its evolution, represents the necessary change in values required for lasting improvement.

A word of caution is in order. If there is an attempt to aggregate these small communities into larger units without regard to the individual tendency for each of them to be self-sufficient, the effort will probably fail. The delegations of responsibility must be clearly explained to the presently cohesive community. Patience must be applied in generous proportions to assure that the community can and desires to cultivate a level of mutual trust with one or more additional communities.

MEASUREMENT OF COST EFFECTIVENESS. A *community health index* in some form is mandatory if cost effectiveness is to be measured and assured. A research instrument for experimental assessment of health status is currently being created through research work by Dr. Alex Leighton, School of Public Health, Harvard University. Research is being done with a rural community in Nova Scotia (1). The rural health care systems within the United States present a rich resource for field testing and the extension of that study. Such field testing would do much to advance the purposes of cost effectiveness as well as to improve the acceptance of new health care processes. The "work ethic" of the rural community enhances the probability that it will accept and implement an index that requires productivity as one dimension of health. As an aside, productivity is not measured in this study as employment but as an estimate of the capacity of the individual to make a contribution to society in accord with his and society's expectation. Such an instrument will not be available for general use in the immediate future, but it is the type of device that will most likely first appear in rural communities as an invaluable aid in the evaluation of priorities.

An available indirect measurement now partially in use is the developing Cooperative Federal, State, and Local Health Statistical System. Under the sponsorship of the National Center for Health Statistics, this program intends to assure that health data, both of the vital statistic and the operational variety, will be collected only once and will then be shared throughout the total system. Such an approach not only makes data collecting less expensive (therefore making more data available at the same cost), but, more importantly, it assures comparability between the data collected locally and those collected nationally or in similar communities. This is essential for the establishment of both national and local priorities and guidelines. It is crucial if national priorities are to effectively relate to local priorities.

CREDIBILITY. The most difficult task in altering a health care process centers about the credibility (or mutual trust) of the suggested change, not its technical viability.

The executive branch of the federal government during the middle 1970s has unfortunately provided a substantial number of illustrations for the difficulties incurred in maintaining credibility at a national level. The rural health care system is and will be no exception. There is good reason to believe that credibility may be easiest to induce when the greatest initiative is left at the local level. Participation in decision-making will increase the probability of understanding the reasons for the decisions, whether or not the participant agrees with the final selection. He will be more likely to cooperate if he feels the process used in developing the selection was equitable. It may well be that a system less scientifically precise with a higher degree of credibility and mutual confidence between the participants will in the long run be the most cost-effective system. In our vigorous search for "objective" data, we have tended to forget how small a portion of the total activities has been described by those data. Our decisions have focused on the measurable forces and considerations, to the exclusion of those more important but currently immeasurable. In so doing, we may well have paralyzed a great part of the system that we cannot analyze and cannot administratively manipulate, even if we understood it. Credibility is primarily a subjective feeling. Social structures and industries have in the past and will in the foreseeable future be primarily directed through the subjective feelings of those who participate in the decision-making process. To deny the subjective nature of most of our choices or priorities is less "objective" or rational from the viewpoint of logic than to accept the fact that the data objectively available measure too small a part of the total problem to be reliable indicators for decisions currently attributed to them. Infant mortality statistics, for instance, have been distorted and overutilized to describe the success of the health care system. In fact, one of the greatest reductions in infant mortality came with the introduction of refrigerators and sewers. Mortality figures can tell only about death for sure—all other characteristics are correlations or extrapolations. Much misplaced faith has been wasted on arguments related to mortality because it is so measurable. Quality of life is the true objective, only subjectively estimated but infinitely more important. It needs more thought in rural health.

Rural communities offer the first and largest insight into a method by which the maximum amount of initiative and local decision-making can be delegated to the local level while at the same time maintaining a common communications system and an acceptable level of public accountability for the content of the planned service process. Credibility, while not measurable in objective terms, may certainly be observed, understood, and commonly agreed to exist or not to exist even in the absence of objective measurements. The factor of credibility needs more specific attention and thought than it has enjoyed in the past; that attention should begin with willingness on the part of those who would plan to trust those whom they would serve, as full partners in the design of change. It will be most clearly studied and understood in the context of the rural community.

Most of the look at the future has dealt with the types of processes to be put in place. This is appropriate. It is the validity of the process, not the specific design of any detailed change, that in the long run will determine what the future will be. A rediscovery of the need for mutual trust between the various segments of society seems inevitable and essential for any other part of the planning process to be effective in rural and urban areas.

REFERENCES TO CHAPTERS

CHAPTER ONE

1. Anderson, Nancy N. 1968. *Comprehensive Health Planning in the States: A Study and Critical Analysis.* Minneapolis: American Rehabilitation Foundation.
2. *Annual Report.* 1940. New York: Rockefeller Foundation.
3. Bodenheimer, Thomas S. 1969. Regional medical programs: No road to regionalization. *Med. Care Rev.* 26: 1125–66.
4. Cater, Douglas, W. R. Willard, E. D. Sax, and P. G. Rogers. 1968. Comprehensive health planning. *Am. J. Public Health* 58: 1022–1038.
5. Coggeshall, Lowell T. 1965. *Planning for Medical Progress through Education.* Evanston, Ill.: Association of American Medical Colleges.
6. *Hospital Care in the United States.* 1946. Chicago: Commission on Hospital Care.
7. de la Chapelle, Clarence E., and Frode Jensen. 1964. *A Mission in Action— The Story of the Regional Hospital Plan of New York University.* New York: New York University Press.
8. Elinson, Jack, and Conrad E. A. Herr. 1970. A sociomedical view of neighborhood health centers. *Med. Care* 8: 97–103.
9. Emerson, Haven. 1945. *Local Health Units for the Nation.* New York: Commonwealth Fund.
10. Falk, I. S. 1970. National health insurance: A review of policies and proposals. *Law Contemp. Probl.* 35: 669–96.
11. Feingold, Eugene. 1966. *Medicare: Policies and Politics.* San Francisco: Chandler.
12. Field, Mark G. 1967. *Soviet Socialized Medicine.* New York: Free Press.
13. Goldman, Franz. 1945. *Public Medical Care: Principles and Problems.* New York: Columbia University Press.
14. Hall, W. W. 1863. Farmers' homes. *Report: Commissioner of Agriculture for 1862.* Washington, D.C., p. 313 ff.
15. ———. 1863. Health of farmers' families. *Report: Commissioner of Agriculture for 1862.* Washington, D.C., p. 453.
16. Harris, Richard. 1966. *A Sacred Trust.* New York: New American Library.
17. Health personnel will be assigned to critical manpower-lacking areas. 1972. *Medical Tribune,* June 28.
18. Jordan, E. P. 1958. *The Physician in Group Practice.* Chicago: Yearbook Publishers.
19. Klarman, Herbert E. 1971. Analysis of the HMO proposal—Its assumptions, implications, and prospects. *Health Maintenance Organizations: A Reconfiguration of the Health Services System.* Chicago: University of Chicago Center for Health Administration Studies, pp. 24–38.

20. Kratz, F. W. 1943. Status of full-time local health organizations at the end of fiscal year 1941–42. *Public Health Rep.* 48: 345–51.
21. Lumsden, L. L. 1930. Extent of rural health service in the U.S. 1926–30. *Public Health Rep.* 45: 1065–81.
22. Madison, Donald L. 1972. A rural health care stategy for the Robert Wood Johnson Foundation. Chapel Hill: University of North Carolina, Rural Health Serv. Res. Unit (processed).
23. Marston, Robert W. 1967. A nation starts a program: Regional medical programs, 1965–66. *J. Med. Educ.* (Jan.): 17–27.
24. Massie, William A. 1957. *Medical Services for Rural Areas: The Tennessee Medical Foundation.* Cambridge, Mass.: Harvard University Press.
25. McNerney, Walter J., and Donald C. Riedel. 1962. *Regionalization and Rural Health Care.* Ann Arbor: University of Michigan Bureau of Hospital Administration.
26. M.D.'s obtained for rural areas. *AMA News*, Feb. 27, 1967.
27. Mott, F. D., and M. I. Roemer. 1945. Federal program of public health and medical services for migratory farm workers. *Public Health Rep.* 60: 229–49.
28. _____. 1948. *Rural Health and Medical Care.* New York: McGraw-Hill, pp. 389–431.
29. Moore, Harry H. 1927. *American Medicine and the People's Health.* New York: Macmillan, p. 195.
30. Mountin, Joseph W., E. H. Pennell, and V. M. Hoge. 1945. *Health Service Areas—Requirements for General Hospitals and Health Centers.* Washington, D.C.: PHS Bull. 292.
31. Munts, Raymond. 1967. *Bargaining for Health: Labor Unions, Health Insurance, and Medical Care.* Madison: University of Wisconsin Press, p. 141.
32. Mustard, Harry S. 1945. *Government in Public Health.* New York: Commonwealth Fund, pp. 73–77.
33. _____. 1936. *Rural Health Practice.* New York: Commonwealth Fund, p. 4 ff.
34. Myers, Robert J. 1970. *Medicare.* Homewood, Ill.: Richard D. Erwin.
35. National Advisory Commission on Health Facilities. 1968. *A Report to the President.* Washington, D.C.: USGPO.
36. Reed, Louis S. 1965. *The Extent of Health Insurance Coverage in the United States.* Washington, D.C.: U.S. Social Security Administration, Res. Rep. 10.
37. *Report of the National Advisory Commission on Health Manpower.* 1967. Washington, D.C.: USGPO, Vol. 1.
38. Rice, Dorothy P., and Barbara S. Cooper. 1971. National health expenditures, 1929–70. *Soc. Secur. Bull.* (Jan.): 3–18.
39. Roemer, Milton I. 1951. Approaches to the rural doctor shortage. *Rural Sociol.* 16: 137–47.
40. _____. 1960. The distribution of hospital beds needed in a region. *J. Health Hum. Behav.* 1: 94–101.
41. _____. 1968. Health needs and services of the rural poor. *Rural Poverty in the United States.* Washington, D.C.: National Commission on Rural Poverty, pp. 311–32.
42. _____. 1948. Historic development of the current crisis of rural medicine in the United States. *Victor Robinson Memorial Volume: Essays on Historical Medicine.* New York: Froben Press, pp. 333–42.
43. Roemer, Milton I., and Barbara Faulkner. 1951. The development of public health services in a rural county: 1838–1949. *J. Hist. Med. Allied Sci.* 1:22–43.
44. Rosen, George. 1946. Fees and fee bills: Some economic aspects of medical practice in the 19th-century America. *Bull. Hist. Med.*, Suppl. 6, pp. 16–18.
45. Rosenfeld, Leonard S., and Henry B. Makover. 1956. *The Rochester Regional Hospital Council.* Cambridge, Mass.: Harvard University Press.
46. Ross, Austin, and Robert L. Boyle, Jr. 1972. Urban-rural exchange programs. *Hospitals* (July 16): 55–19.
47. Schorr, L. B., and J. T. English. 1968. Background, context and significant issues in neighborhood health center programs. *Milbank Mem. Fund Quart.* 46: 289–96.
48. Schottland, Charles I. 1963. *The Social Security Program in the United States.* New York: Appleton-Century-Crofts.

49. Shadid, Michael A. 1947. *Doctors of Today and Tomorrow*. New York: Co-operative League of America.
50. Shanholts, Mark I. 1967. Virginia State Department of Health, personal communication, Apr. 3.
51. Shattuck, Lemuel. 1948. *Report of the Sanitary Commission of Massachusetts, 1850* (reprinted). Cambridge, Mass.: Harvard University Press.
52. Somers, Anne R. 1969. *Hospital Regulation: The Dilemma of Public Policy*. Princeton, N.J.: Princeton University, Industrial Relations Section.
53. Somers, Herman M., and Anne R. Somers. 1961. *Doctors, Patients, and Health Insurance*. Washington, D.C.: Brookings Institution.
54. Southmayd, Henry J., and Geddes Smith. 1944. *Small Community Hospitals*. New York: Commonwealth Fund.
55. Stewart, William H. 1967. *New Dimensions of Health Planning*. Chicago: University of Chicago, Graduate School of Business Administration.
56. *Report for the year ending June 30, 1972*. 1972. Washington, D.C.: United Mine Workers of America Welfare and Retirement Fund.
57. Inter-Bureau Committee on Post-War Programs. 1945. *Better Health for Rural America*. Washington, D.C.: USDA.
58. *Inventory of Federal Programs That Support Health Manpower Training*. 1971. Washington, D.C.: HEW.
59. *To Improve Medical Care—A Guide to Federal Financial Aid for the Development of Medical Care Services, Facilities, Personnel*. 1966. Washington, D.C.: HEW, p. 49.
60. U.S. National Center for Health Statistics. 1964. *Health Insurance Coverage, United States, 1962–63*. Washington, D.C.: PHS Publ. 1000, Ser. 10, No. 11.
61. U.S. Public Health Service. 1964. *Directory of Local Health Units, 1964*. Washington, D.C.: PHS Publ. 118 (rev.).
62. ———. 1957. *Health Services for American Indians*. Washington, D.C.: PHS Publ. 531.
63. ———. 1963. *Medical Groups in the United States*. Washington, D.C.: PHS Publ. 1063.
64. ———. 1966. *Two Decades of Partnership: Hill-Burton Program 1946–1966*. Washington, D.C.: PHS Publ. 930-F-9.
65. U.S. Senate, Committee on Finance. 1970. *Medicare and Medicaid: Problems, Issues, and Alternatives*. Washington, D.C.: USGPO.
66. U.S. Senate, Committee on Labor and Public Welfare. 1965. *The Migratory Farm Labor Problem in the United States, 1965*. Washington, D.C.: USGPO, No. 155.
67. *The Impact of Medicare: An Annotated Bibliography of Selected Sources*. 1969. Washington, D.C.: U.S. Social Security Administration.
68. Vaughan, Henry F. 1972. Local health services in the United States: The story of the CAP. *Am. J. Public Health* 62: 95–111.
69. Wagner, Carruth J., and Erwin F. Rabeau. 1964. Indian poverty and Indian health. *HEW Indicators* (Mar.): 24–44.
70. Williams, Pierce. 1932. *The Purchase of Medical Care through Fixed Periodic Payment*. New York: National Bureau of Economic Research.

CHAPTER TWO

1. Bowring, James R., and Nelson L. LeRay. 1969. *The New Hampshire Older Poor*. Durham: Univ. New Hampshire Coop. Ext. Serv. Ext. Circ. 389.
2. Crecink, John C., and Roosevelt Steptoe. 1970. *Human Resources in the Rural Mississippi Delta—With Emphasis on the Poor*. Washington, D.C.: USDA, ERS, Agr. Econ. Rep. 170.
3. U.S. Senate, Committee on Government Operations. 1971. *The Economic and Social Condition of Rural America in the 1970's*. Washington, D.C.: USDA, ERS.

4. Ellenbogen, Bert L. 1967. Health status of the rural aged. In E. Grant Youmans, ed., *Older Rural Americans: A Sociological Perspective.* Lexington: University of Kentucky Press, pp. 195–220.
5. Grebler, Leo, Joan W. Moore, and Ralph C. Guzman. 1970. *The Mexican-American People: The Nation's Second Largest Minority.* New York: Free Press.
6. Hoover, Herbert, and Bernal L. Green. 1970. *Human Resources in the Ozarks Region—With Emphasis on the Poor.* Washington, D.C.: USDA, ERS, Agr. Econ. Rep. 182.
7. Johnson, Helen W. 1969. *Rural American Indians in Poverty.* Washington, D.C.: USDA, ERS, Agr. Econ. Rep. 167.
8. Moynihan, Daniel P. 1972. The schism in black America. *Public Interest* 27: 3–24.
9. Mott, Frederick D., and Milton I. Roemer. 1948. *Rural Health and Medical Care.* New York: McGraw-Hill.
10. National Center for Health Statistics. 1974. Acute conditions: Incidence and associated disability, United States, July 1971–June 1972. *Vital and Health Statisics,* Ser. 10, No. 88. Washingon, D.C.: HEW.
11. ———. 1972. Disability days: United States, 1968. *Vital and Health Statistics,* Ser. 10, No. 67. Washington, D.C.: HEW.
12. ———. 1974. Health characteristics by geographic region, large metropolitan areas, and other places of residence, United States, 1969–70. *Vital and Health Statistics,* Ser. 10, No. 86. Washington, D.C.: HEW.
13. ———. 1972. Hospital and surgical insurance coverage, United States, 1968. *Vital and Health Statistics,* Ser. 10, No. 66. Washington, D.C.: HEW.
14. ———. 1972. Infant mortality rates: Socioeconomic factors, United States. *Vital and Health Statistics,* Ser. 22, No. 14. Washington, D.C.: HEW.
15. ———. 1970. Motor vehicle accident deaths in the United States, 1950–67. *Vital and Health Statistics,* Ser. 20, No. 9. Washington, D.C.: HEW.
16. ———. 1970. Need for dental care among adults, United States, 1960–1962. *Vital and Health Statistics,* Ser. 11, No. 36. Washington, D.C.: HEW.
17. ———. 1970. Persons injured and disability days due to injury, United States, July 1965–June 1967. *Vital and Health Statistics,* Ser. 10, No. 58. Washington, D.C.: HEW.
18. Rowe, Gene A., and Leslie Whitener Smith. 1974. *Income of Farm Wageworker Households in 1971.* Washington, D.C.: USDA, ERS, Agr. Econ. Rep. 251.
19. Taft, Earl A., and Flossie M. Byrd. 1972. *Black Families under Stress: A Metropolitan-Nonmetropolitan Comparison of Individual and Family Disability in a Southern Area.* Prairie View, Tex.: Prairie View A & M Univ. Dep. Tech. Rep. 72-1.
20. U.S. Bureau of the Census. 1973. *Census of Population: 1970.* Vol. 1, *Characteristics of the Population.* Washington, D.C.: USGPO, Pt. 1, U.S. Summary, Sect. 1.
21. ———. 1974. *Population of the United States, Trends and Prospects: 1950–1990.* Washington, D.C.: USGPO, Curr. Popul. Rep., Ser. P-23, No. 49.

CHAPTER THREE

1. Bogue, Donald J., and Calvin L. Beale. 1961. *Economic Areas of the United States.* New York: Free Press, p. 1161.
2. Friedman, G. D. 1967. Cigarette smoking and geographic variation in coronary heart disease mortality in the United States. *J. Chronic Dis.* 20:769–79.
3. Grove, Robert D., and Alice Hetzel. 1968. *Vital Statistics Rates in the United States, 1940–1960.* Washington, D.C.: Nat. Health Serv. Publ. 1677, p. 881.
4. Hambright, T. Z. 1968. Comparability of age on the death certificate and

matching census record, United States, May–August 1960. Washington, D.C.: PHS Publ. 1000, Ser. 2, No. 29.

5. Linder, Forrest E., and Robert D. Grove. 1943. *Vital Statistics Rates in the United States, 1900–1940*. Washington, D.C.: USGPO, p. 1051.

6. Moriyama, I. M., D. E. Krueger, and J. Stamler. 1970. *Cardiovascular Diseases*. Cambridge, Mass.: Harvard University Press.

7. Namey, Christy W., and Ronald W. Wilson. 1974. Health characteristics by geographic region, large metropolitan areas, and other places of residence. *Vital and Health Statistics*, Ser. 10, No. 86, pp. 1–14. Washington, D.C.: HEW Publ. (HRA) 74–1513.

8. Sauer, H. I. 1962. Epidemiology of cardiovascular mortality—Geographic and ethnic. *Am. J. Public Health* 52: 94–105.

9. ———. 1974. Geographic variations in mortality and morbidity. In Carl L. Erhardt and Joyce E. Berlin, eds., *Mortality and Morbidity in the United States*. Cambridge, Mass.: Harvard University Press, pp. 105–29.

10. ———. 1974. Is there a water factor? The puzzle of competing factors. *Proc., 7th Intern. Water Quality Symp.*, Washington, D.C., in press.

11. ———. 1967. Migration and the risk of dying. *Proc. Am. Stat. Assoc.*, Washington, D.C., pp. 399–407.

12. Sauer, H. I., and F. R. Brand. 1971. Geographic patterns in the risk of dying. *Geol. Soc. Am. Memoir* 123: 131–50.

13. Sauer, H. I., L. D. Edmonds, and G. H. Land. 1975. Cancer death rates for whites age 35–74 by sex, 1950–1972. *Data for Missouri No. 7803*. Columbia: University of Missouri, Ext. Div., in press.

14. Sauer, H. I., and Darrel W. Parke. 1974. Counties with extreme death rates and associated factors. *Am. J. Epidemiol.* 99 (4): 258–64.

15. Sauer, H. I., Algird J. Valiunas, and Lucia K. Leggette. 1973. Mortality variations among the aged. Presented at Am. Public Health Assoc. convention, Statistics Session, San Francisco.

16. Sauer, H. I., H. T. Wright, and G. H. Land. 1975. Death rates for cardiovascular diseases, whites age 35–74 by sex, 1950–1972. *Data for Missouri No. 7801*. Columbia: University of Missouri, Ext. Div., in press.

17. ———. 1975. Death rates for selected natural causes, whites age 35–74 by sex, 1968–1972. *Data for Missouri No. 7802*. Columbia: University of Missouri, Ext. Div.

18. U.S. Bureau of the Census. 1961. *U.S. Census of Population: 1960. General Population Characteristics*. Washington, D.C.: USGPO, Final Rep. PC(1)-1B to 57B.

19. ———. 1963. *U.S. Census of Population: 1960. Selected Area Reports. State Economic Areas*. Washington, D.C.: USGPO, Final Rep. PC(3)-1A.

20. ———. 1971. *U.S. Census of Population: 1970. General Population Characteristics*. Washington, D.C.: USGPO, Final Rep. PC(1)-B1 to B57.

21. ———. 1972. *U.S. Census of Population: 1970. State Economic Areas*. Washington, D.C.: USGPO, Final Rep. PC (2)-10B.

22. White, Kerr L. 1967. Improved medical care statistics and the health services. *Public Health Rep.* 82: 847–54.

23. Wylie, Charles M. 1970. The definition and measurement of health and disease. *Public Health Rep.* 85: 100–104.

CHAPTER FOUR

1. Aday, LuAnn, and Ronald Andersen. 1975. *Development of Indices of Access to Medical Care*. Ann Arbor: Health Administration Press.

2. Albrecht, Stan L., and Michael K. Miller. 1973. Health service delivery: An assessment of some adequacy indicators. Presented at Ann. Meet. Rural Sociol. Soc., University of Maryland, College Park.

3. Albrecht, Stan L. 1973. The provision of health-related services in rural and urban areas. *Utah Sci.* 34(3): 78–82.
4. Andersen, R., and O. W. Anderson. 1967. *A Decade of Health Services.* Chicago: University of Chicago Press.
5. Anderson, James G. 1973. Causal models and social indicators: Toward the development of social systems models. *Am. Sociol. Rev.* 38(3):285–301.
6. Balfe, B. E., J. H. Lorant, and C. Todd. 1971. *Reference Data on the Profile of Medical Practice.* Chicago: American Medical Association.
7. Ball, David S., and Jack Wilson. 1968. Community health facilities and services: The manpower dimensions. *Am. J. Agr. Econ.* 50(5): 1208–22.
8. Benham, L., A. Maurizi, and M. W. Reder. 1968. Migration, location and remuneration of medical personnel: Physicians and dentists. *Rev. Econ. Stat.* 50 (3): 332–47.
9. Bestor, Frank H., William R. Jeffries, and Roberta Minnis. 1971. Are you listening, neighbor? *Report of the Indian Affairs Task Force,* Olympia, Wash.: Secretary of State's Office, pp. 51–55.
10. Bible, Bond L. 1970. Physicians' views of medical practice in nonmetropolitan communities. *Public Health Rep.* 85 (1): 11–17.
11. *Michigan Physician Trainee Survey.* 1974. Detroit: Blue Shield of Michigan.
12. Borhani, Nemat O., and Jess F. Kraus. 1973. Use of health services in a rural community. *Health Serv. Rep.* 88 (3): 275–88.
13. Breisch, William F. 1970. Impact of medical school characteristics on location of physician practice. *J. Med. Educ.* 45: 1068–70.
14. Busek, Linda C. 1973. A doctor who specializes in doctorless towns. *Medical Economics,* Apr. 16, p. 130.
15. Butter, Irene, and Richard Schaffner. 1971. Foreign medical graduates and equal access to medical care. *Med. Care* 9(2):136–43.
16. Caudill, Harry M. 1972. Appalachia: The corporate fiefdom. In Helen Ginsburg, ed., *Poverty, Economics, and Society.* Boston: Little, Brown, pp. 223–27.
17. Champion, Dean J., and Donald B. Olsen. 1971. Physician behavior in southern Appalachia: Some recruitment factors. *J. Health Soc. Behav.* 12: 245–52.
18. Christenson, James A., and Vance E. Hamilton. 1974. *Through Our Eyes: Rural-Urban Health Care in North Carolina.* Raleigh: N.C. Agr. Ext. Serv. Misc. Ext. Publ. 115.
19. Cordes, Sam Meade. 1973. *The General Practitioner in Rural Washington: Opinions, Characteristics, and Comparative Productivity among Practice Sizes.* Ph.D. diss. Pullman: Washington State University.
20. Cordes, Sam Meade, and Paul W. Barkley. 1974. *Physicians and Physician Services in Rural Washington.* Pullman: Wash. State Univ. Agr. Exp. Sta. Bull. 790.
21. Cordes, Sam Meade, and Charles O. Crawford. 1974. Health care needs and resources in Pennsylvania: A guide for studying community health services. University Park: Pennsylvania Cooperative Extension Service.
22. Crawford, Ronald L., and Regina C. McCormack. 1971. Reasons physicians leave primary care. *J. Med. Educ.* 46:263–68.
23. Department of Community Affairs. 1971. *Final Summary Report: The Pennsylvania Panel on Rural Poverty.* Harrisburg, Penn.: Department of Community Affairs, pp. 19–23.
24. Detweiler, David. 1971. Dr. Huerta C. Neals: He takes his office to the patient. *Parade,* Jan. 24, pp. 14–16.
25. DeVise, Pierre. 1973. Physician migration from inland to coastal states: Antipodal examples of Illinois and California. *J. Med. Educ.* 48:141–51.
26. Diehl, Harold S. 1951. Physicians for rural areas: A factor in their procurement. *J. Am. Med. Assoc.* 145: 1134.
27. Dubé, W. F., and Davis G. Johnson. 1974. Study of U.S. medical school applicants, 1972–73. *J. Med. Educ.* 49 (8): 849–69.
28. Elesh, David, and Paul T. Schollaert. 1972. Race and urban medicine: Factors affecting the distribution of physicians in Chicago. *J. Health Soc. Behav.* 13 (3): 236–50.

29. Fahs, Ivan, and Osler L. Peterson. 1968. The decline of general practice. *Public Health Rep.* 83 (4): 267–70.
30. ———. 1968. Towns without physicians and towns with only one—A study of four states in the upper Midwest, 1965. *Am. J. Public Health* 58 (7): 1212–29.
31. Fein, Rashi. 1967. *The Doctor Shortage: An Economic Diagnosis.* Washington, D.C.: Brookings Institution.
32. Ficker, Victor B., and Herbert S. Graves, eds. 1971. *Deprivation in America.* Beverly Hills, Calif.: Glencoe Press, pp. 1–7, 52–65.
33. Garrison, Glen E., Warren H. Gullen, and Connie M. Connell. 1974. Migration of urbanites to small towns for medical care. *J. Am. Med. Assoc.* 227 (7): 770–73.
34. Gottlieb, P. M. 1971. The migration and distribution of physicians. *Reference Data on the Profile of Medical Practice.* Chicago: American Medical Association, pp. 88–90.
35. Grigg, M. R. 1969. *A Demographic and Ecological Analysis of the Rural-Urban Distribution of Physicians in North Carolina.* M. S. thesis. Chapel Hill: University of North Carolina.
36. Hassinger, Edward W. 1963. *Background and Community Orientation of Rural Physicians Compared with Metropolitan Physicians in Missouri.* Columbia: Univ. Mo. Agr. Exp. Sta. Res. Bull. 822.
37. Haug, J. N., G. A. Roback, C. N. Theodore, and B. E. Balfe. 1970. *Distribution of Physicians, Hospitals, and Hospital Beds in the U.S., 1968.* Chicago: American Medical Association.
38. Health professions student loans. 1974. *Fed. Regist.* 39 (38): 7446–66.
39. Joroff, Sheila, and Vicente Navarro. 1971. Medical manpower: A multivariate analysis of the distribution of physicians in urban United States. *Med. Care* 9 (5): 428–38.
40. Klarman, Herbert E. 1969. Economic aspects of projecting requirements for health manpower. *J. Hum. Resour.* 4 (s): 360–76.
41. Knowles, John H. 1969. The quantity and quality of medical manpower: A review of medicine's current efforts. *J. Med. Educ.* 44:81–118.
42. Kosa, John, A. Antonovsky, and I. K. Zola. 1969. *Poverty and Health: A Sociological Analysis.* Cambridge, Mass.: Harvard University Press.
43. Marden, Parker G. 1966. A demographic and ecological analysis of the distribution of physicians in metropolitan America, 1960. *Am. J. Sociol.* 72(3): 290–300.
44. Marguiles, Harold, and Lucille Stephenson Bloch. 1969. *Foreign Medical Graduates in the United States.* Cambridge, Mass.: Harvard University Press.
45. Marshall, Carter L., Khatab M. Hassanein, Ruth S. Hassanein, and Carol L. Marshall. 1971. Principal components analysis of the distribution of physicians, dentists, and osteopaths in a midwestern state. *Am. J. Public Health* 61 (8): 1556–64.
46. Mason, Henry R. 1971. Effectiveness of student aid programs tied to a service commitment. *J. Med. Educ.* 46:575–83.
47. ———. 1972. Manpower needs by specialty. *J. Am. Med. Assoc.* 219 (12): 1621–26.
48. Mattson, Dale E., Donald E. Stehr, and Roy E. Will. 1973. Evaluation of a program designed to produce rural physicians. *J. Med. Educ.* 48: 323–31.
49. McFarland, John. 1973. The physician's location decision. *Reference Data on the Profile of Medical Practice.* Chicago: American Medical Association, pp. 89–96.
50. Mullner, Ross, and Thomas W. O'Rourke. 1974. A geographic analysis of counties without an active non-federal physician, United States, 1963–71. *Health Serv. Rep.* 89 (3): 256–62.
51. Nolan, Robert L., and Jerome L. Schwartz, eds. 1973. *Rural and Appalachian Health.* Springfield, Ill.: Charles C Thomas.
52. Parker, Ralph C., Richard A. Rix, and Thomas G. Tuxill. 1969. Social, economic, and demographic factors affecting physician population in upstate New York. *N.Y. State J. Med.* 69: 706–12.

53. Parker, Ralph C., and Thomas G. Tuxill. 1967. The attitudes of physicians toward small-community practice. *J. Med. Educ.* 42: 327–44.
54. Paxton, Harry T. 1973. Doctor shortage? It's narrowing down to primary care. *Medical Economics*, Mar. 19, pp. 104–7.
55. Perkinson, Leon B. 1974. Distance traveled to obtain medical services in a selected rural area. Presented at Ann. Meet. Am. Agr. Econ. Assoc., Texas A & M University, College Station, Texas.
56. Perkinson, Leon B. 1972. *Health Service Differentials in Michigan.* East Lansing: Mich. State Univ. Dep. Agr. Econ. Rep. 213.
57. Peterson, Gary R. 1968. *A Comparison of Selected Professional and Social Characteristics of Urban and Rural Physicians in Iowa.* Iowa City: University of Iowa Graduate Program in Hospital and Health Administration, Health Care Res. Ser. 8.
58. Ploch, Louis A., and Nancy A. Black. 1974. *A Study of Health Related Factors: Bucksport, Orland, Verona, Maine 1973.* Orono: Univ. Maine Dep. Agr. Resour. Econ. Misc. Rep. 238.
59. Radtke, Hans D. 1974. *The Allocation of Health-Producing Resources in the Pacific Northwest.* Corvallis: Oregon State Univ. Agr. Exp. Sta. Spec. Rep. 406.
60. ———. 1974. Benefits and costs of a physician to a community. *Am. J. Agr. Econ.* 56 (3): 586–93.
61. Reul, Myrtle R. 1974. *Territorial Boundaries of Rural Poverty: Profiles of Exploitation.* East Lansing: Michigan State University, Center for Rural Manpower and Public Affairs and Coop. Ext. Serv.
62. Richardson, Elliot L. 1972. Meeting the nation's health manpower needs. *J. Med. Educ.* 47: 3–9.
63. Roback, G. A. 1974. *Distribution of Physicians in the U.S., 1972.* Chicago: American Medical Association
64 Roth, Russell 1974. Countryside needs health services: What kind and where? *Modern Medicine,* Apr. 1, pp. 26–30.
65. Royce, Paul C. 1972. Can rural health education centers influence physician distribution? *J. Am. Med. Assoc.* 220 (6): 847–49.
66. Scheffler, R. M. 1971. The relationship between medical education and the statewide per capita distribution of physicians. *J. Med. Educ.* 46: 995–99.
67. Schonfeld, Hyman K., Jean F. Heston, and Isidore S. Falk. 1972. Number of physicians required for primary medical care. *New Engl. J. Med.* 286 (11): 571–76.
68. Senior, Boris, and Beverly A. Smith. 1972. The number of physicians as a constraint on delivery of health care: How many physicians are enough? *J. Am. Med. Assoc.* 222 (2): 178–83.
69. Seventy-third annual report on medical education. 1973. *J. Am. Med. Assoc.* 226 (8): 894–89.
70. Steele, Henry B., and Gaston V. Rimlinger. 1965. Income opportunities and physician location trends in the United States. *West. Econ. J.* 3 (2): 182–94.
71. Steinwald, Bruce. 1974. Physician location: Behavior versus attitudes. *Reference Data on the Socioeconomic Issues of Health.* Chicago: American Medical Association, pp. 34–41.
72. Stevens, Carl M. 1971. Physician supply and national health care goals. *Ind. Relat.* 10 (2): 119–44.
73. Taylor, Mark, William Dickman, and Robert Kane. 1973. Medical students' attitudes toward rural practice. *J. Med. Educ.* 48: 885–95.
74. U.S. Senate, Committee on Labor and Public Welfare. 1969. *Migrant Health Services.* Washington, D.C.: USGPO.
75. U.S. Senate, Committee on Government Operations. 1969. *Health Care in America.* Washington, D.C.: USGPO.
76. Rural Development Service. 1973. *Health Services in Rural Areas.* Washington, D.C.: USDA, Agr. Inf. Bull. 362.
77. Bureau of Community Health Services. 1973. *Background Paper: Health Service Scarcity Area Identification Program.* Washington, D.C.: HEW.
78. National Center for Health Statistics. 1973. *Health Resource Statistics: Health Manpower and Health Facilities, 1972-73.* Washington, D.C.: HEW, PHS.

79. Bureau of Health Professions Education and Manpower Training. 1969. *Health Manpower Source Book*. Washington, D.C.: HEW, Sec. 20, PHS Publ. 263.
80. Vahovich, Steve G., and Phil Aherne, eds. 1973. *Reference Data on the Profile of Medical Practice*. Chicago: American Medical Association.
81. Wennberg, John, and Alan Gittelsohn. 1973. Small area variations in health care delivery. *Science* 182: 1102–8.
82. Whieldon, David. 1967. How specialism is affecting G.P.s. *Medical Economics*, Oct. 30, pp. 139–47.
83. Willie, Charles V. 1972. Health care needs of the disadvantaged in a rural-urban area. *HSMHA Health Rep.* 87 (1): 81–86.
84. Yett, Donald E., and Frank A. Sloan. 1974. Migration patterns of recent medical school graduates. *Inquiry* 11 (2): 125–42.

CHAPTER FIVE

1. Baxter, W. Eugene. 1969. An economical ambulance plan for the small community. *Hospitals* 43: 72–74.
2. Bierman, Leland, and Mark Powers. 1970. *Ambulance-Services in Northwest South Dakota*. Brookings: South Dakota State University Press, Bull. 569, pp. 3–4.
3. Blumenfeld, Arthur. 1967. *Heart Attack: Are You a Candidate?* New York: Paul S. Erickson, p. 2.
4. Bodenheimer, Thomas S. 1969. Mobile units: A solution to the rural health problem? *Med. Care* 7 (2): 145.
5. Rural health care on wheels (editorial). 1971. *South. Hosp.* (June):22.
6. Fischer-Murray, Inc. 1970. SOS from patient alone. *Emergency Med.* 6: 68–70.
7. *Funk and Wagnalls New Encyclopedia*. 1972. New York: Funk and Wagnalls, Vol. 1, pp. 471–72.
8. Haddon, William J., Jr. 1967. Highway safety: A progress report. *J. Med. Assoc. Louisiana* 52: 456–59.
9. Huntley, Henry C. 1972. The first hours are critical in medical emergencies. *J. Am. Coll. Emergency Physicians* (March–April): 13–16.
10. Jacobs, Arthur R. 1972. *A Study of Medical Transport Needs in Rural Communities*. Hanover, N.H.: Dartmouth Medical School, Dep. Community Med., p. 1.
11. Jacobs, Arthur R., and Curtis P. McLaughlin. 1967. Analyzing the role of the helicopter in emergency medical care for a community. *Med. Care* 5(5): 343.
12. Luckey, Virginia M. 1960. The first rural public hospital. *J. Iowa State Med. Soc.* (March): 165–66.
13. MAST-Fact Sheet, May 1972.
14. Miller, Clinton, and Randolph Page. 1958. The effect on survival of delay in emergency care in motor vehicle injuries in Louisiana. *J. Louisiana State Med. Soc.* 120: 1–6.
15. Mitchell, Frank L. 1968. Emergency health services. *J. Am. Osteopath. Assoc.* 67:544–46.
16. Reese, James, and Zane Thornton. 1971. A description of the Vermont-New Hampshire medical interactive network. Presented at Nat. Telemetry Conf., Washington, D.C., p. 1.
17. An integrated transportation system to serve health and social service needs. 1972. RRC Corp. paper, Troy, N.Y.
18. Sanders, Irvin. 1972. Public health in the community. In Howard E. Freeman, Sol Levine, and Leo G. Reeder, *Handbook of Medical Sociology*, 2nd ed. Englewood Cliffs, N.J.: Prentice-Hall.
19. Simmerman, David. 1972. If you are going to get hurt, do it in Illinois. *Today's Health* 10: 51–66.

20. Struness, E. B. 1971. Mobile emergency care: Present usage and future potential. Prepared for seminar in Tele-Medicine Promise for 1980, Mass. Med. Soc., p. 3.
21. Taubenhaus, Leon J., and John R. Kirkpatrick. 1967. Analysis of a hospital ambulance service. *Public Health Rep.* 82: 823–27.
22. Turrini, A. 1963. The ambulance for profit or compassion? *Aid* (Nov.–Dec.): 18.
23. Vickens, Allan. 1963. The royal flying doctor service of Australia. *World Med. J.* (May): 171–72.
24. Waller, Julian A. 1969. Emergency health services in areas of low population density. *J. Am. Med. Assoc.* 207 (12): 2255.
25. Wilsen, Robert J. 1970. Ambulance service and emergency rooms: Single unit needed for today's care. *Hosp. Trib.* 4(12):9.

CHAPTER SIX

1. Anderson, W. H. Locke. 1964. Trickling down: The relationship between economic growth and the extent of poverty among American families. *Quart. J. Econ.* (Nov.): 511–24.
2. Board of Governors of the Federal Reserve System. 1974. *Fed. Reserve Bull.* 60 (8): A-55.
3. *Building a National Health-Care System.* 1973. New York: Committee for Economic Development, p. 40.
4. Edwards, Clark, and Calvin L. Beale. 1969. Rural change in the 1960's. Presented at 46th Nat. Agr. Outlook Conf., Washington, D.C., p. 3.
5. Hardy, William E., Jr. 1972. Health care in rural areas. Blacksburg: Virginia Polytechnic Institute and State University, Coop. Ext. Serv., p. 2.
6. Haren, Claude. 1970. Rural industrial growth in the 1960's. *Am. J. Agr. Econ.* (Aug.): 431–37.
7. *Source Book of Health Insurance Data, 1971–1972.* 1972. New York: Health Insurance Institute, p. 16.
8. Kinney, Paul T. 1957. Financing medical care. Ph.D. diss. Los Angeles: University of Southern California, pp. 99–101.
9. Kolodrubetz, W. W. 1968. Employee-benefit plans in 1966. *Soc. Secur. Bull.* 31 (4): 29.
10. Phelps, Charles E., and Joseph P. Newhouse. 1972. Effects of coinsurance: A multivariate analysis. *Soc. Secur. Bull.* 72–11700.
11. Roemer, Milton I., Donald M. Dubois, and Shirley W. Rich. 1970. *Health Insurance Plans, Studies in Organizational Diversity.* Los Angeles: University of California, School of Public Health, passim.
12. Scitovsky, Anne A., and Nelda M. Snyder. 1972. Effect of coinsurance on use of physician services. *Soc. Secur. Bull.* 35(6).
13. Somers, Herman M. 1969. Economic issues in health services. In Neil W. Chamberlain, ed., *Contemporary Economic Issues.* Homewood, Ill.: Richard D. Irwin, pp. 109–44.
14. *Family Economic Review.* 1972. Washington, D.C.: USDA, p. 16.
15. *Developing Rural Communities.* 1971. Washington, D.C.: USDA, ERS, p. 4.
16. *Farm Income Situation.* 1970. Washington, D.C.: USDA, ERS, FIS 216, Table 7 H, p. 50.
17. *Health Care in Rural America.* 1970. Washington, D.C.: USDA, ERS-451, p. 4.
18. U.S. Senate, Committee on Government Operations. 1971. *The Economic and Social Condition of Rural America in the 1970's, Part 1.* Washington, D.C.: USDA, ERS, pp. 48–49 and passim.
19. *The Economic and Social Condition of Rural America in the 1970's, Part 3.* 1971. Washington, D.C.: USDA, ERS.
20. Bureau of the Census. 1972. *Census of Population: 1970 General Social and Economic Characteristics.* Washington, D.C.: USGPO, Final Rep. PC (1)-Cl, U.S. Summary, pp. 401, 413.

21. ———. 1972. Consumer income. *Current Population Reports* P-60 (85): 57. Washington, D.C.: USGPO.
22. ———. 1970. *Current Population Reports* P-20 (233). Washington, D.C.: USGPO.
23. ———. 1971. *Current Population Reports* P-23 (37):34. Washington, D.C.: USGPO.
24. ———. 1971. Number of inhabitants. *Current Population Reports* PC (1)-A1 (26). Washington, D.C.: USGPO.
25. ———. 1971. Social and economic characteristics of population in metropolitan and nonmetropolitan areas: 1970 and 1960. *Current Population Reports* P-23 (37): 34. Washington, D.C.: USGPO.
26. ———. 1970. Trends in social and economic conditions in metropolitan and nonmetropolitan areas. *Current Population Reports, Special Studies* P-23 (33). Washington, D.C.: USGPO.
27. U.S. Bureau of Economic Analysis. 1970. *Survey of Current Business.* Washington, D.C.: USGPO.
28. U.S. Social Security Administration. 1972. *Medical Care Costs and Prices: Background Book.* Washington, D.C.: USGPO.
29. U.S. Bureau of Labor Statistics. 1972. Characteristics of agreements covering 2,000 workers or more. Washington, D.C.: USGPO, Bull. 1729, Table 70, p. 74.
30. ———. 1973. *Handbook of Labor Statistics.* Washington, D.C.: USGPO.
31. ———. 1972. *Three Budgets for an Urban Family of Four Persons, 1969–70.* Washington, D.C.: USGPO, Bull. Suppl. 1570–5.
32. ———. 1969. *Three Standards of Living for an Urban Family of Four Persons, Spring 1967.* Washington, D.C.: USGPO, Bull. 1570–5.
33. U.S. President's National Advisory Commission on Rural Poverty. 1967. *The People Left Behind.* Washington, D.C.: USGPO, p. 70.
34. U.S. Senate, Subcommittee on Health of the Committee on Labor and Public Welfare. 1972. *Health Maintenance Organizations: Questions and Answers Relating to Subcommittee Questionnaire.* Washington, D.C.: USGPO.

CHAPTER SEVEN

1. Robach, G. A. 1972. *Distribution of Physicians in the U.S., 1971.* Chicago: American Medical Association.
2. Benham, L., A. Maurizi, and M. W. Reder. 1968. Migration, location, and remuneration of medical personnel: Physicians and dentists. *Rev. Econ. Stat.* 50:332.
3. Fein, R. 1967. *The Doctor Shortage: An Economic Diagnosis.* Washington, D.C.: Brookings Institution.
4. Fein, R., and G. I. Weber. 1971. *Financing Medical Education: An Analysis of Alternative Policies and Mechanisms.* New York: McGraw-Hill. Prepared for Carnegie Comm. Higher Educ. Commonw. Fund.
5. Held, P. J. 1973. *The Migration of the 1955–1965 Graduates of American Medical Schools.* Berkeley, Calif. Ford Foundation Program Research in University Administration.
6. Joroff, S., and V. Navarro. 1971. Medical manpower: A multivariate analysis of the distribution of physicians in urban United States. *Med. Care* 9:428.
7. Marden, P. G. 1966. A demographic and ecological analysis of the distribution of physicians in metropolitan America, 1960. *Am. J. Soc.* 73: 290.
8. Mountin, J. W., E. H. Pennell, and V. Nicolay. 1942. Location and movement of physicians, 1923 and 1938: General observations. *Public Health Rep.* 57: 1363.
9. ———. 1942. Location and movement of physicians, 1923 and 1938: Turnover as a factor affecting state totals. *Public Health Rep.* 57: 1752.
10. ———. 1942. Location and movement of physicians, 1923 and 1938: Effect of local factors upon location. *Public Health Rep.* 57:1945.

11. Mountin, J. W., E. H. Pennell, and G. S. Brockett. 1945. Location and movement of physicians, 1923–1938: Changes in urban and rural totals for established physicians. *Public Health Rep.* 60: 173.
12. Rimlinger, G. C., and H. B. Steele. 1963. An economic interpretation of the spatial distribution of physicians in the United States. *South. Econ. J.* 30: 1.
13. Steele, H. B., and G. V. Rimlinger. 1967. Income opportunities and physician location trends in the United States. *West. Econ. J.* 3: 182.
14. Kaplan, R. H. 1970. Health care in America: Anachronistic and inequitable. Presented at 65th Ann. Meet. Am. Sociol. Assoc., Washington, D.C.
15. Theodore, C. N., G. E. Sutter, and E. A. Jokiel. 1967. *Distribution of Physicians, Hospitals, and Hospital Beds in the United States, 1966.* Vol. 1, *Regional, State, County.* Chicago: American Medical Association.
16. U.S. Bureau of the Census. 1962, 1963. *U.S. Census of Population: 1960.* Vol. 1, *Characteristics of the Population,* Pts. 2–51, excluding 3 (Alaska), 10 (District of Columbia), 13 (Hawaii), and 48 (Virginia), Washington, D.C.: USGPO.
17. ———. 1967. *County and City Data Book.* Washington, D.C.: USGPO.
18. Pennell, M. Y., and K. I. Baker. 1965. *Health Manpower Source Book.* Sect. 19, Location of Manpower in 8 Occupations. Washington, D.C.: USGPO.
19. Mayhew, B. H., and W. A. Rushing. 1973. Occupational structure of general hospitals: The harmonic series model. *Soc. Forces* 52: 455.
20. Brown, D. L. 1972. The redistribution of professional medical personnel in nonmetropolitan Wisconsin, 1950–1970. Presented at Ann. Meet. Rural Sociol. Soc., Baton Rouge, La.
21. Pennell, M. Y., and M. E. Altenderfer. 1954. *Health Manpower Source Book.* Sect. 4, County Data from 1950 Census and Area Analysis. Washington, D.C.: USGPO.
22. U.S. Bureau of the Census. 1963. *U.S. Census of Population: 1960.* Vol. 1, *Characteristics of the Population,* Pt. 44, Tennessee. Washington, D.C.: USGPO.
23. American Hospital Association. 1950. *Hospitals,* Vol. 24, Pt. 2, Guide Issue.
24. ———. 1967. *Hospitals,* Vol. 41, Pt. 2, Guide Issue.
25. Rushing, W. A. 1971. Public policy, community constraints, and the distribution of medical resources. *Soc. Prob.* 19:30.
26. Hansen, N. M. 1970. *Rural Poverty and the Urban Crisis: A Strategy for Regional Development.* Bloomington: Indiana University Press.
27. Thompson, W. R. 1969. The Economic Base of Urban Problems. In N. W. Chamberlain, ed., *Contemporary Economic Issues.* Homewood, Ill.: Richard D. Irwin.
28. Stewart, W. H., and M. Y. Pennell. 1960. *Health Manpower Source Book.* Sect. 10, Physicians' Age, Type of Practice, and Location. Washington, D.C.: USGPO.
29. Haug, J. N., G. A. Roback, C. N. Theodore, and B. E. Balfe. 1970. *Distribution of Physicians, Hospitals, and Hospital Beds in the U.S.: Regional, State, County, Metropolitan Areas.* Chicago: American Medical Association.
30. Roback, G. 1972. *Distribution of Physicians in the United States, 1971.* Chicago: American Medical Association.
31. U.S. Bureau of the Census. 1951. *Census of Population: 1950. General Population Characteristics: United States Summary.* Washington, D.C.: USGPO.

CHAPTER EIGHT

1. Adamson, T. E. 1971. Critical issues in the use of physician associates and assistants. *Am. J. Public Health* 64: 1765–69.
2. Allan, G. W. 1971. Our health care crisis: Critique of a service tradition. In C. O. Crawford, ed., *Health and the Family: A Medical-Sociological Analysis.* New York: Macmillan, pp. 81–110.
3. Health care delivery in rural areas: Selected models. 1972. Chicago: American Medical Association.
4. The National Health Service Corps. 1972. *Rural Health News* (July/Aug.).

5. Primary health care delivery in central Pennsylvania. 1972. *Rural Health News* (Jan./Feb.).
6. Rural health care delivery in Washington State. 1971. *Rural Health News* (Nov./Dec.).
7. Anderson, O. W. 1968. Health services in a land of plenty. In W. R. Ewald, Jr., ed., *Environment and Policy: The Next Fifty Years.* Bloomington: Indiana University Press, pp. 59–92.
8. Appel, J. Z. 1970. Health care delivery. In B. Jones, ed., *The Health of Americans.* Englewood Cliffs, N.J.: Prentice-Hall, pp. 141–66.
9. Baker, F., and G. O. O'Brien. 1971. Intersystems relations and coordination of human service organizations. *Am. J. Public Health* 61: 130–37.
10. Bishop, F. M., et al. 1969. The family physician—Ideal and real. *Gen. Pract.* 60: 169–77.
11. Blum, H. L. 1966. Research into the organization of community health services agencies: An administrator's review. *Milbank Mem. Fund Quart.* 64: 25–93.
12. Bodenheimer, Thomas S. 1969. Mobile units: A solution to the rural health problem? *Med. Care* (Mar.): 144–53.
13. Brunetto, Eleanor, and P. Birk. 1972. The primary care nurse—The generalist in a structured health team. *Am. J. Public Health* 62:785–94.
14. Health maintenance organizations: A reconfiguration of the health services system. 1971. Chicago: University of Chicago, Center for Health Administration Studies.
15. Collins, M. C., and G. C. Bonnyman. 1971. Physician's assistants and nurse associates: A review. Washington, D.C.: Institute for the Study of Health and Society.
16. Cordes, Sam M. 1973. The general practitioner in rural Washington: Opinions, characteristics, and comparative productivity among practice sizes. Ph.D. diss. Pullman: Washington State University.
17. Cordes, Sam M., and Charles O. Crawford. 1974. Health care needs and resources in Pennsylvania: A guide for studying community health services. University Park: Pennsylvania Cooperative Extension Services.
18. Crawford, Charles O. 1969. Variables related to a referendum vote on creating a county health department. *Public Health Rep.* 84: 639–46.
19. Doherty, N. J. G. 1970. Rurality, poverty and health: Medical problems in rural areas. Washington, D.C.: USDA, Agr. Econ. Rep. 172.
20. Donabedian, Avedis. 1974. Models for organizing the delivery of personal health services and criteria for evaluating them. In Irving K. Zola and John B. McKinlay, eds., *Organizational Issues in the Delivery of Health Services.* A selection of articles from *Milbank Mem. Fund Quart.*, pp. 127–78.
21. Elinoff, C. A. 1971. Three tier therapy. *Bus. Rev.* (Sept.): 16–24.
22. Furlong, W. B. 1972. You and your dangerous health practices. *Today's Health* 50: 560–65.
23. Garfield, S. R. 1970. The delivery of medical care. *Sci. Am.* 222: 15–23.
24. Green, L. W. 1970. Status identity and preventive health behavior. Berkeley: University of California, School of Public Health, Pac. Health Educ. Rep. 1.
25. Hassinger, E. W. 1965. Changing health facilities in a changing society. Raleigh, N.C.: Agricultural Policy Institute.
26. ———. 1971. Health services for rural areas. In *A Good Life for More People: 1971 USDA Yearbook.* Washington, D.C.: USDA.
27. Hassinger, E. W., and R. J. McNamara. 1971. Rural health in the United States. *The Quality of Rural Living: Proceedings of a Workshop.* Washington, D.C.: National Academy of Sciences, pp. 8–22.
28. Hazell, Joseph W., Fred Hodges, and George C. Cunningham. 1972. Intermediate benefit analysis—Spencer's dilemma and school health services. *Am. J. Public Health* 62: 560–65.
29. Jacobs, Arthur R., et al. 1974. Comparison of tasks and activities in physician-Medex practices. *Public Health Rep.* 89: 339–44.
30. Kohn, R. 1965. *Emerging Patterns in Health Care.* Ottawa, Canada: Queen's Printer.
31. Litman, Theodor. 1972. Public perceptions of the physician's assistant—A

survey of the attitudes and opinions of rural Iowa and Minnesota residents. *Am. J. Public Health* 62: 343–47.
32. Matthews, Tresa H. 1974. Health services in rural America. Washington, D.C.: USDA AIB-362.
33. McCorkle, Thomas. 1961. Chiropractic: A deviant theory of disease and treatment in contemporary western culture. In W. Richard Scott and Edmund H. Volkhart, eds., 1966, *Medical Care: Readings in Sociology of Medical Institutions.* New York: John Wiley and Sons, pp. 247–58.
34. McNerney, Walter J., and Donald C. Reidel. 1962. Regionalization and rural health care: An experiment in three communities. Ann Arbor: University of Michigan, Graduate School of Business Administration.
35. Mechanic, David. 1972. Human problems and the organization of health care. *Ann. Am. Acad. Polit. Soc. Sci.* 339: 1–11.
36. ———. 1968. *Medical Sociology.* New York: Free Press, p. 187.
37. Merton, Robert K. 1957. *Social Theory and Social Structure.* Glencoe: Free Press, pp. 19–84.
38. Mierynk, William H. 1974. Economic characteristics of Appalachia and potential for financing health care improvement. In Robert L. Nolan and Jerome L. Schwartz, eds., *Rural and Appalachian Health.* Springfield, Ill.: Charles C Thomas, pp. 45–55.
39. Milio, Nancy. 1971. Health care organizations and innovations. *J. Health Soc. Behav.* 12: 163–73.
40. Mott, F. D., and Milton I. Roemer. 1948. *Rural Health and Medical Care.* New York: McGraw-Hill.
41. University medical care programs. 1971. Washington, D.C.: HEW, National Center for Health Services Research and Development, DHEW Publ. (HSM) 72–3010.
42. Characteristics of patients and selected types of medical specialists and practitioners. 1966. Washington, D.C.: HEW, National Center for Health Statistics, Ser. 10, No. 28, Tables 21–22.
43. Health resources statistics, 1972–73. 1973. Washington, D.C.: HEW, DHEW Publ. (HSM) 73–1059.
44. National Commission on Community Health Services. 1966. *Health Is a Community Affair.* Cambridge, Mass.: Harvard University Press.
45. Manpower supply and educational statistics for selected health occupations. 1969. *Health Manpower Source Book.* Washington, D.C.: HEW, Sec. 20, PHS Publ. 263.
46. Selected training programs for physician support personnel. 1972. Washington, D.C.: HEW, DHEW Publ. (NIH) 72–183.
47. Phillips, G. H., and Albert Pugh. 1970. Selected health practices among Ohio's rural residents. Wooster: Ohio Agr. Res. Dev. Center Res. Bull. 1038.
48. Roemer, Milton I. 1968. Health needs and services of the rural poor. In *Rural Poverty in the United States.* Washington, D.C.: USGPO, pp. 311–32.
49. ———. 1971. An ideal health care system for America. *Transaction* 11: 31–36.
50. Rogers, David E. 1974. A private sector view of public health today. *Am. J. Public Health* 64: 529–33.
51. Roth, Julius A. 1971. Utilization of hospital emergency department. *J. Health Soc. Behav.* 12: 312–30.
52. Rothman, R. A., and A. M. Schwartzbaum. 1971. Physicians and a hospital merger: Patterns of resistance to organizational change. *J. Health Soc. Behav.* 12:46–55.
53. Rubin, Irwin M., and Richard Beckhard. 1972. Factors influencing the effectiveness of health teams. In Irving K. Zola and John B. McKinlay, eds., 1974, *Organizational Issues in the Delivery of Health Services.* A selection of articles from *Milbank Mem. Fund Quart.*
54. Schultz, Dodi. 1972. When you should (and shouldn't) call the doctor. *Today's Health* 50: 20–23, 59–61.
55. Somers, Anne R. 1971. Health care in transition. Chicago: Hospital Research and Educational Trust.
56. Voight, John R. 1973. Foundation for medical care. Presented at Conf. Nat. Health Trends and Local Opportunities, State College, Pa.

57. Wang, Virginia L. 1971. Role of extension in consumer health education. In Charles O. Crawford and Carolyn Schrock, eds., *Proceedings of Health In-Service Training Conference*. University Park: Pennsylvania Cooperative Extension Services, pp. 28–33.
58. Wardwell, Walter I. 1972. Limited, marginal and quasi practitioners. In Howard E. Freeman, Sol Levine, and Leo G. Reeder, eds., *Handbook of Medical Sociology*, 2nd ed. Englewood Cliffs, N.J.: Prentice-Hall, pp. 250–73.
59. Warren, R. L. 1971. Alternative strategies of inter-agency planning. In Paul E. White and G. Vlasak, eds., *Interorganizational Research in Health: Conference Proceedings*. Washington, D.C.: HEW, pp. 114–29.
60. White, Kerr L. 1967. Primary care for families: Organization and evaluation. *New Engl. J. Med.* 277: 847–52.
61. White, Marjorie, and J. K. Skipper, Jr. 1971. The chiropractic physician: A study of career contingencies. *J. Health Soc. Behav.* 12: 300–306.
62. White, Paul E., and George Vlasak, eds. 1971. *Interorganizational Research in Health: Conference Proceedings*. Washington, D.C.: HEW.
63. Wilson, Vernon E. 1971. Rural health care systems. *J. Am. Med. Assoc.* 216: 1623–26.
64. Wysong, Jere A., and R. L. Eichhorn. 1971. The health services complex: Inter-agency relations in the delivery of health services. In Ray Elling, ed., *National Health Care*. Chicago: Aldine-Atherton, pp. 229–44.

CHAPTER NINE

1. Agger, Robert, Daniel Goldrich, and Bert E. Swanson. 1972. *The Rulers and the Ruled*. Duxbury, Mass.: Duxbury Press.
2. Anderson, Ronald, and Odin W. Anderson. 1967. *A Decade of Health Services*. Chicago: University of Chicago Press, p. 41.
3. Anderson, Ronald, R. M. Greeley, J. Kravits, and O. W. Anderson. 1972. *Health Service Use*. Washington, D.C.: HEW, Health Services and Mental Health Administration, pp. 33–34.
4. Bashshur, R. L., G. W. Shannon, and C. A. Metzner. 1970. The application of three-dimensional analogue models to the distribution of medical care facilities. *Med. Care* 8(5):395–407.
5. ———. 1971. Some ecological differentials in the use of medical services. *Health Serv. Res.* (Spring): 61–75.
6. Bollen, John. 1971. *American County Government*. Beverly Hills, Calif.: Sage Publications.
7. Campbell, A., P. E. Converse, W. E. Miller, and D. E. Stokes. 1960. *The American Voter*. New York: John Wiley and Sons (see Chap. 15, Agrarian political behavior, pp. 402–40).
8. Clark, Terry N. 1968. *Community Structure and Decision-Making*. San Francisco: Chandler, pp. 91–126.
9. ———. 1971. Community structure, decision-making, budget expenditure and urban renewal. In C. N. Bonjean, T. N. Clark, and R. L. Lineberry, eds., *Community Politics*. New York: Free Press, pp. 293–313.
10. Cnudde, Charles F., and Donald J. McCrone. 1969. Party competition and welfare policies in the American states. *Am. Polit. Sci. Rev.* (Sept.): 858–66.
11. Cummings, Milton C., Jr. 1971. Reapportionment in the 1970's: Its effect on Congress. In Nelson W. Polsby, ed., *Reapportionment in the 1970's*. Berkeley: University of California Press, pp. 209–41.
12. David, Paul T., and Ralph Eisenberg. 1961. *Devaluation of the Urban and Suburban Vote*. Charlottesville: University of Virginia Press.
13. Dawson, Richard E., and James E. Robinson. 1963. Inter-party competition, economic variables, and welfare policies in American states. *J. Polit.* (May): 265–87.
14. Doherty, Neville. 1970. *Rurality, Poverty and Health: Medical Problems in Rural Areas*. Washington, D.C.: USDA, Agr. Econ. Rep. 1972, p. iv.

15. Dohrenwend, Bruce and Barbara. 1969. *Social Status and Psychological Disorder*. New York: John Wiley and Sons.
16. Dye, Thomas R. 1966. *Politics, Economics and the Public: Policy Outcomes in the American States*. Chicago: Rand McNally, p. 293.
17. Forrester, Jay W. 1969. *Urban Dynamics*. Cambridge, Mass.: M.I.T. Press, pp. 9–10.
18. Fry, Brian R., and Richard F. Winters. 1970. The politics of redistribution. *Am. Polit. Sci. Rev.* 64 (June): 508–22.
19. Gilbert, Claire. 1972. *Community Power Structure*. Gainesville: University of Florida Press.
20. Greenberg, Selig. 1971. *The Quality of Mercy*. New York: Atheneum, p. 348.
21. Grumm, John G. 1971. The effects of legislative structure on legislative performance. In Richard I. Hofferbert and Ira Sharkansky, eds., *State and Urban Politics*. Boston: Little, Brown, pp. 298–322.
22. Health Policy Advisory Center. 1971. *The American Health Empire: Power, Profits and Politics*. New York: Random House, p. 232,
23. Kaufman, Herbert. 1973. The political ingredient of public health services. In John B. McKinlay, ed., *Politics and Law in Health Care Policy*. New York: Prodist, p. 23.
24. Kennedy, Edward M. 1972. *The Critical Condition*. New York: Simon and Schuster.
25. Lasswell, Harold D. 1971. *A Pre-view of Policy Sciences*. New York: American Elsevier.
26. Lerner, Monroe, and Odin Anderson. 1963. *Health Progress in the United States—1900–1960*. Chicago: University of Chicago Press.
27. Lowie, Theodore J. 1964. American business public policy, case studies, and political science. *World Polit.* 16: 677–715.
28. Marmor, Theodore. 1973. *The Politics of Medicare*. Chicago: Aldine, pp. 95–124.
29. Martin, Roscoe C. 1957. *Grass Roots*. University: University of Alabama Press, pp. 91–92.
30. Mayhew, David R. 1966. *Party Loyalty among Congressmen*. Cambridge, Mass.: Harvard University Press.
31. National Commission on Community Health Services. 1966. *Health Is a Community Affair*. Cambridge, Mass.: Harvard University Press, pp. 209–10.
32. National Health Assembly. 1949. *America's Health*. New York: Harper and Brothers, p. 139.
33. President's Commission on the Health Needs of the Nation. 1951. *Building America's Health* 2: 80.
34. Presthus, Robert. 1964. *Men at the Top*. New York: Oxford Press, pp. 368–404.
35. Ribicoff, Abraham. 1972. *The American Medical Machine*. New York: Saturday Review Press, p. 135.
36. Roemer, Milton. 1968. Health needs and services of the rural poor. *Rural Poverty in the United States*. Report by the President's National Advisory Commission on Rural Poverty, May, p. 311.
37. Rubenstein, Robert, and Harold D. Lasswell. 1966. *The Sharing of Power in a Psychiatric Hospital*. New Haven, Conn.: Yale University Press, pp. 273–75.
38. Schwartz, Harry. 1972. *The Case for American Medicine*. New York: David McKay.
39. Sharkansky, Ira. 1970. *Regionalism in American Politics*. Indianapolis, Ind.: Bobbs-Merrill.
40. Shipman, George A. 1971. *Designing Program Action*. University: University of Alabama Press.
41. Somers, Anne. 1971. *Health Care in Transition*. Chicago: Hospital Research and Educational Trust.
42. Swanson, Bert E. Changing decision-making arrangements in urban education: Their relevance to health (forthcoming).
43. ———. 1974. Citizen participant input in varying decision-making systems. In

The Citizenry and the Hospital. Report of the 1973 National Forum. Durham, N.C.: Duke University, Dep. Health Adm., pp. 39–58.

44. ———. 1972. The politics of health. In Howard E. Freeman, Sol Levine, and Leo G. Reeder, eds., *Handbook of Medical Sociology*, 2nd ed. Englewood, N.J.: Prentice-Hall, pp. 443–55.

45. U.S. Bureau of the Census. 1972. *Compendium of Government Finances.* Washington, D.C. USGPO, Vol. 4, No. 5.

46. ———. 1972. *1970 General Social and Economic Characteristics.* Washington, D.C.: USGPO, U.S. Summary.

47. ———. 1972. *The Statistical Abstract of the U.S.* Washington, D.C.: USGPO.

48. Walker, Jack L. 1971. The diffusion of innovations among the American states. In Richard I. Hofferbert and Ira Sharkansky, eds., *State and Urban Politics.* Boston: Little, Brown, pp. 377–412.

49. Remarks of President Richard M. Nixon. 1969. *Wkly. Compil. Pres. Doc.* 5 (July 14): 963. Washington, D.C.: Office of the President.

50. Williams, Walter. 1971. *Social Policy Research and Analysis.* New York: American Elsevier.

CHAPTER TEN

1. Aday, Lu Ann. 1972. *The Utilization of Health Services: Indices and Correlates.* Lafayette: Purdue University, Dep. Sociol., Health Serv. Res. and Training Program.

2. Andersen, Ronald. 1968. *A Behavioral Model for Families' Use of Health Services.* Chicago: Center for Health Administration Studies, Res. Ser. 25.

3. Anderson, Anton H. 1961. *The Expanding Rural Community.* Lincoln: Univ. Nebraska Agr. Exp. Sta. SB 464.

4. ———. 1950. Space as a social cost. *J. Farm Econ.* 32 (3): 419.

5. Anderson, Odin A. 1963. The utilization of health services. In Howard E. Freeman, Sol Levine, and Leo G. Reeder, eds., *Handbook of Medical Sociology.* Englewood Cliffs, N.J.: Prentice-Hall, p. 364.

6. Battistella, Roger M. 1971. Factors associated with delay in the initiation of physicians' care among late adulthood persons. *Am. J. Public Health* 61 (7): 1357.

7. ———. 1968. Limitations in use of the concept of psychological readiness to institute health care. *Med. Care* 4: 313.

8. Beale, Calvin L. 1969. Demographic and social considerations for U.S. rural economic policy. *Am. J. Agr. Econ.* 51(2): 417.

9. ———. 1966. The Negro in American agriculture. In John P. Davis, *The American Negro Reference Book.* Englewood Cliffs, N.J.: Prentice-Hall. See also [48].

10. Belcher, John C. 1958. Acceptance of the Salk polio vaccine. *Rural Sociol.* 23 (2): 158–70.

11. Bennett, John W. 1967. Microcosm-macrocosm, relationships in North American agrarian society. *Am. Anthropol.* 69 (5): 441–54.

12. Bible, Bond L. 1970. Physicians' view of medical practice in nonmetropolitan communities. *Public Health Rep.* 85 (1): 13.

13. Bice, Thomas W., Robert L. Eichhorn, and Peter D. Fox. 1972. Socioeconomic status and use of physicians' services: A reconsideration. *Med. Care* 10 (3): 261–71.

14. Bishop, C. E. 1967. The urbanization of rural America: Implications for agricultural economics. *J. Farm Econ.* 49(5): 999–1008.

15. Booth, Alan, and Nicholas Babchuk. 1972. Seeking health care from new resources. *J. Health Soc. Behav.* 13(1):90–99.

16. Fahs, Ivan J., and Osler L. Peterson. 1968. Towns without physicians and towns with only one—A study of four states in the upper Midwest, 1965. *Am. J. Public Health* 58 (7): 1206.

17. Feldman, Jacob J. 1966. *The Dissemination of Health Information.* Chicago: Aldine, p. 66.
18. Ford, Thomas R. 1969. Rural poverty in the United States. In Task Force on Economic Growth and Opportunity, *Rural Poverty and Regional Progress in an Urban Society.* Washington, D.C.: U.S. Chamber of Commerce.
19. Fox, Karl A. 1967. Discussion of Brian J. L. Berry's paper, "Generalization of the Metropolitan Area Concept." *Proc. Am. Stat. Assoc., Social Statistics Section,* Washington, D.C., pp. 93–94.
20. Fox, Karl A., and T. Krishna Kumar. 1966. Delineating functional economic areas. In Iowa State University Center for Agricultural and Economic Development, *Research and Education for Regional and Area Development.* Ames: Iowa State University Press, pp. 13–55.
21. Freidson, Eliot. 1961. *Patients' Views of Medical Practice.* New York: Russell Sage Foundation, p. 146.
22. ———. 1971. *Profession of Medicine.* New York: Dodd, Mead, pp. 226–52.
23. Fuguitt, Glenn V. 1968. Some characteristics of villages in rural America. In National Advisory Commission on Rural Poverty, *Rural Poverty in the United States.* Washington, D.C.: USGPO, p. 55.
24. Glenn, Norval D., and Jon Alston. 1967. Rural-urban difference in reporting attitude and behavior. *Southwest. Soc. Sci. Quart.* 47: 381–400.
25. Gordon, Gerald. 1966. *Role Theory and Illness: A Sociological Perspective.* New Haven, Conn.: College and University Press.
26. Hall, Oswald. 1946. The informal organization of the medical profession. *Can. J. Econ. Polit. Sci.* 12 (1): 30–44.
27. Hartman, Joel A., and Emory J. Brown. 1970. *Evaluation of a Five-Year Demonstration Farm Program in Two Pennsylvania Counties.* University Park: Penn. State Univ. Ext. Stud. 43, pp. 23–42.
28. Hassinger, Edward W. 1963. *Background and Community Orientation of Rural Physicians Compared with Metropolitan Physicians in Missouri.* Columbia: Univ. Missouri Agri. Exp. Sta. Res. Bull. 822.
29. Hassinger, Edward W., and Daryl J. Hobbs. 1967. *Distribution of Health Services in Missouri.* Columbia: Univ. Missouri Agr. Exp. Sta. Res. Bull. 917, p. 19.
30. Hassinger, Edward W., Daryl J. Hobbs, F. Marian Bishop, and A. Sherwood Baker. 1970. *Extent, Type and Pattern of Use of Medical Services in a Rural Ozark Area.* Columbia: Univ. Missouri Agr. Exp. Sta. Res. Bull. 965.
31. ———. 1971. *Perception of Health Practitioners by Respondents in a Rural Area.* Columbia: Univ. Mo. Agr. Exp. Sta. Res. Bull. 964, pp. 6–9.
32. Hathaway, Dale E., J. Allan Beegle, and W. Keith Bryant. 1968. *People of Rural America: A 1960 Census Monograph.* Washington, D.C.: USGPO, p. 148.
33. Hay, Donald G. 1960. *That They May Have Health Care.* Ann Arbor, Mich.: Edwards Brothers, p. 22.
34. Heinzelmann, Fred. 1962. Factors influencing prophylaxis behavior with respect to rheumatic fever: An exploratory study. *J. Health Hum. Behav.* 3 (2): 73–81.
35. Hochbaum, Godfrey A. 1958. *Public Participation in Medical Screening Programs: A Socio-psychological Study.* Washington, D.C.: PHS Publ. 572, p. 8.
36. Hollingshead, August B., and Frederick C. Redlich. 1958. *Social Class and Mental Illness: A Community Study.* New York: John Wiley and Sons.
37. Jones, Gwyn E. 1967. The adoption and diffusion of agricultural practices. *World Agr. Econ. Rural Sociol. Abstr.* (3): 1–34.
38. Kassebaum, Gene G., and Barbara O. Bauman. 1965. Dimensions of the sick role in chronic illness. *J. Health Hum. Behav.* (Spring): 16–27.
39. Kegeles, S. S. 1963. Why people seek dental care: A test of a conceptual formulation. *J. Health Hum. Behav.* 4:166–72.
40. Koos, Earl L. 1954. *The Health of Regionville.* New York: Columbia University Press.
41. Kraenzel, Carl K. 1953. Sutland and Yonland: Settings for community organization in the plains. *Rural Sociol.* 18 (4): 344–58.

42. Levitan, Sar A. 1969. *The Great Society's Poor Law: A New Approach to Poverty*. Baltimore: Johns Hopkins Press, p. 227.
43. Lionberger, Herbert L. 1960. *Adoption of New Ideas and Practices*. Ames: Iowa State University Press.
44. Loomis, Charles P., and J. Allan Beegle. 1950. *Rural Social Systems*. Englewood Cliffs, N.J.: Prentice-Hall.
45. Lowry, Sheldon G., Selz C. Mayo, and Donald G. Hay. 1958. Factors associated with the acceptance of health care practices among rural families. *Rural Sociol.* 23 (2): 198–202.
46. McKinlay, John B. 1972. Some approaches and problems in the study of the use of services—An overview. *J. Health Soc. Behav.* (2): 118.
47. Menzel, Herbert, and Elihu Katz. 1955. Social relations and innovation in the medical profession: The epidemiology of a new drug. *Public Opin. Quart.* 19 (4): 337–52.
48. Moore, Joan, and Alfredo Cuellar. 1970. *Mexican Americans*. Englewood Cliffs, N.J.: Prentice-Hall.
49. Munk, Michael. 1967. *Rural youth-work programs: Problems of size and scope*. New York: New York University, Graduate School of Social Work, Center for the Study of Unemployed Youth, pp. 21–22.
50. Nall, Frank C., II, and Joseph Speilberg. 1967. Social and cultural factors in responses of Mexican-Americans to medical treatment. *J. Health Soc. Behav.* 8 (4): 303.
51. National Advisory Commission on Rural Poverty. 1967. Hearings before the Commission, Memphis, Tenn. Washington, D.C.: USGPO, pp. 124–35.
52. ———. 1967. *The People Left Behind*. Washington, D.C.: USGPO, pp. 3–9.
53. National Center for Health Statistics. 1964. *Medical Care, Health Status, and Family Income in the United States*. Washington, D.C.: USGPO, Ser. 10, No. 9.
54. ———. 1971. *Persons Hospitalized by Number of Hospital Episodes and Days in a Year, United States 1968*. Washington, D.C.: USGPO, ser. 10, No. 64, p. 10.
55. ———. 1972. *Physicians, Visits Volume and Interval since Last Visit, United States, 1969*. Washington, D.C.: USGPO, Ser. 10, No. 75, p. 7.
56. North Central Rural Sociological Subcommittee for the Study of Diffusion of Farm Practices. 1955. *How Farm People Accept New Ideas*. Ames: Iowa Agr. Ext. Serv. Spec. Rep. 15.
57. Padfield, Harland, and William E. Martin. 1965. *Farmers, Workers and Machines: Technological and Social Change in Farm Industries of Arizona*. Tucson: University of Arizona Press.
58. Parsons, Talcott. 1951. *The Social System*. Glencoe, Ill.: Free Press, pp. 436–37.
59. Pedersen, Harold A., and Earl B. Peterson. 1963. *Market and Trade Center Patronage Patterns in Central Montana*. Bozeman: Mont. State Coll. Agr. Exp. Sta. Bull. 578.
60. Petroni, Frank A. 1969. Significant others and illness behavior: A much neglected sick role contingency. *Sociol. Quart.* 10 (1): 32–41.
61. Rogers, Everett M., and F. Floyd Shoemaker. 1971. *Communication of Innovation: A Cross-Cultural Approach*. New York: Free Press.
62. Rosenstock, Irwin M. 1961. Acceptance of vaccination. *Am. Rev. Respir. Dis.* 83 (2).
63. ———. 1969. Prevention of illness and maintenance of health. In John Kosa, Aaron Antonovsky, and Irving Zola, eds., *Poverty and Health: A Sociological Analysis*. Cambridge, Mass.: Harvard University Press.
64. Rosenstock, Irwin M., Mayhew Derryberry, and Barbara K. Carriger. 1959. Why people fail to seek poliomyelitis vaccination. *Public Health Rep.* 74 (2): 98–103.
65. Stephens, Jack J. 1970. *Socioeconomic Status and Related Variables That Influence the Initiation of Professional Medical Care among Montana Families*. Bozeman: Mont. State Univ. Agr. Exp. Sta. Bull. 631, pp. 20–21.
66. Stephenson, John B. 1968. *Shiloh, a Mountain Community*. Lexington: University of Kentucky Press, p. 93.

67. Suchman, Edward A. 1966. Health orientation and medical care. *Am. J. Public Health* 56 (1).
68. ———. 1965. Social patterns of illness and medical care. *J. Health Hum. Behav.* 6: 2–16.
69. ———. 1964. Sociomedical variations among ethnic groups. *Am. J. Sociol.* (3): 329.
70. Taylor, Lee, and Arthur R. Jones, Jr. 1964. *Rural Life and Urbanized Society.* New York: Oxford University Press.
71. U.S. Bureau of the Census. 1969. Poverty in the United States, 1956–1968. *Curr. Popul. Rep.,* Ser. P-60, No. 68, p. 4.
72. U.S. Department of Commerce. 1972. *Statistical Abstract of the U.S., 1972.* Washington, D.C.: USGPO, p. 323.
73. Vidich, Arthur J., and Joseph Bensman. 1958. *Small Town in Mass Society.* Princeton, N.J.: Princeton University Press, pp. 95–97.
74. Weller, Jack E. 1965. *Yesterday's People: Life in Contemporary Appalachia.* Lexington: University of Kentucky Press.
75. Zborowski, Mark. 1952. Cultural components in response to pain. *J. Soc. Issues* 8 (1): 16–30.
76. Zeller, Frederick, and Robert W. Miller. 1968. *Problems of Community Action in Appalachia.* Morgantown: West Virginia University, Office of Research and Development, Appalachian Center, Res. Ser. 4.
77. Zola, Irving K. 1966. Culture and symptoms—An analysis of patients' presenting complaints. *Am. Sociol. Rev.* 31 (5): 615–30.

CHAPTER ELEVEN

1. Ardell, Donald B. 1974. The demise of CHP and the future of planning. *Inquiry* 11: 233–35.
2. Arnstein, Sherry R. 1969. A ladder of citizen participation. *J. Am. Inst. Planners* 35: 216–24.
3. Arthur Young and Company. 1974. Guide to comprehensive health planning. Rockville, Md.: HEW, Division of Comprehensive Health Planning.
4. Burke, Edmund M. 1968. Citizen participation strategies. *J. Am. Inst. Planners* 34: 287–94.
5. Clark, Weldon E., Virginia A. Clark, and James J. Souder. 1968. Data for planning from health information system sources. *Inquiry* 5(3): 5–16.
6. Comprehensive health planning expectations project final report. 1972. Rockville, Md. HEW, Division of Comprehensive Health Planning.
7. Health planning issue paper. 1972. New York: Community Health, Inc., Issue Paper 7.
8. Health planning memorandum. 1972. New York: Community Health, Inc., Health Planning Memo. 29.
9. Regulation of the health care system and the emerging role of comprehensive health planning. 1973. New York: Community Health, Inc., Issue Paper 9.
10. The review and comment responsibilities of state and areawide comprehensive health planning agencies—Some principles and guides. 1971. Rockville, Md.: HEW, Division of Comprehensive Health Planning, Pub. HSM 71-6100.
11. Frazier, Todd M. 1970. The questionable role of statistics in comprehensive health planning. *Am. J. Public Health* 60 (9): 1701–5.
12. Galinski, Thomas P. 1972. Memorandum. Chicago: American Hospital Association, Oct. 26.
13. Hilleboe, Herman E. 1968. Health planning on a community basis. *Med. Care* 6 (3): 203–14.
14. Lubin, Jerome W., Junior K. Knee, Royal A. Crystal, and Valeda Slade, eds. 1972. Statistics for comprehensive health planning. Washington, D.C.: HEW, National Center for Health Statistics.

15. May, Joel. 1974. Is planning worth the price? *Hospitals* 48:51–55.
16. McClure, Walter. 1974. Federal control: National health insurance and health planning. Ann. Meet. Am. Public Health Assoc., New Orleans, La. Los Angeles: On the Spot Duplicators.
17. Michael, Jerrold M., George Spatafore, and Edward R. Williams. 1968. A basic information system for health planning. *Public Health Rep.* 83 (1): 21–28.
18. National Center for Health Statistics. 1972. The cooperative federal-state-local health statistics system. Rockville, Md.: HEW, DHEW Publ. (HSM) 72-1209.
19. Circ. A-95, rev. 1971. Washington, D.C.: White House, Office of Management and Budget.
20. What it is—How it works. N.D. Washington, D.C.: White House, OMB Circ. A-95, rev.
21. Olson, Linda, and John Michael Daly, Jr. 1973. Comprehensive health planning: The drift toward federal control. New York: Community Health, Issue Paper 10.
22. Public Law 89-749.
23. Public Law 92-603, Sect. 1122.
24. Roemer, Milton I. 1969. Comprehensive health planning in rural areas. Seminar, Health Problems of the Great Plains. Lincoln, Nebr. Great Plains Agricultural Council.
25. Rosenfeld, Eugene E. 1972. Areawide planning controls costs. *Hospitals* 46:36–38 and passim.
26. Wallace, Helen M., Victor Eisner, and Samuel Dooley. 1967. Availability and usefulness of selected health and socioeconomic data for community planning. *Am. J. Public Health* 57(5): 762–71.
27. Willie, Charles V., Edward Noroian, Gregory Simms, and James Harris. 1970. Why and how to involve people. Dallas: HEW, Regional Office of Comprehensive Health Planning.

CHAPTER TWELVE

1. Doherty, Neville J. G. 1970. The economic structure and performance of the medical industry in Michigan's Grand Traverse region. Ph.D. diss. East Lansing: Michigan State University.
2. Doherty, Neville J. G., David Halkola, William Hanson, Shyamalendu Sarkar, and Glenn Johnson. 1972. Health care industries in the Michigan Grand Traverse and copper country regions: Case studies in community resource development. East Lansing: Mich. State Univ. Agr. Exp. Sta. Res. Rep. 177.
3. Johnson, Glenn L., Albert N. Halter, Harald R. Jensen, and D. Woods Thomas. 1961. *Managerial Processes of Midwestern Farmers*. Ames: Iowa State University Press.
4. Johnson, Glenn L., Orlin J. Scoville, George K. Dike, and Carl K. Eicher. 1969. Strategies and recommendations for Nigerian rural development 1969/1985. Consortium for the study of Nigerian rural development.
5. Manetsch, Thomas J., Marvin L. Hayenga, Albert N. Halter, Tom W. Carroll, Michael H. Abkin, Kwong-Yuan Chong, Gloria Page, Earl Kellogg, and Glenn L. Johnson. 1971. A generalized simulation approach to agricultural sector analysis. Consortium for the study of Nigerian rural development.
6. Rossmiller, G. E., Tom W. Carroll, Sang Gee Kim, Young Sik Kim, Thomas J. Manetsch, Han Hyeck Suh, Dong Hi Kim, and Glenn Johnson. 1972. Korean agricultural sector analysis and recommended development strategies 1971–1985. Korean Agricultural Sector Study Team.
7. Sarkar, Shyamalendu. 1969. The copper country medical industry in Michigan as it serves rural people. Ph.D. diss. East Lansing: Michigan State University.

CHAPTER THIRTEEN

1. Agrawal, R. C., and Earl O. Heady. 1972. *Operations Research Methods for Agricultural Decisions.* Ames: Iowa State University Press, pp. 54–78.
2. Comprehensive Health Planning Council. 1974. Comprehensive health plan for the state of Iowa. Des Moines: Office of Planning and Programming, State of Iowa.
3. ———. 1974. *Fact Sheet on Partnership for Health,* CHPC working paper. Des Moines: Office of Planning and Programming, State of Iowa, p. 3.
4. Coughlin, Robert E., Walter Isard, and Jerry Schneider. 1964. *The Activity Structure and Transportation Requirements of a Major University Hospital.* Philadelphia: Regional Science Research Institute.
5. Dowling, William Laine. 1970. A linear programming approach to the analysis of hospital production. Ph.D. diss. Ann Arbor: University of Michigan.
6. Feldstein, M. S. 1968. Cost benefit analysis and health program planning for developing countries. Presented at 2nd Conf. on Economic Health, Baltimore, Md.
7. ———. 1967. *Economic Analysis for Health Service Efficiency.* Amsterdam: North Holland Publishing Co., pp. 168–83.
8. Gurfield, B. 1968. *Planning Hospital Services.* Santa Monica, Calif.: Rand Corp.
9. Heady, Earl O., and Wilfred Candler. 1958. *Linear Programming Methods.* Ames: Iowa State University Press, pp. 333–77.
10. Isard, Walter. 1960. *Methods of Regional Analysis: An Introduction to Regional Sciences.* Cambridge, Mass.: MIT Press, pp. 413–92.
11. Johnson, Richard L. 1974. The specter of bankruptcy over building of hospital facilities. *Hospitals* 48: 6, 39–42.
12. Long, M. F. 1964. Efficient use of hospitals. In *The Economics of Health and Medical Care.* Ann Arbor: University of Michigan Press, pp. 211–26.
13. Matthews, Tresa H. 1974. Health services in rural America. Washington, D.C.: USDA, Agr. Inf. Bull. 362, pp. 4–7.
14. Navarro, Vicente. 1969. Systems analysis in the health field. *Socio-Econ. Plan. Sci.* 3: 179–89.
15. Newell, D. J. 1964. Problems in estimating the demand for hospital beds. *J. Chronic Dis.* (Sept.): 756.
16. Office of Comprehensive Health Planning. 1974. Iowa Operating Procedures, Public Law 92–603, Sec. 1122, Health Facilities Construction Review. Des Moines: Office of Planning and Programming, State of Iowa, p. c-23.
17. Phillips, Donald F. 1974. Hospitals and cost controls: Road to crisis. *Hospitals* 48: 4, 24–26.
18. Public Health Service. 1974. Inpatient facilities as reported from the 1971 MFI survey, Ser. 14, No. 12. Rockville, Md.: HEW, pp. 12–14.
19. Revelle, W., and F. Feldmann. 1967. Mathematical models for the economic allocation of tuberculosis control activities in developing countries. Geneva: World Health Organization, Tech. Inf. Bull. 59.
20. Stevens, C. N. 1970. Hospital market efficiency: The anatomy of the supply responses. In *Empirical Studies in Health Economics.* Baltimore: Johns Hopkins Press, pp. 229–48.

CHAPTER FOURTEEN

1. Cooper, Barbara S., and Mary F. Magee. 1970. Health care outlays for the young, intermediate, and older age groups. Washington, D.C.: USGPO, Note 17, Oct. 23.
2. Doherty, Neville. 1970. Rurality, poverty, and health: Medical problems in rural areas. Washington, D.C.: USGPO, Agr. Econ. Rep. 172.

3. DuVal, Merlin K., M.D. 1972. The responsibility of being free. *Mod. Med.* (Nov. 13): 88–89.
4. Edwards, Representative Don. 1972. *Washington Post and Times Herald* 95 (July 22): 4A.
5. Finch, Robert A. 1970. Letter from Secretary of HEW to U.S. Senate Committee on Government Operations, Hearings on Intergovernmental Cooperation Act of 1969 and related legislation. 91st Congr. 1st Sess., p. 28.
6. *Group Health and Welfare News.* 1972. 2:13.
7. Health Management Corporation. 1972. *New York-Penn News.* Oct. 1.
8. Horty, John F. 1972. Health care: Is it a legal right? *Hosp. Med. Staff* 1:8.
9. Johnson, Robert H., M.D. 1972. Ambulatory care centers—Patterns and pitfalls. *Hosp. Med. Staff*, Aug., pp. 28–34.
10. Jones, Robert P. 1972. Press release. Washington, D.C.: HEW, July 7.
11. Kennedy, Senator Edward. 1972. Emergency health service personnel act amendments of 1972. *Congressional Record* 118:S12151. Washington, D.C.
12. ———. 1972. Health services for migrant workers. *Congressional Record* 118:S13951. Washington, D.C.
13. Maddox, D. 1971. Samaritan health service: Arizona's voluntary chain may be the model for the future. *Mod. Hosp.* 116: 89.
14. *Medical Group News.* 1972. 5:13.
15. *Medical World News.* 1974. Sept. 13, p. 45.
16. Millis, John S. 1972. Inter action: Physicians, the hospital, and society. *Hosp. Med. Staff* 1:4.
17. Morris, Stephen M. 1971. *Hospitals* 45: 40.
18. ———. 1972. Inaugural Address, AHA House of Delegates, Feb. 7, Washington, D.C.
19. Mountin, J. W., E. H. Pennell, and V. M. Hoge. 1945. Health service areas—Requirements for general hospitals and health centers. Washington, D.C.: USGPO, Public Health Bull. 292.
20. National Center for Health Services Research and Development. 1971. *Fact Sheet,* Experimental Health Services Delivery Systems. Washington, D.C.: HEW, Health Serv. Mental Health Adm.
21. RMP doctors are going to the people. 1972. *Medical World News,* Sept. 1.
22. Somers, Anne R. 1971. Health care in transition—Directions for the future. Chicago: Hospital Research and Educational Trust.
23. Special Committee on the Provision of Health Services. 1970. Ameriplan—A proposal for the delivery and financing of health services in the United States. Chicago: American Hospital Association.
24. Spitzer, Walter O. 1970. Small general hospital. Problems and solutions. *Milbank Mem. Fund Quart.* 48: 413–47.
25. Toomey, R. E. 1971. Community vs. specialized medicine. *Hospitals* 45: 43.
26. Experimental health services delivery systems. 1972. Washington, D.C.: HEW. Press release, July 27.

CHAPTER FIFTEEN

1. Geiger, H. Jack. 1972. A health center in Mississippi—A case study in social medicine. In Lawrence Corey, Steven E. Saltman, Michael F. Epstein, eds., *Medicine in a Changing Society.* St. Louis, Mo.: C. V. Mosby.
2. Hatch, John W. 1971. A review of the efforts of the A.P.H.A. task force on public education and participation in health care. Minneapolis: A.P.H.A. Ann. Conf.
3. Heller, Frank A. 1970. Group feedback analysis as a change agent. *Hum. Relat.* 23 (4): 319–33.
4. Omran, Abdel. 1971. The epidemiologic transition. *Milbank Mem. Fund Quart.* 49: 509–38.

5. Organ, Dennis. 1971. Some variables affecting boundary role behavior. *Sociometry* 34 (4): 524–37.
6. Reynolds, Richard. 1970. The university and rural health. *J. Am. Med. Assoc.* 214 (3): 540–46.
7. Schwartz, Jerome L. 1970. Early histories of selected neighborhood health centers. *Inquiry* 7 (4): 3–16.
8. Seipp, Conrad. 1965. The role of the community in rural health. In E. Croft Long, ed., *Health Objectives for the Developing Society: Responsibility of Individual, Physician, and Community*. Durham, N.C.: Duke University Press.
9. Stewart, William H. 1965. Health problems of rural communities. In E. Croft Long, ed., *Health Objectives for the Developing Society: Responsibility of Individual, Physician, and Community*. Durham, N.C.: Duke University Press.

CHAPTER SIXTEEN

1. Beiser, Morton, Robert C. Benfari, Alex Leighton, and Jane N. Murphey. 1975. Further explorations in social psychiatry. Burton Kaplan, Alex Leighton, Robert N. Wilson (eds.). Basic Books.
2. Ginzberg, Eli. Address delivered at National Conference on Medical Costs. Washington, D.C., June 1967.
3. Van Peenan, John, M.D. 1969. Unpublished data, RMP research, Columbia: University of Missouri.
4. Wilson, Vernon E., M.D. 1967. The medical school of a land grant university and its relation to the health care of a state. *J. Am. Med. Assoc.* 202 (5): 102–4.

INDEX

Access to health care services, 13, 31–36, 67, 71, 75, 160, 164, 178, 230–35
and changes in health care systems, 217–18, 263–65
effect of social group identification on, 184
through family physician, 185–86
financial, 95, 100, 104–5
and utilization of health services, 177
Accidents, 6, 29–31, 42, 84, 89, 147. *See also* Emergency medical care; Ambulance service
Age, 20–21, 35, 39–52, 74, 104–5, 143, 144, 149. *See also* Medicare
and access to health care, 83, 231
and communication systems, 268
and community health care systems, 256
and income, 196
of rural population, 33, 40, 55, 165–66
in simulation example, 206–10
and Tufts-Delta health project, 247
and utilization of health services, 127, 176, 182, 218–21, 223–24
Agricultural Workers Health and Medical Association, 13. *See also* Farm population
Aid to Families with Dependent Children, 18
Air Evac, 92
Air transportation, 83, 85–86, 88–89, 92–94
Aliens, illegal, 34
Ambulance service, 82–94. *See also* Emergency medical care; Transportation
Ambulatory care, 12, 14, 130, 239. *See also* Hospital, outpatient care in
American Academy of General Practice, 18
American Board of Family Practice, 233
American College of Emergency Physicians, 85
American College of Surgeons, 89
American Hospital Association, 110, 116, 240
American Indians. *See* Indians, American

American Medical Asssociation, 8–9, 20, 66
and consumer education, 133
data on distribution of physicans, 107, 116, 119
data on ratio of hospital beds to physicians, 113
Medicredit plan, 139, 162
American Public Health Association, 5–6. *See also* Public Health
Ameriplan, 240–41. *See also* Health Care Corporations
Amish, 167–68
Appalachia, 12, 15, 33, 67, 103, 166–68, 170
Appalachian Regional Development Act, 12
Area Health Education Centers, 18
Areawide health planning agencies (B agencies), 189–90, 193, 196–98

Behavioral factors. *See* Psychosocial factors
Beliefs and values. *See* Psychosocial factors
Benefits, health, 196
and consumer involvement, 254–55
Bingham Associates Fund, 15–16
Blacks, 32, 67, 144, 149–53, 158–60, 165–68. *See also* Race and health; South
and Tufts-Delta health project, 245–54
Blue Cross–Blue Shield, 13, 19, 98, 139, 141, 231–32
and utilization of health care services, 177
British health care system, 265–66
Bureau of Community Health Services, 74
Bureau of Health Manpower Education, 237
Bureau of Labor Statistics, 97

Central Virginia Community Health Center, 88

Utilization of health services, 98, 122,
146–48, 158–63, 175–87
and age, 33, 127, 176, 182, 218–21, 223–
24
and changes in services, 218
and cost, 177, 215–16
of hospital beds, 241
and income, 125–27, 177
and insurance, 71, 177
and legislation, 216–17
in linear programming example, 219,
221–24, 226–29

Vermont–New Hampshire Medical Interactive Network, 90

Welfare. *See* Aid to Families with Dependent Children; Medicaid; Poverty
White House Commission reports on
health, 157
Workman's compensation, 21